A Practical Manual to Labor and Delivery

Second Edition

T0273782

A Practical Manual to Labor and Delivery

Second Edition

Edited by

Shad Deering, MD
Uniformed Services University of the Health Sciences, Maryland, USA

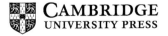
CAMBRIDGE
UNIVERSITY PRESS

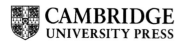

Shaftesbury Road, Cambridge CB2 8EA, United Kingdom

One Liberty Plaza, 20th Floor, New York, NY 10006, USA

477 Williamstown Road, Port Melbourne, VIC 3207, Australia

314–321, 3rd Floor, Plot 3, Splendor Forum, Jasola District Centre, New Delhi – 110025, India

103 Penang Road, #05–06/07, Visioncrest Commercial, Singapore 238467

Cambridge University Press is part of Cambridge University Press & Assessment,
a department of the University of Cambridge.

We share the University's mission to contribute to society through the pursuit of
education, learning and research at the highest international levels of excellence.

www.cambridge.org
Information on this title: www.cambridge.org/9781108407830
DOI: 10.1017/9781108291323

First published by Xlibris 2009
Second edition published by Cambridge University Press 2018 (version 7, January 2025)

Printed in Mexico by Litográfica Ingramex, S.A. de C.V., January 2025

A catalog record for this publication is available from the British Library.

Library of Congress Cataloging-in-Publication Data
Names: Deering, Shad, editor.
Title: A practical manual to labor and delivery / [edited by] Shad Deering.
Description: New York, NY : Cambridge University Press, 2018. | Includes bibliographical
references and index.
Identifiers: LCCN 2018014370 | ISBN 9781108407830 (alk. paper)
Subjects: | MESH: Labor, Obstetric | Delivery, Obstetric
Classification: LCC RG651 | NLM WQ 300 | DDC 618.4–dc23
LC record available at https://lccn.loc.gov/2018014370

ISBN 978-1-108-40783-0 Paperback

....

This book would not have been possible without the constant support of my wife and three sons. Katie has supported our family and my career in obstetrics through the long days and longer nights while completing her Master's in Education degree and continuing to teach. It was seeing her experience complications in labor with our first child that inspired me to write this book. And, every day since then, Tyler, Conner, and Jake are a constant reminder of why this book is needed.

Contents

Contributors

Noelle Breslin, MD
Department of Obstetrics and Gynecology
Columbia University Medical Center –
New York Presbyterian Hospital
New York, NY, USA

Ashley S. Coggins, MD
Department of Obstetrics and Gynecology
Walter Reed National Military Medical
Center
Bethesda, MD, USA

Mary Kathryn Collins, MD
Department of Obstetrics and Gynecology
Walter Reed National Military Medical
Center
Bethesda, MD, USA

Shad Deering, MD
Department of Obstetrics and Gynecology
Uniformed Services University of the
Health Sciences
Bethesda, MD, USA

Elise Diamond, MD
Department of Obstetrics and Gynecology
MedStar Washington Hospital Center
Washington, DC, USA

Kristen Elmezzi, DO
Department of Obstetrics and Gynecology
Walter Reed National Military Medical
Center
Bethesda, MD, USA

Allison Eubanks, MD
Department of Obstetrics and Gynecology
Walter Reed National Military Medical
Center
Bethesda, MD, USA

Morgan Light, DO
Department of Obstetrics and Gynecology
Walter Reed National Military Medical
Center
Bethesda, MD, USA

Devon M. Rupley, MD
Department of Obstetrics and Gynecology
Columbia University Medical Center –
New York Presbyterian Hospital
New York, NY, USA

Sierra Seaman, MD
Department of Obstetrics and Gynecology
New York Presbyterian – Columbia
University Medical Center
New York, NY, USA

Emily Sheikh, MD
Department of Obstetrics and Gynecology
Walter Reed National Military Medical
Center
Bethesda, MD, USA

Kelsey J. Simpson, MD
Department of Obstetrics and Gynecology
Walter Reed National Military Medical
Center
Bethesda, MD, USA

Irina U. Tunnage, DO, MHS
Department of Obstetrics and Gynecology
MedStar Washington Hospital Center
Washington, DC, USA

Meghan Yamasaki, DO
Department of Obstetrics and Gynecology
Walter Reed National Military Medical
Center
Bethesda, MD, USA

Preface

There are few experiences in medicine that are more emotionally charged than the delivery of a child, and almost nothing is more rewarding than taking care of a pregnant patient and being able to place a healthy baby into her arms. To achieve this, every person on the labor and delivery unit must do their job. Every resident, nurse, staff member, and student plays a critical part in ensuring the best outcome possible.

On obstetric rotations, however, providers are placed in a fast-paced environment where there is often minimal time for instruction in the procedures performed and little explanation of why certain treatment plans are made. Similarly, when first working on labor and delivery, providers are expected to be able to perform many "basic" tasks and examinations for which there are no good teaching references available – or, if there are, they are buried in the middle of a large and cumbersome reference book. When you add to this the common variations in clinical practice patterns, you have the perfect setup for confusion as you try to learn how to take care of laboring patients.

This book is intended to bridge the gap between small handbooks that do not contain enough material to understand why you are doing certain things and large textbooks that lack the practical information you need for how to do specific procedures, and write notes, orders, and dictations. After reading it, you will be prepared to care for an obstetric patient from the moment she arrives in triage until the time she is discharged. You will understand not only how to perform both simple and complicated procedures, but why they are necessary. The most up-to-date literature and evidence-based recommendations have been used to create simple treatment algorithms for the most common issues you will face, and numerous illustrations are included for clarity as well.

This book should also be a valuable resource for staff physicians who need an updated text on current obstetric care, as well as for those who regularly interact with and teach residents, medical students, and nursing students.

In just the past few years, since the publication of the first edition of this book, there have been important changes in the practice of obstetrics. Some of the most notable include expanding the use of steroids for fetal lung maturity, new definitions for progress in labor, and more evidence-based guidelines for cesarean section techniques. For these reasons, the second edition has been updated to include the most recent literature and evidence for these and many other facets of obstetrics. What has not changed, however, are the basic principles that are included in this manual. The need for a solid foundation of practical knowledge will never go away, and this new edition retains this mission at its core.

You have the opportunity and privilege to be part of one of the most important moments in your patients' lives on every shift, and also the responsibility to do your job well. This book is the place to begin. Welcome to the adventure, and thank you for all you do for each and every patient.

Acknowledgments

A project of this magnitude does not happen without a dedicated team. I would like to thank each of the authors who gave of their time and energy to assist in updating this book. Despite their busy schedules, they each made it a priority to take part in this important project. I know that every provider who reads it and all the patients they take care of will be grateful for it as well.

I have greatly appreciated the feedback of many students, residents, nurses, and other staff since the first edition was published, and they have provided the impetus for many of the improvements that have been made in this second edition. Receiving all their comments has not only reinforced the notion that the book is needed more than ever, but it has demonstrated how important it is to keep it firmly grounded in the experiences of the providers who are working on labor and delivery every day.

I would also like to recognize the team at Cambridge University Press. Whether helping me to navigate through the process or gently reminding me of deadlines, they were instrumental in bringing this book to its final publication.

Abbreviations

ABD	abdomen
ACOG	American College of Obstetricians and Gynecologists
AFI	amniotic fluid index
ALL	allergies
ALT	alanine transaminase
AROM	artificial rupture of membranes
ART	assisted reproductive technologies
AST	aspartate transaminase
AV	arteriovenous
BMI	body mass index
BP	blood pressure
bpm	beats per minute
BPP	biophysical profile
CBC	complete blood count
CNS	central nervous system
CPAP	continuous positive airway pressure
CSF	cerebrospinal fluid
CST	contraction stress test
CTA	clear to auscultation
Ctx	contractions
D&C	dilation and curettage
DIC	disseminated intravascular coagulation
DM	diabetes mellitus
DBP	diastolic blood pressure
DTR	deep tendon reflexes
DVT	deep venous thrombosis
EBL	estimated blood loss
ECG	electrocardiogram
ECV	external cephalic version
EDD	estimated date of delivery
EFW	estimated fetal weight
EGA	estimated gestational age
ETT	endotracheal tube
EXT	extremities
FAVD	forceps-assisted vaginal delivery
fFN	fetal fibronectin
FGR	fetal growth restriction
FHR	fetal heart rate
FKC	fetal kick counts
FM	fetal movement
FSE	fetal scalp electrode
GABA	gamma-aminobutyric acid

GBS	group B streptococcus
GC	gonorrhea
GHTN	gestational hypertension
GU	genitourinary
H&P	history and physical examination
Hct	hematocrit
HEENT	head, eyes, ears, nose, and throat
HELLP	hemolysis, elevated liver enzymes, low platelet count
Hgb	hemoglobin
HIV	human immunodeficiency virus
HR	heart rate
HSV	herpes simplex virus
HTN	hypertension
IM	intramuscular
I/O	intake/output
IUD	intrauterine device
IUFD	intrauterine fetal demise
IUP	intrauterine pregnancy
IUPC	intrauterine pressure catheter
IV	intravenous
LARC	long-acting reversible contraception
LDH	lactate dehydrogenase
LE	lower extremity
LF	low forceps
LFT	liver function test
LMP	last menstrual period
LOA	left occiput anterior
LOP	left occiput posterior
LR	lactated Ringer's
MDI	metered-dose inhaler
MLE	midline episiotomy
MSV	Mauriceau–Smellie–Veit
MTP	massive transfusion protocol
MVP	maximum vertical pocket
MVUs	Montevideo units
NICU	neonatal intensive care unit
NKDA	no known drug allergies
NPO	nil by mouth (*nil per os*)
NRNST	non-reactive NST
NS	normal saline
NSAID	non-steroidal anti-inflammatory drug
NST	non-stress test
NTTP	non-tender to palpation
OA	occiput anterior
OCP	oral contraceptive pill
OF	outlet forceps
OP	occiput posterior

OR	operating room
PCA	patient-controlled analgesia
PCN	penicillin
PDS	polydiaxanone (suture)
PE	pulmonary embolism
PID	pelvic inflammatory disease
PLTCS	primary low transverse cesarean section
PMH	past medical history
PNV	prenatal vitamin
PO	by mouth (*per os*)
PPH	postpartum hemorrhage
PPV	positive-pressure ventilation
PR	per rectum
PRBCs	packed red blood cells
Pre-E	preeclampsia
PRN	as needed (*pro re nata*)
PROM	premature rupture of membranes
PPROM	preterm premature rupture of membranes
PSH	past surgical history
PT	prothrombin time
PTL	preterm labor
PTT	partial thromboplastin time
RBC	red blood cell
RLTCS	repeat low transverse cesarean section
RNST	reactive NST
ROA	right occiput anterior
ROM	rupture of membranes
ROP	right occiput posterior
RRR	regular rate and rhythm
RUQ	right upper quadrant
SAA	same as above
SBP	systolic blood pressure
S/P	status post
SQ	subcutaneous
SROM	spontaneous rupture of membranes
SSE	sterile speculum exam
STAT	urgent priority
SVD	spontaneous vaginal delivery
SVE	sterile vaginal exam
SVT	supraventricular tachycardia
TAP	transversus abdominis plane
TOLAC	trial of labor after cesarean
UO	urinary output
US	ultrasound
VAC	vacuum delivery
VAVD	vacuum-assisted vaginal delivery
VBAC	vaginal birth after cesarean

VS	vital signs
VTE	venous thromboembolism
WBC	white blood cell
WNL	within normal limits
WPW	Wolff–Parkinson–White

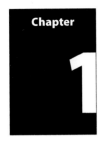

Introduction and Basic Principles

Shad Deering

Introduction

Managing patients on a labor and delivery suite can be a daunting task for any provider. It is an intimidating place to learn, where the clinical situation is constantly changing and more blood is being lost in a shorter amount of time than nearly anywhere else in the hospital. The care team is charged with taking care of two patients at the same time and must take into account how the care of one affects the other. Add to this the fact that you are dealing with all the expectations that nine months of pregnancy brings to the new parents, and that decisions must often be made quickly to ensure the best outcome when emergencies arise, and you have the modern labor and delivery ward.

Too often in obstetric training, the management of laboring patients is learned by being thrust onto labor and delivery without the benefit of adequate preparation for what will be encountered. While there is much that can only be learned by actually doing, such as cervical exams and deliveries, it is imperative to understand certain basic principles of labor and delivery management up front. This book is intended to provide a simple, structured overview of how to manage laboring and postpartum patients and function on a labor and delivery unit. While senior physicians and nurses must continue to teach and mentor junior staff, residents, and students how to perform obstetric exams and procedures, this book will provide a solid framework and background to work from.

The following is a concise set of general principles and information about labor and delivery that every provider should know.

General Principles

1. **Understand the basics.** The goal of this text is to help you to know the basic concepts you will need to manage laboring patients, as well as to recognize when problems occur. If you don't understand why a complication occurs, it is difficult to anticipate or correct it. You also need to know what medications, doses, and instruments to ask for during emergencies, because there are situations where even a short delay can make the difference between life and death. This knowledge is critical to responding to urgent situations in a calm and appropriate manner. While taking care of patients is a team

effort, junior or inexperienced staff may not know what you need in an emergency, and you must be very specific in terms of medication doses, instruments needed, and where to find them.

2. **Never be afraid to ask for help.** The best providers, when they are unsure of the proper course of action, will ask for another opinion. When, not if, a situation arises and you do not know what to do, think through the problem and have an idea of what you would like to do, and then ask for guidance. It is a sign of maturity, not weakness, to ask for help, and it will protect your patients.

3. **Do not make decisions without examining the patient.** When you first start to work on a labor and delivery ward, it is imperative to look at the patient before making decisions about management. As you progress and your clinical skills improve, you will have an idea of exactly what to do before you see the patient. But if there is ever a question in your mind about what action to take, then go and see the patient. This especially applies to the interpretation of fetal heart rate (FHR) tracings, which always look slightly different at the bedside, sometimes more reassuring, sometimes less.

4. **Communicate with your team.** Nothing you will learn from this book can help you if you don't work well with the rest of the care team. More than half of poor outcomes in obstetrics are related to breakdowns in communication and teamwork. Make it a point to know all of their names. At the beginning of every shift, be clear on who is the staff, charge nurse, anesthesia staff, etc. Keep them informed when you are expecting patients on labor and delivery, when you decide to admit a patient, and whenever you write an order or the plan of care changes. Doing these simple things will make your job of working on and managing a busy labor and delivery unit infinitely easier, and will keep your patients safe.

5. **Know where supplies are located.** If you are faced with an emergency, e.g., a postpartum hemorrhage, an eclamptic seizure, or fetal bradycardia, and everyone is busy with other patients, it is imperative that you know where to get the appropriate medications, instruments, or forceps in a timely manner. Remember that even if it isn't your role to go and get the medication, you may have to tell a new person where to find it.

6. **Practice with simulation when possible.** In the past, much of what you would do in labor and delivery was learned by the "see one, do one, teach one" method, but there are now simulators available for many procedures. You can practice performing a vaginal delivery, repairing vaginal lacerations, and even managing complications without any risk to actual patients. There is clear evidence that working with simulators can improve outcomes in real life. For an example and explanation of this, you can watch the TEDx talk "Why Doctors Should Play with Dolls," which can be seen at www.youtube.com/watch?v=rnuNft5sWUg.

7. **Assume the worst and hope for the best.** Whenever you evaluate a patient for a complaint, even one as simple as a headache, think of the worst thing it could be and work backward to the most benign. This will prevent you from missing the diagnosis of something uncommon but serious in favor of a more common and minor problem. An example of this is a headache in pregnancy. While it may be due to lack of sleep,

a migraine, or a simple cold, you should think of preeclampsia first and convince yourself that this is not the cause. It is usually an easy thing to rule out severe problems, but at least you will have considered them and not missed something that could have significant consequences for the patient.

An important part of this last basic concept is not to unnecessarily worry the patient. Do not tell every woman who has a headache, "I just want to make sure you don't have a tumor or bleeding in your head." You must consider everything to be thorough, but you do not need to mention the very serious but rare possibilities if you can rule them out.

Summary

By choosing to work on the labor and delivery unit, you assume an awesome responsibility. There is no greater reward or feeling than helping to bring life into the world, and no greater guilt than when things go poorly and you wonder if you could have done better. This book is written with the weight of this in mind. It will help you both to manage the normal, uncomplicated laboring patient, and to respond quickly and appropriately to common obstetric emergencies. Thank you for taking the time to prepare and do the best for your patients.

Common Examinations and Procedures

Ashley S. Coggins and Shad Deering

Introduction

Labor and delivery involve numerous examinations and procedures. While many of the examinations are learned only by actually performing them on patients, some basic instruction in how and when to perform the examinations and procedures is essential. You must understand not only what to do during an examination, but also when it is necessary and why you are doing it.

Brief Overview of Labor

Central to learning how to take care of laboring patients is understanding exactly what labor is. Labor is defined as regular uterine contractions that result in the progressive effacement (thinning) and dilation (opening) of the cervix. This is accompanied by the fetus moving down through the birth canal.

Effacement is usually described as a percentage. The cervix is approximately 4 cm long before labor, and this is said to be 0% effaced, or "long." If it shortens to 2 cm then it is described as 50% effaced. This is determined by digital exam, and it takes practice to become consistent. When the cervix is completely thinned out, it is said to be 100% or completely effaced.

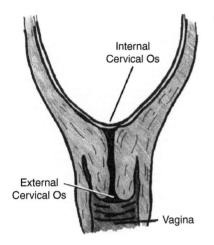

Figure 2.1 Internal and external cervical os.

Internal
Cervical Os

External
Cervical Os

Vagina

Dilation of the cervix describes how open the internal cervical os is in centimeters, between 0 and 10 cm. It is important to note that in multiparous women the external os may be dilated 1–2 cm normally, but the internal os is usually closed until labor begins (Figure 2.1). At 10 cm, the cervix is completely dilated. Judging the degree of dilation is another skill that is learned through practice.

The term "station" is used to describe how far down in the pelvis the fetus is. When the leading fetal body part, most often the head, is at the level of the maternal ischial spines, which can be felt on digital exam, the fetus is said to be at zero station. Everything is relative to this landmark, and station is measured in centimeters with a range of 5 cm in either direction.

Fetal station is important because when certain interventions such as rupturing the amniotic membranes or applying forceps or vacuum devices can be performed safely is dependent on this (see Chapter 9, *Operative Vaginal Delivery*). A complete description of how to perform a cervical exam is found later in this chapter.

Labor is divided into three stages:

Stage 1 begins with regular uterine contractions and ends when the cervix is fully dilated (10 cm) and completely effaced (100%).

Stage 2 begins when the cervix is completely dilated and effaced and ends with delivery of the fetus. This is the stage when the woman will push to deliver the infant.

Stage 3 begins after the fetus is delivered and ends with delivery of the placenta.

Each of these stages, as well as their management, is discussed in detail in subsequent chapters.

Exams

Admission History and Physical Exam

When a woman is admitted to the labor and delivery unit, a thorough physical exam should be performed. While the physical exam of a pregnant patient is essentially the same as for a non-pregnant patient, there are some important differences, and some findings that would be abnormal outside of pregnancy. Going through the exam:

History

A thorough history should be taken, to include the following:

Patient's age, gravidity, and parity. The patient's current age should be recorded. Gravidity and parity require more of an explanation.

Gravidity. This is the total number of times the patient has been pregnant. This includes all pregnancies, even those that ended in a miscarriage or abortion. This is written as "G" in the chart. If a patient has been pregnant three times, she is a gravida 3, or G3. (Note: If a patient is pregnant with twins or other multiple gestations, this only counts as one pregnancy.)

Parity. This refers to the number of births a woman has had, and how far along she was when they occurred. It is written as four numbers, which take into account the following events:

- Full-term births (37 weeks and up)
- Preterm births (20–36 weeks gestation)
- Abortions (this includes spontaneous and elective abortions)
- Living children (this is the number of children currently living)

Note: One part of this nomenclature that is tricky is that, in a woman with twins who delivers, this only counts as one delivery. The following are two examples to demonstrate how to write gravidity and parity.

Example 2.1. A 25-year-old woman is currently pregnant, and this is her third pregnancy. She has had one previous full-term delivery and one spontaneous miscarriage. Her gravidity and parity would be written as G3P1011.

Example 2.2. A 25-year-old woman is currently pregnant, and this is her second pregnancy. She had twins at 35 weeks with the previous pregnancy. Her gravidity and parity would be written as G2P0102. (She has one preterm delivery and two living children.)

Gestational age. It is imperative that the gestational age is recorded accurately, as decisions about augmenting or attempting to stop labor are largely based on this.

When writing the gestational age in the chart, it is written as the number of weeks completed plus the number of days of the next week. For instance, if the patient has completed 34 weeks and 4 days of her pregnancy, this is written as "34^{+4} weeks." A full discussion of how to calculate and check the gestational age can be found in Chapter 4, *Management of the First Stage of Labor*.

Both the gestational age and the criteria it is based on should be recorded in the chart. If it is based on a sure last menstrual period (LMP) then the chart should say the patient is "__ weeks by sure LMP." If the patient had an ultrasound that agreed with the estimated date of delivery (EDD), then both the LMP and ultrasound, as well as the gestational age the ultrasound was performed at, should be listed. For example, a patient with an ultrasound done at 8 weeks' gestation that agreed with her EDD from her LMP would be recorded in the chart as "__ weeks by sure LMP and 8-week ultrasound." If a patient's EDD was changed based on an ultrasound performed at 8 weeks' gestation, then this should be written as "the patient is *n* weeks by 8-week ultrasound."

Chief complaint. Always list the reason that the patient has presented for evaluation.

The 4 OB questions. Every patient who shows up to labor and delivery should be asked the following four questions:

1. Are you having any **BLEEDING?**
2. Are you having any **CONTRACTIONS?** (include time of onset/frequency/ intensity)
3. Do you feel like you broke your **WATER?** (include time/color of fluid)
4. Have you felt your baby **MOVING** today? (if not, then how long since the baby moved?)

Prenatal complications. All complications occurring during this pregnancy should be listed. Some of these may include gestational diabetes, Rh-negative status, group B streptococcus (GBS) status, preterm labor, etc.

Past medical history. All pertinent medical conditions should be listed. While this is no different than in non-pregnant patients, some common problems that have obstetric implications include diabetes, hypertension, asthma, thrombophilias, and thyroid disease.

Past surgical history. All previous surgeries must be recorded. Ask specifically regarding abdominal surgery, as this can make a cesarean delivery more difficult because of adhesions, and certain abdominal operations (such as a myomectomy) may mean that a vaginal delivery is contraindicated (see Chapter 10).

Past gynecologic history. Make a note of any history of abnormal Pap smears or sexually transmitted diseases. Especially important are HIV and herpes simplex virus (HSV), as they may require a cesarean delivery depending on the situation.

Past obstetric history. List all previous pregnancies as well as the year they occurred and what the outcomes were. Include the gestational age at delivery and the infant's birth weight and route of delivery (vaginal, cesarean, forceps, or vacuum). Also note any complications that occurred, such as shoulder dystocia or postpartum hemorrhage.

Social history. Ask about alcohol or tobacco use in pregnancy as well as illicit or recreational drugs.

Allergies. List all allergies a patient claims, as well as what reactions occurred with each.

Family history. Ask about a family history of diabetes, hypertension, preeclampsia, and cancer.

Medications. List all current medications being taken by the patient.

Prenatal laboratory results. Make a list of all prenatal laboratory results from the patient's chart in your history and physical. These will typically include the following:

- Hematocrit
- Hemoglobin
- Platelets
- Pap smear
- Rubella/varicella titers
- Hepatitis B surface antigen
- Blood type
- Antibody screen
- Gonorrhea/chlamydia cultures
- HIV

- GBS culture (see Chapter 4)
- Urinalysis and culture
- Genetic/cystic fibrosis screening results

An example outline and sample notes can be found in Appendix B, *Sample Notes and Orders*.

Physical Examination

Neurologic exam. The patient should be alert and oriented to person, place, and time. She may be in mild distress because of labor, but no focal neurologic deficits should be present.

Head, eyes, ears, nose, and throat (HEENT). A general inspection is done and any abnormalities noted. Make sure to note any significant facial edema, as this can be a sign of preeclampsia (see Chapter 14). Often, since you may not have seen the patient previously, it is easier to simply ask the woman or her partner if her face looks swollen.

Lungs. The lungs should be clear to auscultation, although at term there may be slightly decreased breath sounds noted in the bases of both lungs secondary to elevation of the hemi-diaphragm by the pregnancy.

Heart. A systolic ejection murmur is a normal finding, and nearly 95% of pregnant women will have one at term.

Abdomen. The abdomen will be gravid, which near term makes palpation of other abdominal organs essentially impossible. The fundal height should be determined and Leopold's maneuvers performed to assess both the position and estimated weight of the fetus. Both exams are explained later in this chapter.

Genitourinary. The perineum should be visually inspected for evidence of lesions, especially active herpes lesions, as these will preclude a vaginal delivery. A digital vaginal exam is performed and the cervix checked to determine dilation, effacement, fetal station, and what the presenting part of the fetus is (see *Cervical Exam* below). During the exam, the adequacy of the pelvis can also be examined by performing clinical pelvimetry, also explained later in this chapter. A rectal exam is not usually performed as part of the standard admission exam. If collecting a GBS culture then do this now with a rectal/vaginal swab.

Extremities. Examine the extremities for evidence of edema. Some edema, especially bilaterally in the lower extremities, is common and a normal finding during pregnancy. If unilateral edema is present, especially accompanied by pain, then the diagnosis of a deep venous thrombosis must be considered and additional studies pursued.

Other. Obviously, if the patient has specific complaints, such as flank pain or breast pain, then the physical examination should focus more attention on these areas.

Outline. A sample outline note of an admission physical exam can be found in Appendix B, *Sample Notes and Orders*.

Cervical Exam

Digital cervical exams are performed to assess a patient's labor progress and to help you decide when a woman needs to be admitted to the hospital. They are performed on almost every woman who will be admitted to labor and delivery, and it takes practice to become consistent in your exams. When starting out, it is easiest to examine laboring patients who have an epidural in place, as they are generally less uncomfortable during the exam.

Indications

A cervical exam is indicated during the initial evaluation of a laboring patient, during labor to evaluate progression, and when evaluating fetal distress or a non-reassuring fetal heart rate tracing (see Chapter 3).

Contraindications

The most important contraindications to a cervical exam are vaginal bleeding and preterm premature rupture of membranes (PPROM).

Bleeding. If a patient presents with vaginal bleeding, then an ultrasound should be performed to determine the location of the placenta. If the placenta is overlying the cervical os, then a cervical exam can cause catastrophic hemorrhage and should not be performed. A transvaginal sonogram is done if the abdominal ultrasound is unclear as to exactly where the placenta is located.

Another possibility is a vasa previa, which occurs when the fetal blood vessels abnormally run through the membranes before inserting into the placenta. If the membranes rupture and the vessels are lacerated, then fetal hemorrhage may occur and, because of the small fetal blood volume, this can be life-threatening to the fetus in a very short time.

If you feel the patient has either of these problems, then additional evaluation and stabilization may be required. Interventions include monitoring both fetal and maternal vital signs and attempts to stabilize the patient and fetus while being prepared to effect delivery by an urgent cesarean section if indicated.

Premature preterm rupture of membranes (PPROM). This occurs when the membranes rupture before 37 weeks' gestation. The most recent American College of Obstetricians and Gynecologists (ACOG) Practice Bulletin on the topic recommends delivery at 34 weeks for all women with PPROM (ACOG 2016a). Because cervical exams can increase

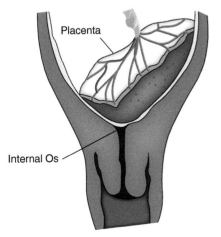

Figure 2.2 Placenta previa.

the chance of infection, a sterile speculum exam is performed in place of a cervical exam and the dilation and effacement of the cervix are determined visually. PPROM is discussed in more detail in Chapter 14.

Before Performing the Exam

1. Make sure there are no contraindications to the exam.
2. Ensure you have a chaperone standing by. (This is sometimes difficult on a busy labor and delivery unit, but is extremely important.)

Performing the Exam

The exam begins by informing the patient that you are going to check her cervix and explaining the indication. After this, position the patient for the exam. If stirrups are available for the feet, then assist the woman in placing her feet into them. If not, then have the patient place her heels together and let her legs fall outward. There are several components that should be evaluated during the exam and then recorded on the patient's chart. These include:

Cervical dilation. The cervix is normally closed prior to the onset of labor. Cervical dilation describes how dilated the internal cervical os is in centimeters, from 0 cm (closed) to 10 cm. It is important to recognize that the external os may be several centimeters dilated while the internal os is closed or 1 cm dilated. This is especially true for multiparous patients. Ten centimeters means the cervix is fully dilated, and the first stage of labor is complete.

Determining exactly how dilated the cervix is takes practice, and checking a laboring patient after a more senior provider and comparing your exam with theirs will help you to learn this skill. In general, if you can fit one finger into the internal os, the cervix is 1 cm dilated. If your two fingers on top of each other fit tightly into the internal os, this is 2 cm, and if you can insert two fingers side by side, this is 3 cm. (Obviously, these measurements will vary slightly depending on the size of the examiner's hands.) From this point, it becomes slightly more difficult and will take practice to become consistent.

Cervical effacement. Prior to the onset of labor, the cervix is approximately 4 cm long by digital exam. The cervix is usually referred to as being "long" in this case. As the cervix shortens with labor, the effacement is described as a percentage of the original length. So if the cervix shortens from 4 cm to 3 cm, it is said to be 25% effaced. When it is only 1 cm long, it is 75% effaced, and when it is completely thinned out it is "completely" effaced. This part of the exam also requires significant practice and will seem extremely subjective at first.

Fetal station. The fetal station usually refers to the leading bony part of the fetal head. (In the case of a frank breech presentation, it is the station of the fetal buttocks.) The reference point for this measurement is the ischial spines. When the fetal head is at the level of the ischial spines (Figure 2.3), this is referred to as "zero (0) station." The measurements then go for 5 cm on either side of this, with positive numbers as the fetus is further down into the birth canal and negative numbers when the fetal head is above the level of the ischial spines (Figure 2.4). When the fetus is at 0 station, the head is said to be "engaged."

- This measurement is important because, when the fetus is not engaged, and especially when the head is above –2 station, performing an amniotomy can result

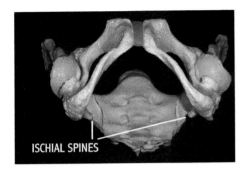

Figure 2.3 Ischial spines.

ISCHIAL SPINES

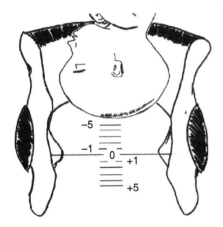

Figure 2.4 Fetal station.

−5

−1

0

+1

+5

in a prolapsed umbilical cord, which requires an urgent cesarean section (see Chapter 14). It is also important in determining when an operative vaginal delivery can be safely performed (see Chapter 9). In general, an operative vaginal delivery is rarely performed when the fetus is above +2 station.

• When starting to perform cervical exams, you may not appreciate the ischial spines at first. Again, performing exams on patients with epidural anesthesia will allow you to do a more thorough exam when starting out, and help you to find these landmarks.

Presenting part. Always document what the presenting part is, which will usually be the fetal head. If you are unsure that what you are palpating is the fetal head, then perform an abdominal ultrasound to confirm the presentation. Many institutions now perform an ultrasound to confirm fetal presentation for every woman who is admitted in labor.

Fetal head position (if vertex). During the cervical exam, you should always try and determine the fetal head position. This is done by palpation of the fetal sutures. A diagram of the fetal sutures is shown in Figure 2.5.

First, determine the location of the sagittal suture, which will tell you the axis of the fetal head. Then, palpate the fontanelles on either side. The anterior fontanelle is shaped like a diamond, and the posterior fontanelle as a triangle. After determining the axis of the

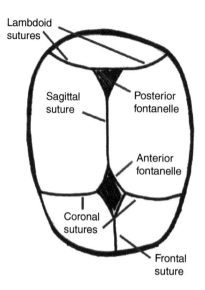

Figure 2.5 Fetal sutures.

fetal head and where the anterior/posterior fontanelles are facing, you can then record the fetal head position.*

The fetal head position is described in terms of the fetal occiput's relationship to the maternal left and right. If the fetus is facing the floor (Figure 2.6a), then it is said to be in the occiput anterior (OA) position. If the fetus is facing up, then it is in the occiput posterior (OP) position (Figure 2.6b). If the fetal head is rotated such that the occiput is anterior and to the maternal left, then the fetus is in the left occiput anterior (LOA) position. An example of this is shown in Figure 2.6c, and Figure 2.6d shows the left occiput posterior (LOP) position. If the sagittal suture runs in a horizontal plane, then the fetus is said to be either left or right occiput transverse (LOT or ROT), depending on which way the fetus is facing. A diagram demonstrating all the possible head positions is shown in Figure 2.7. Always remember that this is in reference to the maternal left and right.

It is helpful to identify the fetal head position early in labor because later on, after a long labor or with pushing, molding and scalp edema (or caput) can make this very difficult to determine. Remember that many malpositioned infants will spontaneously rotate during the labor process and will not cause a problem.

Recording the Exam

When describing the examination in the chart, it is typically written in shorthand. One common way this is represented is:

Dilation (cm) / Effacement (%) / Station (−5 to +5) / Head position

---

* If caput makes it difficult to define the fontanelles, but you can tell which way the sagittal suture is running, then palpation of an ear can assist you by determining which way the fetus is facing. Additionally, an abdominal sonogram may be performed to help better assess the fetal head position. If the fetus is in an OP or OT position, you will be able to visualize the ocular socket(s).

(a)

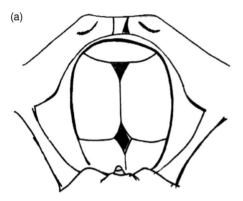

Figure 2.6a Occiput anterior (OA) position.

(b)

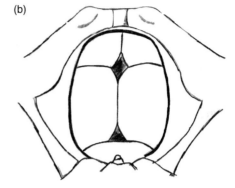

Figure 2.6b Occiput posterior (OP) position.

(c)

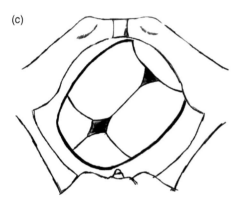

Figure 2.6c Left occiput anterior (LOA) position.

(d)

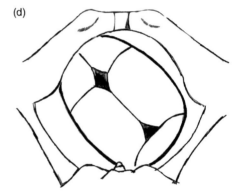

Figure 2.6d Left occiput posterior (LOP) position.

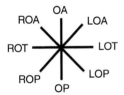

Figure 2.7 Diagram of possible fetal head positions (based on fetal occiput).

So, if a patient was 4 cm dilated, 75% effaced at 0 station, and in the left occiput anterior position, the exam would be recorded in the chart as:

Cervix exam: 4 / 75% / 0 / LOA

If the cervix has not started to efface, it is referred to as "long" in this shorthand. Also, when the cervix is completely dilated or completely effaced, it is characterized as "C" for "complete" in this shorthand. An example of a patient who is 10 cm dilated, 100% effaced, at +1 station in the occiput anterior position would be written as:

Cervix exam: C / C / +1 / OA

Hint: If you have difficulty reaching the cervix, which will happen at times because of how posterior it can be, then you can have the patient make fists with her hands then lift up her hips and put her hands underneath her hips. Doing this will sometimes make the cervix more accessible by tilting it forward.

Clinical Pelvimetry

Clinical pelvimetry is a series of exam maneuvers to determine if the patient's pelvis feels "adequate" or large enough to allow for vaginal delivery. This is a helpful examination, but is frequently not done in its entirety on labor and delivery because of patient discomfort or lack of provider training in recent years. Pelvimetry is not an exact science, and a truly contracted and inadequate pelvis can rarely be determined without a trial of labor. When a contracted pelvis is suspected, however, you can monitor more closely for evidence of obstructed labor. This initial exam may also affect your decision to attempt an operative vaginal delivery later in the labor process. Radiographic pelvimetry has been shown to increase C-section rates, and there is insufficient evidence for its use; thus it is not recommended (Pattinson *et al.* 2017).

In order to appreciate why this exam matters, and how to perform it, some knowledge of pelvic anatomy and a few basic definitions are necessary.

Anatomy

The important anatomic structures that must be assessed with clinical pelvimetry include the following (Figure 2.8):

- Coccyx
- Ischial spines
- Pelvic sidewalls
- Pubic arch
- Sacral prominence

Pelvic Shapes

It is also necessary to understand that there are different pelvic shapes, some of which can result in obstructed labor, or a baby that will persistently remain in the occiput posterior

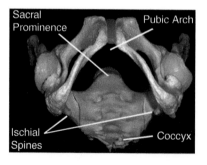

Figure 2.8 Pelvic bony anatomy.

position. In general, there are four types of pelvic shape described, although most women will have one that falls in between these.

Gynecoid. This is the most common pelvic shape (> 50% of women) and is generally compatible with vaginal delivery. The inlet of the pelvis tends to be round, which allows for the fetus to descend and rotate for delivery. The sidewalls are straight and the pubic arch is wide (> 90 degrees). The distance between the ischial spines is also usually adequate for vaginal delivery (Figure 2.9a).

Anthropoid. An anthropoid pelvis differs from a gynecoid pelvis in that there is more room for the fetal head in the posterior portion of the pelvis, which can allow the fetus to engage in the occiput posterior position. The sidewalls may be slightly convergent, and the pubic arch may also be just less than 90 degrees. This type is more common in non-white females, and usually allows for a vaginal delivery (Figure 2.9b).

Android. This type of pelvis is heart-shaped, with the anterior portion being very narrow. The ischial spines are very prominent, which may hinder internal rotation, and the sidewalls are convergent. The sacrum also tends to be angled anteriorly with very little curve present. The pubic arch is narrow and usually much less than 90 degrees. While vaginal delivery is possible with this type of pelvis, it can be associated with difficult operative vaginal deliveries as well as obstructed labor (Figure 2.9c).

Platypelloid. A platypelloid pelvis is the least common pelvic shape. The pelvic inlet is very wide in the transverse diameter. The sidewalls are straight and the ischial spines are not prominent. The pubic arch is also very wide (Figure 2.9d).

Definitions

Diagonal conjugate. This is the distance from the symphysis pubis to the sacral promontory (Figure 2.10). It can be measured during a vaginal exam by inserting two fingers into the vagina and directing them to the sacral prominence and then measuring how far in your hand was inserted at this point. An adequate diagonal conjugate is 11.5 cm or greater. The easiest way to do this is, with your hand in the same position as during the exam, to measure a distance of 11.5 cm from the tip of your middle finger back toward your hand. When you perform your exam, if the distance is greater than this, it is considered adequate.

Obstetric conjugate. Although we measure the diagonal conjugate, we must also take into account the width of the pubic symphysis. The obstetric conjugate is the actual measurement that the fetus must pass through, and it is calculated by subtracting 1.5 cm from the diagonal conjugate. So an obstetric conjugate of 10.0 cm or greater is generally adequate for a vaginal delivery.

Bi-ischial diameter. This is simply the distance between the ischial spines. A normal measurement for this is 8 cm or greater. It is measured by placing a closed fist against the perineum. The ischial spines will be palpable on either side of the fist. Again, measure your fist prior to performing the exam so you know how wide it is in relation to what a normal bi-ischial diameter should measure (Figure 2.11).

Pubic arch. The pubic arch is palpated during a vaginal exam. In most women, the arch will be at least 90 degrees, which should be adequate for a vaginal delivery. With certain pelvic shapes, most notably the android pelvis, this arch may be less than 90

(a)

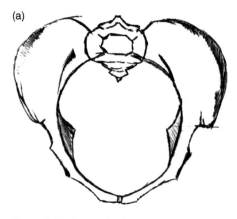

Figure 2.9a Gynecoid pelvis.

(b)

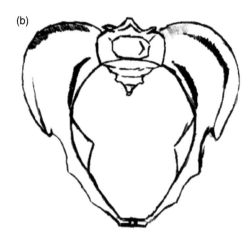

Figure 2.9b Anthropoid pelvis.

(c)

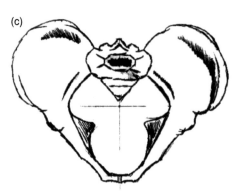

Figure 2.9c Android pelvis.

(d)

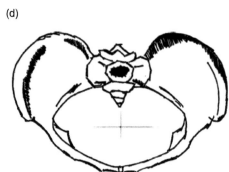

Figure 2.9d Platypelloid pelvis.

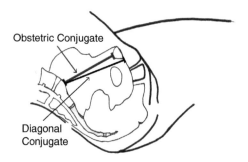

Obstetric Conjugate

Diagonal
Conjugate

Figure 2.10 Diagonal and obstetric conjugates.

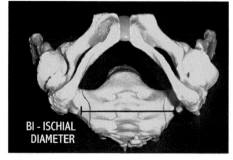

BI - ISCHIAL
DIAMETER

Figure 2.11 Bi-ischial diameter.

degrees. While this does not preclude a vaginal delivery, it should be noted and taken into consideration if an operative vaginal delivery is considered (Figure 2.12).

Performing the Measurements

When you perform the exam and measurements, having a mental checklist will help prevent you from omitting any part. The following is a checklist for clinical pelvimetry.

Place the patient in the dorsal lithotomy position and assess the following:

1. Bi-ischial diameter (normal > 8 cm)
2. Pubic arch (> or < 90 degrees)
3. Coccyx mobility (mobile vs. not mobile / prominent vs. not prominent)
4. Sacrum (curved vs. straight)
5. Diagonal conjugate (> or < 11.5 cm)
6. Ischial spines (prominent vs. not prominent)
7. Sidewalls (convergent vs. not convergent)

Recording the Examination

You should note a description of your clinical pelvimetry in your admission physical exam. If the pelvis is adequate by your exam, you can simply state "Pelvis appears adequate for labor by clinical pelvimetry." If there is an abnormality on exam, such as a narrow pubic arch or convergent sidewalls, it should also be noted.

Fundal Height

The fundal height is checked at each antepartum visit as well as when a patient is admitted in labor. If the fundal height is within 2 cm of the gestational age in weeks (i.e., 34 cm ± 2 cm at 34 weeks EGA), then the fetus is assumed to be growing appropriately. It is measured from the pubic symphysis to the top of the fundus (Figure 2.13). This is obviously easier in some patients than in others, depending on the body habitus. Some reasons for an increased fundal height include fetal macrosomia, multiple gestation, and polyhydramnios. A fundal height that is lagging can be caused by ruptured membranes, oligohydramnios, a growth-restricted fetus, or labor as the fetus descends into the pelvis.

On the postpartum ward, the fundal height is checked on a daily basis and is described in relation to the umbilicus. If the top of the fundus is palpable at the umbilicus, it is said to be at "U," whereas if it is 2 cm below, it is at "U–2." If the fundus is above U+2, then you should look for a reason, such as retained clots in the uterus or, more commonly, a distended

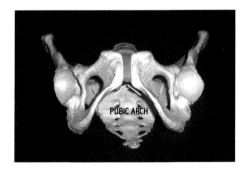

Figure 2.12 Pubic arch.

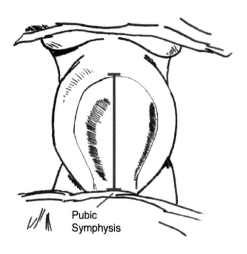

Figure 2.13 Fundal height.

Pubic
Symphysis

bladder. Having the patient void and then rechecking will often result in a normal measurement.

Leopold's Maneuvers

At the time of admission, you should perform Leopold's maneuvers, both to determine the fetal lie (i.e., vertex, breech, or transverse) and to get an estimate of the fetal weight. While it is obviously easier to perform on patients who are not obese, they should still be attempted on every patient. The first three maneuvers are done facing the head of the woman from whichever side of the bed is the easiest for the examiner. For the fourth maneuver it is best to turn and face the woman's feet.

First maneuver. Using both hands, palpate the fundal portion of the uterus. A head should feel much harder than the buttocks (Figure 2.14a). Don't worry if the fetal position is not completely clear with the first maneuver, as the others will usually make things more clear.

Second maneuver. Move your hands from the fundus down on both sides of the uterus. On one side you should feel a firm, relatively straight structure, which corresponds to the fetal back, while the other side should have multiple small and irregular parts, which are the fetal limbs. If the back is directly anterior, then you may not feel any of the fetal extremities (Figure 2.14b).

Third maneuver. Using one hand, grasp just superior to the pubic symphysis with the thumb and fingers and determine again what the presenting part is. When the head is palpated, it is noted to be a hard, round mass, and if it is the buttocks, it will be softer and nodular.

If the fetus is not engaged, then the presenting part will be mobile. If this is the case and the fetus is vertex, you can attempt to determine if the head is flexed or extended by determining if the cephalic prominence is on the same side as the extremities (which would imply that the head is flexed) or on the same side as the back (which means the head is extended). If the presenting part is deeply engaged, then it will be fixed in the pelvis and not mobile, and you will not be able to determine flexion/extension of the fetal head (Figure 2.14c).

Fourth maneuver: Turn and face the patient's feet and place your hands on either side of the presenting part and push down toward the pelvis with your fingers. If the fetus is in a vertex presentation, then the hand on the back of the fetal head should go farther before resistance is encountered, as the other hand will be stopped by the cephalic prominence (Figure 2.14d). Remember that if the fetus is deeply engaged, this will be difficult or impossible to determine. If the fetus is breech, then you will not palpate the cephalic prominence.

These maneuvers, while they require practice, will allow you to determine the fetal position with a reasonable degree of certainty. One study reported that abnormal presentations were correctly identified 88% of the time with just these maneuvers (Lydon-Rochelle *et al.* 1993).

Many factors such as provider skill, patient habitus, and placenta location can make these maneuvers difficult to perform. Nearly all labor and delivery units will have a portable ultrasound available for evaluation. It is common practice to confirm fetal position with an ultrasound after performing Leopold's maneuvers to avoid potentially committing a woman to labor with a breech fetus.

Estimating Fetal Weight

While performing the maneuvers and determining the fetal lie, you should attempt to estimate the fetal weight. As you palpate the fetus, imagine that you are palpating 1-liter bags of normal saline and try and decide how many bags would be equal to the fetus. For every 1 liter bag, assume the weight would be 1000 grams. Keep in mind that normal birth weight is highly

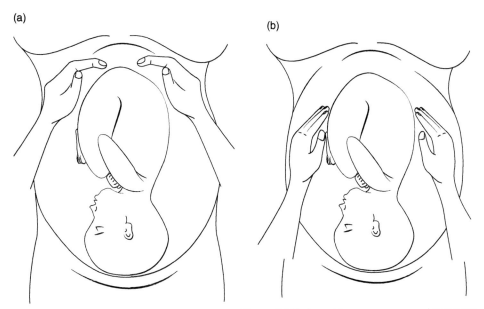

(a)   (b)

Figure 2.14a Leopold's maneuvers: first maneuver.

Figure 2.14b Leopold's maneuvers: second maneuver.

(c) (d)

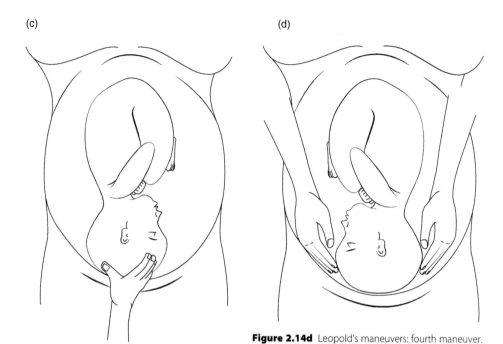

Figure 2.14d Leopold's maneuvers: fourth maneuver.

Figure 2.14c Leopold's maneuvers: third maneuver.

variable and dependent on multiple factors, but the average birth weight at term in the United States is somewhere between 3000 and 3500 grams (Cunningham *et al.* 2014).

Exam for Patients on Magnesium Sulfate

Whenever patients are on magnesium sulfate, whether for neuroprotection or for seizure prophylaxis for preeclampsia (see Chapter 14), they should be examined on a regular basis by a physician to monitor for magnesium toxicity. Check with your institution's policy, but usually a physician should write a note every 2–4 hours for patients undergoing treatment with magnesium sulfate. The exam and note should focus on the following:

Vital signs. These should include the patient's pulse, blood pressure, temperature and pulse oximeter reading if there is any complaint of shortness of breath.

Urine output. Since magnesium sulfate is excreted in the urine, a decrease in urine output can result in accumulation of toxic amounts of magnesium sulfate. The amount of urine output over both the past hour and the past 6–12 hours should be recorded.

Heart. This part of the exam is usually normal, as cardiovascular collapse occurs only with extreme toxicity.

Lungs. Monitor for evidence of decreased breath sounds as well as crackles that can be the first signs of pulmonary edema.

Reflexes. Deep tendon reflexes (DTRs) should be monitored. DTRs disappear when the serum level of magnesium sulfate is 10 mEq/L, and since respiratory failure can occur at serum levels of 12 mEq/L, you must be extremely vigilant when DTRs are not present. (See Chapter 14 for a discussion of magnesium sulfate toxicity and treatment.)

Assessment. The note should report whether the patient is stable or unstable.

Plan. The plan should include any changes to the magnesium sulfate regimen being given (see Appendix B for a sample magnesium sulfate note).

Rule Out Ruptured Membranes (ROM)

This is one of the most common complaints of women who present to labor and delivery for evaluation. After taking a standard history, as described earlier in this chapter, if the patient complains of any suspicious leakage of fluid, then a sterile speculum exam should be performed. There are four things you are looking for during the exam:

Pooling. A very sensitive marker of ruptured membranes is pooling of amniotic fluid in the vagina. It can often be seen on the labia and perineum even before placement of the speculum when the membranes are grossly ruptured. (Even if this is seen, the speculum should still be placed to evaluate the rest of the parameters as well as to determine cervical dilation.)

Valsalva. With the speculum in place and the cervix in view, have the patient Valsalva. If you see fluid come from the cervical os, this is evidence of ruptured membranes.

Ferning. After obtaining a sample of fluid from the vagina and allowing it to dry on a slide, observe the slide under a microscope. Amniotic fluid will demonstrate a pattern that looks like the leaf of a fern (or like the tree on the back of the Connecticut state quarter) whereas vaginal fluid will not.

Nitrazine. The normal pH of vaginal fluid is between 4.5 and 5.5, and amniotic fluid usually has a pH of between 7.0 and 7.5. If the fluid obtained from the vagina during the exam demonstrates a pH above 6.5, it will cause the nitrazine paper to change color, and this is suggestive of ruptured membranes. Some things that can cause a false-positive nitrazine test include blood and semen.

Before Performing the Exam

Before starting the exam, make sure you have the following:

1. Sterile speculum
2. Sterile gloves
3. Nitrazine paper
4. Sterile cotton-tipped swab
5. Glass slide
6. Chaperone/assistant

Performing the Exam

The steps to performing the exam include the following:

1. Put on sterile gloves and have your assistant open the sterile speculum in a sterile manner so that you can grasp it.
2. Place the speculum into the vagina and visualize the cervix and note how dilated it appears.
3. Look for **pooling** of fluid in the vagina.

4. Take a sterile swab and obtain a sample of whatever fluid is present.
5. Apply the swab to both **nitrazine** paper and the blank slide.
6. Have the patient **Valsalva** to see if any fluid comes from the cervix.
7. Remove the speculum.
8. Allow the slide to dry completely and then place it under a microscope to look for **ferning**.
9. Perform an abdominal ultrasound to determine fetal presentation (vertex vs. breech).

It is worthwhile to mention some newer tests available for evaluating rupture of membranes. Due to cost and availability, the type of test offered will vary from hospital to hospital so it is good to review what is available at your institution. These tests can be helpful when the basic ROM exam is equivocal, but should not take the place of the basic ROM evaluation.

AmniSure. Detects placental alpha-microglobulin-1 (PAMG-1) in vaginal secretions. A benefit of this test is that it is not affected by semen or small amounts of blood that might alter a nitrazine test. The sterile swab must be twirled in the vagina for 1 minute and then twirled in the kit solution vial for 1 minute. A test strip is then placed in the vial for 10 minutes, with a positive result demonstrated by two visible lines. This is a highly sensitive and specific test but might not be offered in some hospitals because of its cost.

Actim PROM. Detects placental protein 12 in vaginal secretions. Similarly, this test is not affected by semen or small amounts of blood. A dipstick method is used, with a positive result demonstrated by two lines on the dipstick. This test is more accurate the sooner it is used after rupture of membranes. In a meta-analysis this test has been shown to be less accurate than AmniSure; it is used more often in Europe than in the United States (Ramsauer *et al.* 2013).

ROM Plus. This is a combined monoclonal/polyclonal antibody test detecting placental protein 12 and alpha-fetoprotein. The sterile swab is placed in the vagina for 15 seconds, then in the provided solution. Some of this fluid is then placed on a test strip. This test is not affected by trace amounts of blood.

After evaluating for ROM, a sterile digital vaginal exam can be performed if the patient is at term, and there was difficulty in visualizing the cervix because of the presence of a significant amount of amniotic fluid. If, however, the patient is preterm, then you should refrain from performing a digital exam until necessary, as you are trying to prevent infection. If the exam is negative for ruptured membranes, then it is prudent to evaluate the amniotic fluid volume by measuring the maximum vertical pocket (MVP) to demonstrate a normal level of amniotic fluid.

Recording the Exam

After performing the exam, write a note on the patient's chart and comment on all four of the criteria as well as recording how dilated the cervix appeared. It is also important to note the color and consistency of the amniotic fluid, which is usually clear, as meconium or blood may be present and require some form of intervention.

Procedures

Amnioinfusion

This refers to the instillation of fluid around the fetus, and it is usually performed during labor when specific situations arise. While in the past this procedure was performed routinely for any evidence of meconium, more recent evidence has shown that an amnio-infusion is not indicated for oligohydramnios or meconium-stained fluid in the absence of fetal heart rate (FHR) abnormalities.

Indications for Amnioinfusion

Oligohydramnios. When a patient with oligohydramnios is laboring, it is important to monitor for variable decelerations and be ready to perform an amnioinfusion, though doing this prophylactically is probably not indicated (Hofmeyr and Lawrie 2012).

Variable decelerations. When variable decelerations are present during labor, performing an amnioinfusion can decrease the severity of the decelerations by preventing cord compression. It may also decrease the risk of cesarean section for FHR abnormalities by up to 80% (Pitt *et al.* 2000, Hofmeyr and Lawrie 2012). ACOG advocates amnioinfusion for repetitive variable decelerations in efforts to reduce the rate of cesarean delivery (ACOG 2014, reaffirmed 2016).

Meconium. In the past, amnioinfusion was routinely done for meconium-stained fluid. The theory behind this procedure is to dilute the meconium in hopes of preventing meconium aspiration syndrome after birth, which can result in significant infant morbidity and mortality. In practice, however, amnioinfusion has been shown to decrease the incidence of meconium below the vocal cords, but not to decrease the risk of meconium aspiration syndrome (Xu *et al.* 2007). Subsequent studies have failed to demonstrate improvements in perinatal outcome with amnioinfusion placed for meconium in most hospital settings (Hofmeyr *et al.* 2014). The most recent ACOG Committee Opinion on the topic agrees with this and recommends that amnioinfusion be performed in the presence of repetitive variable decelerations regardless of amniotic fluid meconium status (ACOG 2006, reaffirmed 2018).

Contraindications for Amnioinfusion

The contraindications to an amnioinfusion are essentially the same as the contraindications to placement of an intrauterine pressure catheter (IUPC) or any condition that makes amniotomy contraindicated (see *Intrauterine Pressure Catheter,* later in this chapter). Intra-amniotic infection is a relative contraindication at some institutions.

Before Performing Amnioinfusion

1. Make sure you have room-temperature normal saline available for the infusion.
2. Have the equipment and tubing in the room and ready to start the infusion.
3. Consider whether there are any contraindications to the procedure.

Procedure

After an IUPC is inserted, either a bolus or continuous infusion of normal saline can be given. The bolus protocol will usually be 500 mL of normal saline (although up to 800 mL may be given) running in at 10–15 mL/minute. The continuous protocol begins with 10 mL/minute for the first hour, followed by 3 mL/minute after this. Monitor how much fluid leaks out during the labor and whether or not the meconium becomes more diluted.

Complications

Complications with amnioinfusion are rare, but the most common ones reported are uterine tachysystole and FHR abnormalities (Wentstrom *et al.* 1995). Additionally, there may be an increase in intrapartum fever with amnioinfusion (Novikova *et al.* 2012). Overall, the procedure is considered very safe.

Amniotomy: Artificial Rupture of Membranes (AROM)

Indications for AROM

An amniotomy may be performed in order to assist in the progress of labor (see Chapter 7) or to allow for better assessment of fetal status and uterine contraction strength by allowing for internal monitors – intrauterine pressure catheter (IUPC) and fetal scalp electrode (FSE) – to be placed.

Contraindications for AROM

Maternal infection. In patients with active herpes (HSV) lesions, amniotomy should not be performed, as it can increase the risk of transmission of the infection to the fetus.
In patients with HIV, care should be taken to minimize fetal exposure to maternal fluids. However, when the viral load is < 1000 copies/mL, patients may elect for a vaginal delivery and appropriate labor interventions can be done at the clinician's discretion (ACOG 2000, reaffirmed 2017).

Fetal head not engaged. If the fetal head is not engaged, or well applied to the cervix, then performing an amniotomy could precipitate a cord prolapse (see Chapter 14).

Non-vertex presentation. If the presenting part is a foot, or the fetus is in a transverse lie, then rupturing the membranes is contraindicated, as labor should not proceed with a fetus in that position, and there is an increased risk of umbilical cord prolapse.

Before Performing AROM

1. Make sure you have sterile gloves and an amniotomy hook.
2. Ensure the patient's nurse or an assistant is in the room in case of fetal distress or a cord prolapse.
3. Make sure there are no contraindications to the procedure.

Procedure

A digital cervical exam is performed. During the exam, you should check to make sure the fetal head is either engaged or well applied and not higher than –2 station, and that no portion of the umbilical cord is palpable. If the fetus is –2 station, then having your assistant apply moderate fundal pressure can help keep the head well applied to the cervix in an attempt to prevent a cord prolapse during the procedure. The amniotomy instrument, often referred to as an "amniohook," is inserted between the index and middle fingers of the hand in the vagina with the sharp hook facing down in order to prevent any trauma to the vagina or cervix. When the amniohook is in place against the fetal vertex, it is rotated 180 degrees and then gently scraped against the membranes until a hole is made, at which point you will both feel and see amniotic fluid. If internal monitors (FSE or IUPC) need to be placed, this can be done at this time.

Recording the Exam

You should make a note in the chart after performing an AROM and include the cervix examination, the time it was performed, if internal monitors were placed, and the color and amount of amniotic fluid that was seen. If meconium is present, comment on whether it is thin, thick, or particulate.

Complications

The most emergent complication that can result from amniotomy is a prolapsed umbilical cord, which requires immediate cesarean delivery (see Chapter 14). Fortunately, this is a rare occurrence when the fetal head is well applied to the cervix at the time of amniotomy. As there will be less amniotic fluid around the fetus after amniotomy, variable decelerations may also occur.

Contraction Stress Test (CST)

A contraction stress test (CST) induces contractions in an attempt to better evaluate fetal status. A well-oxygenated fetus will be able to tolerate the intermittent stress of contractions without difficulty, while a compromised fetus may demonstrate distress with the temporarily decreased oxygenation that occurs normally with contractions. The incidence of a stillbirth occurring within a week of a reassuring, or negative, CST is extremely low at 0.3 per 1000, which is even lower than that for a reassuring non-stress test (NST), which has been reported as 1.9 per 1000 (ACOG 1999, reaffirmed 2014).

Because this test involves inducing contractions, it is rarely used in preterm patients, and because other less invasive tests are now possible on labor and delivery, such as the biophysical profile (BPP), it is not commonly performed. However, when a woman comes to labor and delivery for evaluation of labor, and she is spontaneously contracting at least three times in 10 minutes, this is essentially a spontaneous CST. If this is the case, it should be noted in the chart, as a normal CST is even more reassuring than a reactive NST, as stated previously.

Indications for CST

A CST is usually performed after another less invasive test is equivocal regarding fetal status. For instance, if a patient has a non-reactive NST, a CST can be performed as a follow-up test.

Contraindications for CST

Patients who should not labor should not have this test performed. Some of these conditions include the following:

- Preterm premature rupture of membranes (PPROM)
- Placenta previa or vasa previa
- Previous classical uterine incision or other uterine surgery that makes labor contraindicated (see Chapter 10, *Cesarean Delivery*)
- Preterm labor or patients at risk for preterm labor

Before Performing CST

1. Make sure there are no contraindications to the procedure.
2. Counsel the patient regarding the possibility of fetal distress and the need for urgent delivery.

Procedure

The patient is placed in the recumbent position on her side, and external monitors are placed to continuously monitor both the fetal heart rate and contractions. Peripheral intravenous access is usually obtained even if oxytocin is not used to stimulate contractions. In order for the test to be interpreted, the patient must have at least three contractions in 10 minutes that last at least 40 seconds each and a concurrent tracing of the FHR. If the patient is spontaneously contracting and meets these criteria, then the test may be interpreted, and no uterine stimulation is required. If the patient is not contracting, or her contractions do not meet these criteria, then contractions must be stimulated. Two available methods are intravenous (IV) oxytocin and nipple stimulation.

IV oxytocin. A dilute solution of IV oxytocin is started at a rate of 0.5 mU/minute to stimulate contractions. This rate is doubled every 20 minutes until adequate contractions are achieved.

Nipple stimulation. The patient is instructed to rub one nipple for 2 minutes or until a contraction occurs. If this does not produce adequate contractions, then the stimulation is stopped and repeated in approximately 5 minutes. If this still does not result in adequate contractions, then IV oxytocin is administered.

Stop the test when either an adequate test has occurred, or there is evidence of significant fetal distress.

Interpretation of Results

After adequate contractions and a concurrent tracing of the FHR have been obtained, the results are classified according to the following categories:

1. **Negative.** No late decelerations or significant variable decelerations are present.
2. **Positive.** Late decelerations are present with at least 50% of contractions.*
3. **Equivocal – suspicious.** Intermittent late or intermittent significant variable decelerations are present.
4. **Equivocal – hyperstimulatory.** Uterine tachysystole is present (contractions are lasting > 60 seconds or occur < 2 minutes apart), and decelerations are present as well.
5. **Unsatisfactory.** Fewer than three contractions in 10 minutes or an uninterpretable tracing (ACOG 1999, reaffirmed 2014).

Intervention

If the test is **positive**, then delivery is usually indicated, although it is important to remember that a non-reactive NST and a positive CST when seen together can be associated with congenital anomalies, and that an ultrasound to evaluate this should be performed if possible.

If the test is **equivocal**, then a biophysical profile can be performed, and uterine tachysystole should be corrected if present.

If the test is **negative**, you can tell the patient that this is very reassuring and that the fetus appears stable at this time.

---

* If late decelerations are present after more than half of contractions, this is a positive test even when there are not three contractions in 10 minutes. See Chapter 3, *Intrapartum Fetal Heart Rate Monitoring*, for a discussion/explanation of decelerations.

Complications

When contractions occur in a compromised fetus, then fetal distress may occur, requiring delivery. Uterine hyperstimulation may also occur, and if fetal distress occurs with this, it should be treated in the same manner as if it occurs during spontaneous labor (see Chapter 14).

External Cephalic Version (ECV)

An external cephalic version (ECV) is a procedure during which a baby is externally manipulated from a breech or transverse position to a vertex position. Multiple studies have demonstrated that this procedure can reduce the need for cesarean section for malpresentation without increasing perinatal mortality. Success rates of up to 76% have been reported, though the average success rate is closer to 60% (Hofmeyr *et al.* 2015, ACOG 2016b).

Indications

When the fetus is found to be breech approaching term, an option for avoiding a cesarean section is to attempt to turn the fetus to a vertex position to allow for a vaginal delivery. It is generally attempted at 37 weeks' gestation in order to maximize the chance of success, to minimize the chance that the fetus will revert to a breech or transverse position if the ECV is successful, and to prevent any problems related to prematurity should an emergency delivery be required. It may be attempted during labor as long as the membranes are intact and there are no contraindications present.

Contraindications

There is no consensus about contraindications to ECV. The only absolute contraindication is any condition which would prevent vaginal delivery and would not be resolved by a version. Some of these include the following:

- Placenta previa
- History of certain uterine surgeries (classical C-section, myomectomy, etc.)
- Ruptured membranes
- Non-reassuring fetal heart rate tracing or other evidence of fetal distress
- Placental abruption

Other conditions that are relative contraindications include the following:

- Maternal obesity
- Fetal growth restriction (FGR)
- Oligohydramnios

Previous low transverse C-section is not considered an absolute contraindication to an ECV attempt. However, data are insufficient to determine the risk of uterine rupture in these patients. For this reason, some providers may not offer an ECV to patients with a previous C-section (ACOG 2016b).

Before Performing the Procedure

Prior to attempting an ECV, the following steps should be taken:

1. Ultrasound to assess the following:
   a. Determine placental location and exclude placenta previa
   b. Determine the MVP/AFI (as oligohydramnios is a relative contraindication to ECV)
   c. Confirm fetal position

2. Non-stress test or biophysical profile to document fetal status
3. Informed consent obtained, signed, and placed in the chart
4. Ensure that you have anesthesia and operating room support available in case an emergency cesarean section is needed
5. Obtain anti-D immunoglobulin (Rhogam) if the patient is Rh-negative

Procedure

The patient is placed in a recumbent position after the fetal status has been determined to be reassuring. The uterus must be relaxed, and this is usually accomplished with a single dose of terbutaline 0.25 mg SQ. The abdomen is lubricated with ultrasound lubricant, mineral oil, or powder (cornstarch). The breech is disengaged and elevated from the pelvis by pushing the fingertips of one hand behind the symphysis pubis. If the procedure is being done by a single provider, then the free hand is used to push on the fetal back/head at the same time as the buttocks are manipulated and a forward roll is attempted. If two operators are attempting the ECV, then one physician elevates the breech and the other attempts to move the head and back in the forward roll. The movements should be slow and steady and the fetal heart rate checked at least every 2 minutes. The attempt is aborted if a prolonged deceleration or fetal bradycardia occurs. In general, no more than four attempts are made and no single attempt should last for more than 5 minutes. After the procedure, the fetus should be monitored for at least an hour to ensure there is no evidence of fetal distress. If the patient is Rh-negative, then Rhogam is administered.

Previous studies had demonstrated improved success rates for ECV with the use of epidural anesthesia. Subsequent studies and a meta-analysis also noted increased success with regional anesthesia compared to ECV without anesthesia, but with insufficient data to determine whether spinal or epidural anesthesia is superior. Data are also insufficient to determine if regional anesthesia without tocoloysis is equivalent to regional anesthesia with tocolysis. As a result, it is reasonable to offer regional anesthesia to patients desiring an ECV attempt, but a tocolytic should still be given (ACOG 2016b).

Complications

There are no significant maternal risks, except for the potential for an emergency cesarean section should fetal distress occur. In terms of fetal risks, the exact incidence of complications is not well defined. The FHR tracing may be non-reactive after the procedure, and a transient bradycardia may also occur. Other rare but reported complications include placental abruption and preterm labor at a rate of < 1% (Grootscholten et al. 2008). To date, randomized trials of ECV have not demonstrated any increase in perinatal mortality (Hofmeyr et al. 2015). If significant fetal distress does occur, then an emergency cesarean section is performed.

Fetal Fibronectin Collection

During the workup of preterm labor, a vaginal swab for fetal fibronectin (fFN) is often done for use in the evaluation. While a positive test is associated with an increased risk of preterm delivery, the real value of the test lies in its high negative predictive value of up to 99%. It is important to think about doing this test at the beginning of your workup, because once you have checked the patient's cervix you cannot collect a sample for 24 hours.

Indications

During the workup of a patient with preterm labor, an fFN swab may be done. You should check with your institution about the availability of the test as well as whether it is incorporated into the standard protocol for preterm labor evaluation (if there is one).

Contraindications

This test should not be performed when there is active bleeding or ruptured membranes, or within 12–24 hours of intercourse or a previous vaginal examination when any kind of lubrication was utilized. While some authors list the presence of a cervical cerclage as a contraindication to the procedure, there is now literature to support the use and interpretation of the test when a cerclage is present (Roman *et al.* 2003).

Procedure

A sterile speculum examination is performed during the evaluation of a patient for preterm labor. Samples are taken from the posterior fornix or external os using the swab from the manufacturer's kit.

Before performing the collection, make sure the following conditions are met:

- Cervical dilation < 3 cm
- Intact membranes
- Gestational age between 24^{+0} and 34^{+0} weeks
- No intercourse in the past 24 hours
- No digital or vaginal ultrasound examination in the past 24 hours
- No use of lubricants for the examination

Results

The results are generally reported as either positive or negative. A positive result is returned when a concentration of fFN is greater than 50 nm/mL.

Intervention

A negative result is very reassuring in that it has a very high negative predictive value (up to 99%) in relation to the risk of preterm delivery (Kuhrt *et al.* 2016). On the other hand, a positive result implies an increased risk of delivery within the next 2 weeks although the incidence of this is only approximately 20% (Kuhrt *et al.* 2016). Because of this, there are no evidence-based recommendations for exactly how to use a positive test, and the major value of the fFN test lies in its high negative predictive value and ability to determine which patients will not deliver in the 2 weeks after a negative result. Please refer to the section on preterm labor in Chapter 14 for a discussion of how to interpret the results based on the clinical situation. Many times this will include obtaining a transvaginal ultrasound and cervical length to determine those patients for whom having the fFN result would change management.

Complications

There are no expected complications from the procedure.

Fetal Scalp Electrode (FSE)

During labor, when a fetal heart rate (FHR) tracing is concerning or difficult to monitor with external fetal monitors, a fetal scalp electrode (FSE) may be placed. The FSE gives a more accurate assessment of the FHR as well as serving as a fetal electrocardiogram. It allows for interpretation of FHR variability, which is important in assessing fetal well-being. It can only be placed after the amniotic sac has ruptured, so if the fetus is too high up for the membranes to be ruptured, it should not be placed. An FSE should not be placed if the mother has an infection that could be transmitted to the baby more easily through the small break in the skin created by the FSE. Some examples of this would be HIV, active HSV lesions in the birthing canal, or hepatitis B infection.

Indications for Placement of FSE

- Inability to monitor FHR with external monitors
- Concerning FHR tracing
- Twins in labor with difficulty monitoring both twins

Contraindications to Placement

- HIV infection
- Maternal infection with acute hepatitis B
- Active HSV lesions
- Fetal bleeding disorder
- Contraindications to amniotomy (AROM)

Before Placement

Before placement of an FSE, consider the following questions:

1. What is the indication for placing this? (Complications are extremely rare, but you need to know why you are doing any procedure.)
2. Do you have the cable to hook up the FSE? (It is a different cable than that used for the external fetal monitor.)
3. Are there any contraindications to placement?

Placement

A digital cervical exam is performed with the dominant hand and the fontanelles palpated to determine the fetal head position. The FSE is then inserted into the vagina with the free hand and held between the fingers of the dominant hand. The tip of the FSE is pressed against a bony portion of the fetal skull, and then the end of the probe is rotated in a clockwise fashion, which will attach the FSE to the scalp. Care must be taken to avoid placement over a fontanelle or suture, as this can injure the fetus.

Complications

Complications of FSE placement are very rare but can result from improper placement, such as injury to an eye or over a fontanelle. The risk of infection in the area of placement is low, but there are rare case reports of osteomyelitis and subgaleal abscess at the FSE site (McGregor and McFarren 1989, Onyeama et al. 2009).

Fetal Scalp Sampling

At times during labor you will have an FHR tracing that is not reassuring and does not respond to conservative measures, such as maternal position changes, discontinuing oxytocin infusion, administering oxygen by face mask to the mother, and fetal scalp stimulation (see Chapter 3). When this occurs, and delivery is not imminent, then performing this test can help you determine whether or not the fetus is truly in distress and in need of immediate delivery. (Of note, this procedure is not used at most institutions, so you will need to see if this is an option at your hospital.)

Indications for Fetal Scalp Sampling

This procedure is indicated when there is a non-reassuring FHR tracing that does not respond to conservative measures or scalp stimulation.

Contraindications to Fetal Scalp Sampling

- Contraindications to rupture of the membranes
- Maternal HSV or HIV infection
- Fetal bleeding disorder
- Patient not in active labor or fetus not low enough in the pelvis to safely perform the procedure

Before Performing the Procedure

Before performing fetal scalp sampling, do the following:

1. Ensure there are no contraindications.
2. If the membranes are not ruptured, then make preparations to rupture the membranes (AROM).
3. Make sure you have a fetal scalp sampling kit.
4. Assign one person to take the blood samples obtained to the lab for immediate analysis.
5. Call and inform the laboratory you are going to perform this procedure.
6. Alert the pediatricians that this is being done, and that you will inform them should delivery be required.
7. Counsel the patient regarding the procedure.

Procedure

1. Insert the cylinder that comes in the kit into the vagina and place the tip against the fetal skull.
2. Wipe the scalp clear of blood and amniotic fluid with the sterile swab included in the kit.
3. Coat the area to be incised with the silicone gel from the package (this will cause the blood to form beads rather than running down the scalp).
4. Make an incision approximately 2 mm deep in the area you have prepared with the cutting instrument (this is a long plastic handle with a small blade on the end and is provided in the kit).
5. Collect the beads of blood immediately into the heparinized capillary tubes and send them to the laboratory.
6. Remove the cylinder from the vagina.

Interpretation and Interventions Based on Results

The pH results from this test are assigned to one of three categories:

< 7.20. If the pH is in this range, then immediate delivery is indicated by whatever route is most expedient (vaginal or cesarean).

7.20–7.25. If the pH is between these values, then the procedure is repeated in 30 minutes and the FHR monitored closely until then for evidence of worsening distress.

> 7.25. When the pH is in this range, labor may continue with close monitoring.

Complications

In general, the bleeding from the small incision stops almost immediately, and complications are rare. There is always a small risk of a scalp infection after delivery, and if the fetus has a bleeding disorder, then the bleeding may be more than normal.

Fetal Pulse Oximetry

This method of fetal monitoring measures the oxygen saturation of arterial hemoglobin by utilizing a sensor in a catheter that is similar in appearance to an IUPC catheter and reflects fetal tissue perfusion. It is based on the principle that oxyhemoglobin and hemoglobin differ in their ability to absorb light at different wavelengths (Yam *et al.* 2000a, 2000b). If the fetal oxygen saturation falls below 30%, then fetal distress is present, and intervention should be made. This technology is still being investigated and is not in widespread use at this time.

Intrauterine Pressure Catheter (IUPC)

An intrauterine pressure catheter (IUPC) can be used to determine both the timing and intensity of uterine contractions, and also to perform an amnioinfusion during labor. It can only be inserted when the membranes are ruptured.

Indications for IUPC Placement

- Inability to monitor contractions during labor (often due to maternal obesity)
- Protracted labor with need to document contraction strength
- Need for an amnioinfusion (i.e., for meconium or variable decelerations)

Contraindications to IUPC Placement

- Any contraindication to rupturing the membranes (see *Amniotomy*)
- Cervix completely dilated (placing the IUPC is nearly impossible at this time although it may be attempted)

Before Performing the Procedure

Before placement of IUPC, do the following:
1. Ensure there are no contraindications.
2. If AROM needs to be performed, make preparations for this.
3. Make sure you have the appropriate cables to hook up the IUPC after placement.
4. Get out sterile gloves for the procedure.

Placement of IUPC

Start by putting on a pair of sterile gloves and performing a digital cervical exam. If the membranes need to be ruptured, that is done at this time. After this, insert the tips of the index and middle fingers between the fetal head and the cervix to make room to insert the IUPC. Have your assistant open the IUPC catheter in a sterile fashion and then thread the catheter between the two fingers of the hand that is in the cervix and advance the tip of the catheter to the cervix. The catheter itself will usually have a removable plastic sheath around it that you can insert up the external cervical os. At this point, hold onto the outer plastic sheath and thread the actual catheter between the cervix and the fetal head and up into the uterus. After this is done, carefully remove your hand from the vagina, and the plastic sheath is then removed from around the catheter.

Recording the Exam

Make a note in the patient's chart and describe your cervical exam as well as the fact that you placed an IUPC. If you are starting an amnioinfusion, note this as well.

Complications

Complications of IUPC placement are uncommon, but if it is forced into the placenta, then hemorrhage is possible.

Montevideo Units (MVUs)

This is a way to quantify the actual intensity of contractions. It requires the use of an IUPC, because external monitors can provide information only on the timing and duration of contractions, and not on their actual strength. To determine how many Montevideo units (MVUs) are present, follow this procedure:

1. Count all contractions in a 10-minute period.
2. For each contraction, measure the pressure (listed in mmHg on the tracing) from the baseline to the peak.
3. Add the values for each contraction.

An example of this is seen in Figure 2.15.

An adequate contraction pattern will have at least 200 MVUs. If this is not the case and the patient is not progressing in labor, then you can consider labor augmentation (see Chapter 7).

Non-Stress Test (NST)

Nearly every patient who comes to labor and delivery will be evaluated with a non-stress test (NST). While much of this will become pattern recognition, it is important to have a systematic method to evaluate this test. If contractions are present, and at least three occur in a 10-minute period, then you have a spontaneous contraction stress test (CST) rather than an NST.

Indications for NST

An NST is performed for all patients who present to labor and delivery after 24 weeks' gestation as part of the basic assessment of the fetus. This test is also performed as part of antepartum testing for high-risk pregnancies. The most common patient that will have an NST on labor and delivery is the woman at term (> 37 weeks) who presents to rule out labor.

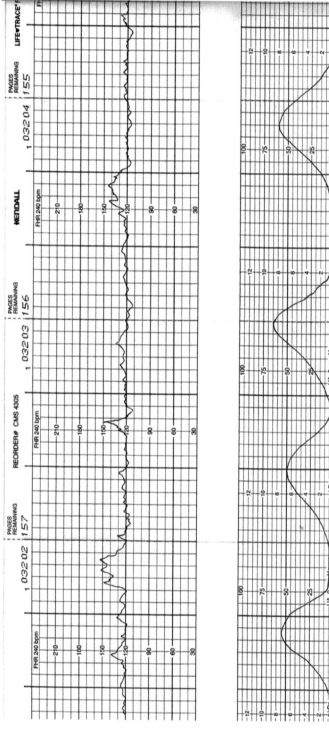

Figure 2.15 Montevideo units.

Contraindications for NST

Because an NST is not invasive, there are no contraindications to performing the test. In cases where significant fetal distress is noted, however, emergency delivery may be indicated and preclude completing the test.

Performing an NST

The patient is placed in either the lateral recumbent or semi-Fowler position with lateral hip displacement to prevent the gravid uterus from compressing the inferior vena cava, and external monitors are placed on the abdomen to record both the FHR and uterine activity for 20–40 minutes. The FHR is monitored for accelerations, which are defined as elevations of the FHR of at least 15 bpm above baseline for at least 15 seconds.* If there are at least two accelerations present in the first 20 minutes, the test may be stopped at this time. If accelerations are not present, then the test can be continued up to 40 minutes.

Interpretation of NST

The results of an NST are classified as either *reactive* or *non-reactive*, depending on whether or not at least two accelerations of adequate size as stated before are present (Figure 2.16). It is important to note that this will be dependent on gestational age, as up to 50% of non-compromised fetuses between 24 and 28 weeks will have a non-reactive NST (Bishop 1981). This number decreases to only 15% between 28 and 32 weeks' gestation, and after this a reactive NST is expected in nearly all cases (ACOG 1999, reaffirmed 2014).

The NST must also be interpreted with consideration given to any decelerations present. If there are late decelerations or significant and repetitive variable decelerations, then the FHR tracing is non-reassuring even if the test is reactive. Please refer to Chapter 3 for a detailed discussion of FHR interpretation.

Interventions

If the NST is reactive, then this is reassuring that the fetus is not felt to be in distress. If, during the NST, there are no accelerations in the first 20 minutes, then vibro-acoustic stimulation with an artificial larynx may be applied to the maternal abdomen for 1–2 seconds in an attempt to elicit accelerations. After 32 weeks, where a reactive NST is expected, a biophysical profile should be performed if the NST is non-reactive.

Recording the Results

A note should be made in the patient's chart regarding the exam. The baseline FHR should be noted, and the test should be recorded as either reactive or non-reactive (these can be abbreviated as RNST and NRNST, respectively). Additional information, such as the presence or absence of decelerations, should be recorded, as well as any additional monitoring that is needed.

---

* If the patient is < 32 weeks' gestation, then the accelerations must only be 10 bpm above baseline for 10 seconds to meet criteria for a reactive tracing.

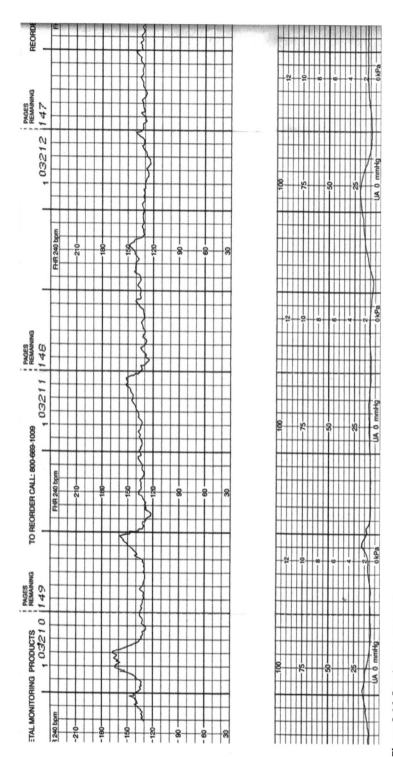

Figure 2.16 Reactive non-stress test.

Ultrasound Evaluation

Estimated Fetal Weight

It is possible to perform measurements utilizing ultrasound to provide an estimated fetal weight. This is more useful with women who are being admitted for preterm labor, where the fetal weight is related to survival in the neonatal intensive care unit (NICU), than for term patients, but is an important skill to have.

The three basic measurements that should be taken to calculate an estimated fetal weight on labor and delivery are:

1. **Biparietal diameter.** This measurement should include the thalamus as well as the falx and the cavum septum pellucidum. The measurement should be taken from the outside edge of the cranium to the internal edge of the skull on the opposite side, as shown in Figure 2.17a.

2. **Abdominal circumference.** The abdominal circumference is a cross-sectional view of the abdomen and should include the spine as well as the stomach and the portal vein. The measurement encompasses the entire circumference, as demonstrated in Figure 2.17b. If the fetal heart is visible, then the ultrasound probe is directed too superiorly.

3. **Femur length.** The femur is measured from one end to the other when the femur is visualized in its greatest length (Figure 2.17c).

All ultrasound machines are different, and you must become familiar with the one at your institution and practice obtaining these measurements. It is also important to learn how to record them on the machine and produce an estimation of the fetal weight.

Interpretation of the Exam

It is important to note whether or not fetal macrosomia, which is often defined as a birth weight of > 4000 grams, is present or if the fetus is growth-restricted, which is defined as

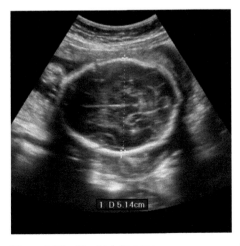

Figure 2.17a Biparietal diameter.

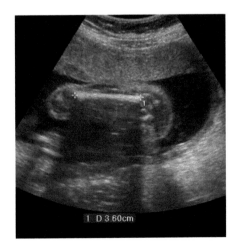

Figure 2.17b Abdominal circumference.

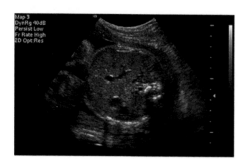

Figure 2.17c Femur length.

below the 10th percentile for gestational age. Table 2.1 lists the 10th percentile cutoffs for different gestational ages.

Recording the Exam

In the chart, you should note the position of the fetus as well as the estimated fetal weight based on your measurements. Make sure to comment on the following:

- Fetal lie (vertex, breech, transverse)
- Position of the placenta (anterior, posterior, low-lying, previa)
- Amount of amniotic fluid (AFI/MVP)
- Estimated fetal weight

Amniotic Fluid Index (AFI)

The amniotic fluid index (AFI) is simply an ultrasound assessment of the amount of amniotic fluid around the fetus/fetuses. An alternative to the AFI is measuring the maximum vertical pocket (MVP). Recent studies suggest that using the MVP rather than the AFI may decrease the number of false diagnoses of oligohydramnios, and this is the preferred method of ACOG (2014, reaffirmed 2016).

Indications for Evaluation of Amniotic Fluid Volume

- Evaluation of a patient who complains of decreased fetal movement
- Evaluation for ruptured membranes
- In conjunction with biophysical profile (BPP)

Contraindications to AFI or MVP

There are no contraindications to AFI or MVP.

Performing an AFI

The AFI is calculated by first dividing the uterus into four quadrants, usually using the umbilicus as the center point and drawing an imaginary line vertically and horizontally from there (Figure 2.18). Ultrasound is then used to measure the largest vertical pocket of amniotic fluid (in centimeters) in each of these four quadrants, and the AFI is the sum of the four measurements. You must make sure that the pockets of fluid do not contain any sections of the umbilical cord, as these cannot be counted in the AFI.

Table 2.1 Cutoff for 10th percentile by gestational age

Gestational age (weeks)	10th percentile (grams)
26	568
27	754
28	765
29	884
30	1020
31	1171
32	1338
33	1519
34	1714
35	1919
36	2129
37	2340
38	2544
39	2735
40	2904
41	3042

(Adapted from Doubilet et al. 1997)

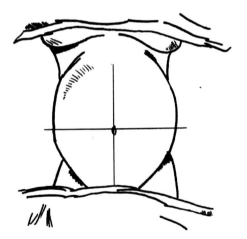

Figure 2.18 Amniotic fluid index (AFI) quadrants.

Performing an MVP

This is similar to an AFI, except the single largest vertical pocket of all quadrants is measured and recorded. This pocket may not contain umbilical cord or fetal parts.

Interpretation and Interventions

In general, an AFI of < 5 cm or an MVP of < 2 cm is classified as oligohydramnios. In the term or post-term patient, oligohydramnios is usually treated with induction of labor. (See Chapter 14 for a discussion of oligohydramnios.) If the patient is preterm, then close monitoring is usually initiated, and an attempt is made to determine the cause, with preterm premature rupture of membranes (PPROM) being one of the more common reasons.

At the other end of the spectrum, polyhydramnios is defined as an AFI of > 25 cm or a MVP of > 8 cm. This complication has been associated with maternal diabetes as well as congenital anomalies and warrants further evaluation.

Biophysical Profile (BPP)

A biophysical profile (BPP) is usually performed after an NST is found to be non-reactive, or as part of a more intensive antepartum testing regimen. It has five separate components, and a score of 0 or 2 points is given for each part of the test (so it is impossible to have an odd number for a BPP result). It is performed with ultrasound, with the exception of the NST, and the test continues until either all components are present or when 30 minutes expires. The five components are:

1. **Non-stress test**: reactive (2 points) or non-reactive (0 points)
2. **Amniotic fluid assessment**: MVP > 2 cm or AFI > 5 cm
3. **Gross fetal body movements**: at least three discrete body or limb movements
4. **Fetal tone**: at least one episode of rapid flexion/extension of extremity or hand/foot
5. **Fetal breathing movement**: at least 30 continuous seconds

BPP Scores and Interpretations

8–10: Reassuring, and correlates well with good fetal outcomes. With a BPP of 8 or higher, the perinatal mortality rate is only 0.8 per 1000 women tested.

6: Equivocal; repeat testing is indicated within 12–24 hours, or consider delivery if the fetus is mature.

2–4: Reflective of fetal compromise, and immediate intervention must be considered.

Modified BPP

Sometimes a modified biophysical profile is performed. Rather than looking for fetal tone, movement, and breathing with the ultrasound, an NST and AFI are done. If the NST is reactive and the AFI is > 5 cm, then the test is normal and reassuring. If the NST is not reactive, or the AFI is < 5 cm, then a full BPP is done as a follow-up test.

References

ACOG (1999). Antepartum fetal surveillance. *ACOG Practice Bulletin #9*, October 1999, reaffirmed 2014.

ACOG (2000). Scheduled cesarean delivery and the prevention of vertical transmission of HIV infection. *ACOG Committee Opinion #234*, May 2000, reaffirmed 2017.

ACOG (2006). Amnioinfusion does not prevent meconium aspiration syndrome. *ACOG Committee Opinion #346*, October 2006, reaffirmed 2018.

ACOG (2014). Safe prevention of the primary cesarean delivery. *ACOG Obstetric Care Consensus #1*, March 2014, reaffirmed 2016.

ACOG (2016a). Premature rupture of membranes. *ACOG Practice Bulletin #172*, October 2016.

ACOG (2016b). External cephalic version. *ACOG Practice Bulletin #13*, February 2016.

Bishop EH (1981). Fetal acceleration test. *Am J Obstet Gynecol* **141**: 905–9.

Cunningham GF, Leveno KJ, Bloom SL, *et al.* (eds.) (2014). *Williams Obstetrics*, 24th edn. New York: McGraw-Hill, p. 874.

Doubilet PM, Benson CB, Nadel AS, Ringer SA (1997). Improved birth weight table for neonates developed from gestations dated by early ultrasonography. *J Ultrasound Med* **16**: 241–9.

Grootscholten K, Kok M, Oei SG, Mol BW, Van der Post JA (2008). External cephalic version-related risks: a meta-analysis. *Obstet Gynecol* **112**: 1143–51.

Hofmeyr GJ, Lawrie TA (2012). Amnioinfusion for potential or suspected umbilical cord compression in labour. *Cochrane Database Syst Rev* (1): CD000013.

Hofmeyr GJ, Xu H, Eke AC (2014). Amnioinfusion for meconium-stained liquor in labour. *Cochrane Database Syst Rev* (1): CD000014.

Hofmeyr GJ, Kulier R, West HM (2015). External cephalic version for breech presentation at term. *Cochrane Database Syst Rev* (4): CD000083.

Kuhrt K, Smout E, Hezelgrave N, *et al.* (2016). Development and validation of a tool incorporating cervical length and quantitative fetal fibronectin to predict spontaneous preterm birth in asymptomatic high-risk women. *Ultrasound Obstet Gynecol* **47**: 104–9.

Lydon-Rochelle M, Albers L, Gorwoda J, Craig E, Qualls C (1993). Accuracy of Leopold maneuvers in screening for malpresentation: a prospective study. *Birth* **20**: 132–5.

McGregor JA, McFarren T (1989). Neonatal cranial osteomyelitis: a complication of fetal monitoring. *Obstet Gynecol* **73**: 490–2.

Novikova N, Hofmeyr GJ, Essilfie-Appiah G (2012). Prophylactic versus therapeutic amnioinfusion for oligohydramnios in labour. *Cochrane Database Syst Rev* (9): CD000176.

Onyeama CO, Srinivasan H, Lotke M, Vickers D (2009). Subgaleal abscess and *E. coli* septicemia following scalp electrode in a preterm newborn: a case report. *J Matern Fetal Neonatal Med* **22**: 1201–3.

Pattinson RC, Cuthbert A, Vannevel V (2017). Pelvimetry for fetal cephalic presentations at or near term for deciding on mode of delivery. *Cochrane Database Syst Rev* **3**: CD000161.

Pitt C, Sanchez-Ramos L, Kaunitz AM, Gaudier F (2000). Prophylactic amnioinfusion for intrapartum oligohydramnios: a meta-analysis of randomized controlled trials. *Obstet Gynecol* **96**: 861–6.

Ramsauer B, Vidaeff AC, Hösli I, *et al.* (2013). The diagnosis of rupture of fetal membranes (ROM): a meta-analysis. *J Perinat Med* **41**: 233–40.

Roman AS, Rebarber A, Sfakianaki AK, *et al.* (2003). Vaginal fetal fibronectin as a predictor of spontaneous preterm delivery in the patient with cervical cerclage. *Am J Obstet Gynecol* **189**: 1368–73.

Wenstrom K, Andrews WW, Maher JE (1995). Amnioinfusion survey: prevalence protocols and complications. *Obstet Gynecol* **86**: 572–6.

Xu H, Hofmeyr J, Roy C, Fraser W (2007). Intrapartum amnioinfusion for meconium-stained amniotic fluid: a systematic review of randomized controlled trials. *BJOG* **114**: 383–90.

Yam J, Chua S, Arulkumaran S (2005a). Intrapartum fetal pulse oximetry. Part I: principles and technical issues. *Obstet Gynecol Surv* **55**: 163–72.

Yam J, Chua S, Arulkumaran S (2005b). Intrapartum fetal pulse oximetry. Part 2: clinical application. *Obstet Gynecol Surv* **55**: 173–83.

Further Reading

DeRosa J, Anderle LJ (1991). External cephalic version of term singleton breech presentations with tocolysis: a retrospective study in a community hospital. *J Am Osteopath Assoc* **91**: 351–2, 355–7.

Freeman RK, Anderson G, Dorchester W (1982). A prospective multi-institutional study of antepartum fetal heart rate monitoring. I. Risk of perinatal mortality and morbidity according to antepartum fetal heart rate test results. *Am J Obstet Gynecol* **143**: 771–7.

Hofmeyr GJ (2017). External cephalic version. *UpToDate*, version 32.0, Jun 2017. www .uptodate.com/contents/external-cephalic-version (accessed May 2018).

Honest H, Bachmann LM, Gupta JK, Kleijen J, Khan KS (2002). Accuracy of cervicovaginal fetal fibronectin in predicting risk of spontaneous preterm birth: systematic review. *BJOG* **325**: 301.

Iams JK (2003). Prediction and early detection of preterm labor. *Obstet Gynecol* **101**: 402–12.

Kehl S, Schelkle A, Thomas A, *et al.* (2016). Single deepest vertical pocket or amniotic fluid index as evaluation test for predicting adverse pregnancy outcome (SAFE trial): a multicenter, open-label, randomized controlled trial. *Ultrasound Obstet Gynecol* **47**: 674–9.

Maharaj D, Teach DT (2010). Assessing cephalopelvic disproportion: back to the basics. *Obstet Gynecol Surv* **387**: 395.

Manning AU, Morrison FA, Harman CR, Lange IR, Menticoglou S (1987). Fetal assessment based on fetal biophysical profile scoring: experience in 19,221 referred high-risk pregnancies: An analysis of false-negative fetal deaths. *Am J Obstet Gynecol* **157**: 880.

Reddy UM, Abuhamad AZ, Levine D, Saade GR (2014). Fetal imaging workshop. *Obstet Gynecol* **123**: 1070–82.

Chapter 3

Intrapartum Fetal Heart Rate Monitoring

Noelle Breslin and Shad Deering

Use of FHR Monitoring

Fetal monitoring and interpretation of fetal heart tracings have become an essential part of labor management. In an attempt to evaluate fetal wellbeing, both in the antepartum period and during labor, there are several tests that may be performed. Doppler ultrasound can be used to measure the fetal heart rate (FHR), FHR variability, and other factors that are an indirect assessment of fetal status.

Continuous FHR monitoring has been in use since the 1970s. It is most often used during labor but can also be used during the antepartum period when monitoring the health of a fetus in a high-risk pregnancy. Doppler ultrasound technology detects the fetal heart motion, which is interpreted to produce a "tracing" of the fetal heart rate over time. The FHR tracing allows close monitoring and evaluation of the fetus and the fetal tolerance of the physiological changes of labor in real time, allowing prompt intervention if signs of compromise arise.

While much of FHR tracing interpretation is basically pattern recognition, understanding the underlying physiology will allow you to make appropriate and timely interventions to ensure the best outcome for the fetus.

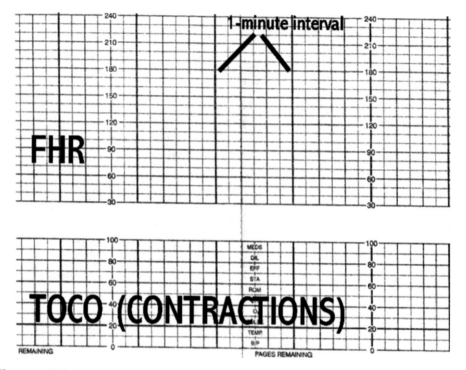

Figure 3.1 FHR tracing paper.

Basics of FHR Monitoring

The FHR is recorded in a continuous manner onto standard FHR tracing paper and/or a digital display that mimics the standard tracing paper. This recording paper moves at approximately 3 cm/minute. Each small block represents 10 seconds, and each large block 1 minute, as shown in Figure 3.1. The top section of the paper is where the FHR is recorded, and the rate is identified by a scale on the paper ranging from 30 to 240 beats per minute (bpm). The bottom portion of the recording paper is where contractions are recorded, represented by pressure changes detected by either an external tocometer or an intrauterine pressure catheter (IUPC). This has a scale that runs from 0 to 100 mmHg and indicates both the timing and magnitude of uterine contractions. (It is important to realize that only an IUPC can give a real measurement of the strength of contractions. If external monitors are used to trace contractions, you cannot comment on their strength, only on how often they are occurring. This is discussed in more detail later.)

Indications for FHR Monitoring

Antepartum

Testing of the fetus in the antepartum period is performed for a multitude of reasons, but in general any condition, maternal or fetal, that places the fetus at increased risk for complications or compromise is an indication for antepartum testing. Examples include fetal growth restriction (FGR), maternal diabetes, multiple gestations, and maternal hypertensive disease, to name a few.

The most commonly performed tests to accomplish this are the non-stress test (NST), biophysical profile (BPP), and amniotic fluid index (AFI). Frequency of antepartum monitoring is dependent on the maternal or fetal condition which places the fetus at risk of compromise. The American College of Obstetricians and Gynecologists (ACOG) gives guidelines as to the frequency of antepartum testing, but local guidelines may also apply. In this chapter, we will focus on the use of FHR testing in the management of labor and delivery. More information on antepartum testing indications and intervals can be found in Chapter 2.

Intrapartum (During Labor)

In some institutions, for low-risk pregnancies, or when labor occurs outside of the hospital environment, intermittent auscultation of the FHR may be used to assess fetal wellbeing when continuous monitoring is not desired or not available. However, it is common practice for FHR monitoring to be initiated when a patient is admitted in labor.

The use of electronic fetal monitoring, compared with intermittent auscultation, has been shown to increase the incidence of cesarean delivery and operative delivery (both vacuum and forceps) with a reduction in the rate of neonatal seizures but no decrease in the risk of cerebral palsy or perinatal mortality (Thacker and Stroup 2001). The false-positive rate of electronic fetal monitoring in predicting cerebral palsy is very high, exceeding 99%, promoting possibly unnecessary intervention for presumed fetal distress when there is none (Kim *et al.* 2003). However, it is critical to understand that this is not a reason for inaction or delay when signs of presumed fetal distress appear to be present, but rather it should help you understand why the fetal outcome is almost always good even when a tracing appears concerning. Despite its flaws, the lack of an alternative method of fetal surveillance in labor makes electronic fetal monitoring the best available non-invasive method of determining fetal wellbeing at the present time.

ACOG recommends that pregnancies with "high-risk conditions" such as fetal growth restriction, preeclampsia, and type 1 diabetes should be continuously monitored during labor (ACOG 2010). Table 3.1 shows current guidelines on how often you should evaluate the FHR during labor.

When intermittent auscultation is used, the FHR should be auscultated/recorded after a contraction for 60 seconds at the time intervals specified in Table 3.1. If at any time during intermittent monitoring the FHR becomes concerning, i.e. category II or III, then continuous

Table 3.1 Recommended frequency of intrapartum fetal heart rate monitoring

	High-risk pregnancy	Low-risk pregnancy
1st stage of labor	(Active phase) q15 minutes	q30 minutes
2nd stage of labor	q5 minutes	q15 minutes

(ACOG 2010)

monitoring should be instigated and interventions taken to restore the tracing to category I. The categorization of FHR tracings is explained below (Table 3.3).

It is imperative that your periodic assessments of the FHR tracing be accurately entered and meticulously documented in the medical record during labor. See the sample notes for this in Appendix B.

Interpretation of FHR Tracings

When evaluating an FHR tracing, it is important to have a systematic approach in order to avoid omitting key information either verbally or in the written record. The critical elements to record are:

1. Identity of patient
2. Internal or external monitors
3. Uterine contractions
4. Baseline FHR
5. FHR variability
6. Presence/absence of accelerations
7. Presence/absence of decelerations
8. Category of FHR tracing
9. Decision and interventions

Each of these elements is discussed in detail in the following sections.

1. Identify the Patient

Make sure the FHR tracing belongs to the appropriate patient. Incorrectly identifying the patient, especially if you are looking at monitors with multiple FHR tracings, can lead to unnecessary interventions or failure to act when action is needed.

2. Internal or External Monitors

The use of internal monitors may be necessary to best assess FHR or uterine contractions if there is concern regarding the accuracy of the FHR tracing or strength of uterine contractions when abnormal labor is suspected. A fetal scalp electrode (FSE) is a small device attached to the scalp of the fetus that allows accurate recording of the FHR where there is concern either that the transabdominal Doppler is unable to detect a continuous heart rate or that the accuracy of that heart rate tracing is in question. An intrauterine pressure catheter (IUPC), which is placed through the cervix and sits in the uterus and detects pressure changes with contractions, provides an accurate assessment of uterine contraction strength. It also allows for titration of synthetic oxytocin to create the optimum strength of contractions to elicit cervical change, and can be used to perform an amnioinfusion in the presence of variable decelerations.

3. Uterine Contractions

Comment on the contraction pattern: for example, are the contractions regular in timing, occurring every 3–4 minutes, or irregular? If an IUPC is in place, how many Montevideo units (MVUs) are present? (See Chapter 2 for how to calculate MVUs.)

It is important to identify if there is evidence of uterine tachysystole, which is defined as a persistent pattern of more than five contractions in 10 minutes averaged over 30 minutes. Uterine tachysystole is important to recognize, because if the uterus is not allowed adequate time to relax between contractions placental blood flow will be reduced, which can lead to fetal compromise.

It is also important to document the baseline uterine tone if an IUPC is in place. Baseline tone is usually less than 20 mmHg. An elevated resting tone may mean that the uterus is not completely relaxing between contractions, which can compromise placental blood flow, or that the dose of oxytocin is too high.

4. Baseline FHR

This is the average FHR rounded to the nearest 5 bpm during a 10-minute period. A normal FHR is between 110 and 160 bpm in the term fetus. If the average FHR changes for > 10 minutes then this is the new baseline and not a prolonged acceleration or deceleration.

Fetal tachycardia is defined as a baseline of > 160 bpm. Tachycardia may be due to maternal fever, cardiac arrhythmias, intrauterine infection, administration of medications such as terbutaline, and/or fetal distress.

Bradycardia is defined as a baseline FHR of < 110 bpm.

5. Describe FHR Variability

Variability of the FHR refers to fluctuations around the baseline. In the past, description of FHR variability was broken down into short-term and long-term variability components, but this is no longer done.

Definitions of baseline variability (ACOG 2010) are:

- Absent: undetectable
- Minimal: ≤ 5 bpm (Figure 3.2a)
- Moderate: 6–25 bpm (Figure 3.2b)
- Marked: > 25 bpm

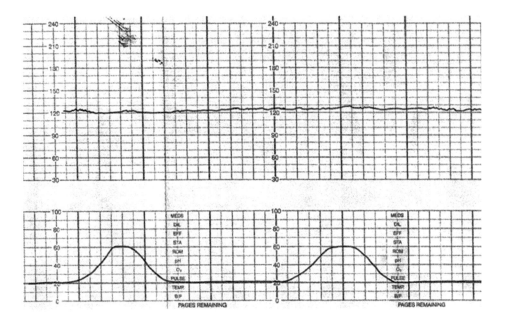

Figure 3.2a Minimal FHR variability.

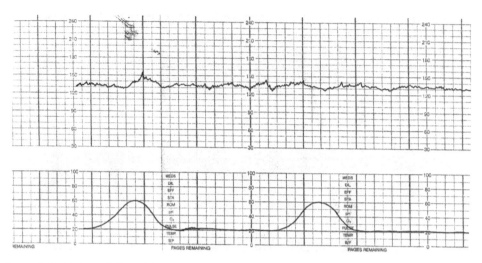

Figure 3.2b Moderate FHR variability.

Variability, when present, is reassuring and reflects adequate oxygenation and a neurologically intact fetus, while its absence requires additional investigation and possibly intervention. Variability can be assessed by external or internal monitors. If there is a question about the variability or there are prolonged periods of absent or minimal variability, it is often necessary to place a fetal scalp electrode (FSE), which is essentially a fetal electrocardiogram. (See Chapter 2 for more information on indications and technique for FSE placement.)

Factors that can affect short-term variability include those shown in Table 3.2.

6. Presence/Absence of Accelerations

When the fetal heart rate demonstrates intermittent, abrupt elevations above the baseline, these are called accelerations and are a reassuring feature. Accelerations have a rapid increase from baseline (< 30 seconds from onset to peak), are at least 15 seconds in duration, and increase by at least 15 bpm from the baseline. If the patient is less than 32 weeks' gestation, a 10 bpm increase for 10 seconds is considered an acceleration.

If the acceleration lasts ≥ 2 minutes it is called a prolonged acceleration. If the increase in the FHR lasts for ≥ 10 minutes, then this is considered a change in baseline and not an acceleration.

7. Presence/Absence of Decelerations

Decelerations are a common occurrence during labor. It is important to recognize the different types of decelerations, as they are treated differently. Types of decelerations that can occur include early decelerations, variable decelerations, and late decelerations. In general, most decelerations last less than 1 minute. If a deceleration lasts for ≥ 2 minutes, then it is defined as a prolonged deceleration, which must always be investigated. If the deceleration lasts ≥ 10 minutes then it is considered a change in the baseline, and if this baseline is < 110 bpm, then it is a bradycardia and not a deceleration.

Table 3.2 Factors that may affect short-term fetal heart rate variability

Increased variability	Decreased variability
Fetal breathing	Narcotics / barbiturates / general anesthesia
Fetal movements	Fetal acidemia
	Maternal acidemia
	Fetal sleep cycle
	Magnesium sulfate

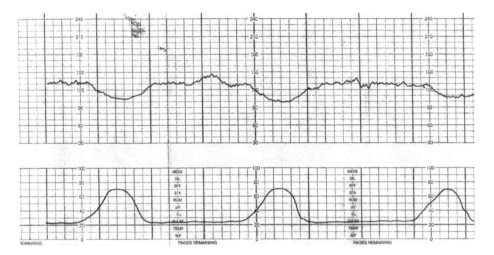

Figure 3.3 Early decelerations.

Early decelerations are the result of fetal head compression. The FHR begins to decrease with the start of a contraction, reaches its lowest point at the peak of the contraction, and then recovers back to normal by the end of the contraction (Figure 3.3). These decelerations rarely fall more than 30 bpm below the baseline, and are common during active labor. They are not indicative of fetal compromise and do not require intervention. However, if there is any question that the decelerations are actually late decelerations, an IUPC may be helpful to distinguish the type of deceleration present by comparing the trough of the deceleration to the peak of the contraction.

Variable decelerations are the most common type of deceleration seen during labor and are the result of intermittent cord compression leading to decreased blood flow to the fetus. Variable decelerations are often associated with contractions, but unlike early decelerations, they do not necessarily begin or end exactly with the contraction. They appear as visually apparent abrupt decreases in the FHR from its baseline and are often accompanied by a small acceleration just before and afterward, which are referred to as shoulders or shouldering (Figure 3.4). In general, variable decelerations are a common

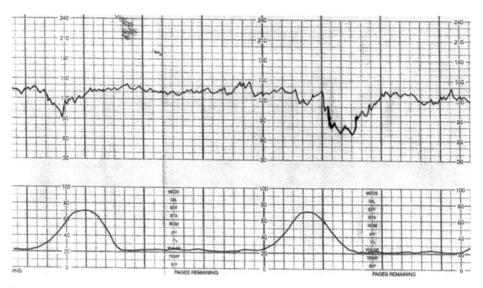

Figure 3.4 Variable decelerations.

occurrence and not associated with poor fetal outcome. However, if these decelerations become recurrent (occurring with ≥ 50% of contractions) and/or are prolonged (≥ 2 minutes), they are concerning for fetal compromise. If there are variable decelerations present with < 50% of contractions, then these are called intermittent variable decelerations. A more urgent cause of variable decelerations is umbilical cord prolapse, which is an emergency situation (this is discussed later in this chapter, and also in Chapter 14).

Late decelerations are similar to early decelerations in appearance in that there is usually a smooth decline (≥ 30 seconds from onset to nadir) in the FHR and a smooth, gradual recovery, but the timing of the deceleration is different. Late decelerations always begin after the peak of the contraction, and do not recover until after the contraction is over (Figure 3.5).

Unlike variable decelerations, the drop in the FHR may only be 10–20 bpm. These decelerations are the result of uteroplacental insufficiency, making the presence of late decelerations an important entity to be rapidly assessed. Uteroplacental insufficiency may be caused by either uterine hyperstimulation or maternal hypotension after conduction anesthesia. Other diseases that result in poor placental perfusion, such as hypertension, preeclampsia, or diabetes, can also lead to poor placental reserve and late decelerations.

While intermittent late decelerations can occur during normal labor, when they occur with most contractions, they are extremely concerning, and intervention must be made to improve uteroplacental blood flow. These interventions are discussed in the next section.

8. Identify the Category of FHR Tracing

In 2008 the National Institute of Child Health and Human Development published recommendations for electronic fetal monitoring (Macones *et al.* 2008). These guidelines have

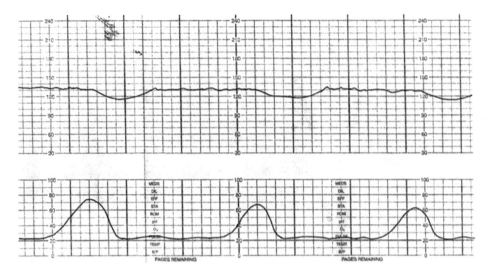

Figure 3.5 Late decelerations.

been integrated into clinical practice and endorsed by ACOG (2009). It is critical to know the definitions, because standardizing communication about FHR tracings is central to good management of all laboring patients. The three-tier system for FHR interpretation defines the categories as shown in Table 3.3.

9. Decision and Intervention as Needed

After evaluation of the FHR tracing, you should classify the tracing as category I, II, or III. If the FHR tracing is category I, then you can continue with your current management or augment labor if needed. If you have decided that you have a category II or III tracing and intervention is necessary, then you may need to attempt to address the underlying problem. An overview of how to manage the different FHR categories can be seen in Figure 3.6. The next section of the chapter will discuss interventions for specific FHR abnormalities.

Interventions for FHR Tracing Abnormalities

What follows are some interventions for these common specific FHR abnormalities:

- Decreased variability
- Fetal tachycardia
- Variable decelerations
- Late decelerations
- Uterine tachysystole
- Prolonged decelerations/fetal bradycardia

Make sure that, after any intervention, you document what you did in the patient's chart as well as the fetal response and current plan. See Appendix B for sample notes for fetal interventions.

Table 3.3 Three-tier fetal heart rate interpretation system

Category I: Considered reassuring and strongly predictive of normal fetal acid–base status
No specific interventions required
Must include **ALL** of the following:
  • FHR baseline between 110 and 160 bpm
  • Moderate FHR variability
  • No late or variable decelerations
May or may not include either of the following:
  • Early decelerations
  • Accelerations

Category II: Includes all FHR tracings that are not categorized as Category I or III
Requires evaluation, continued surveillance and potential intervention
Baseline FHR with
  • Bradycardia (< 110 bpm with *at least* minimal variability)
  • Tachycardia (> 160 bpm)
FHR variability with
  • Minimal baseline variability (> 5 bpm)
  • Absent baseline variability *without* recurrent decelerations
  • Marked baseline variability
Absence of induced accelerations after fetal stimulation
Recurrent variable decelerations with minimal or moderate baseline variability
Prolonged deceleration ≥ 2 minutes but < 10 minutes
Recurrent late decelerations with moderate baseline variability
Variable decelerations with other characteristics, e.g., slow return to baseline, "shoulders" or overshoots

Category III: These FHR tracings are predictive of abnormal fetal acid–base status and require prompt evaluation and intervention
Absent FHR variability with any of the following:
  • Recurrent late decelerations
  • Recurrent variable decelerations
  • Bradycardia
Sinusoidal pattern

Decreased Variability

If the beat-to-beat variability is significantly decreased or absent, and there are no spontaneous accelerations noted, then additional steps should be taken to ensure the fetus is not in distress.

1. **Ask if narcotics have been administered.** If narcotics were given, these can result in a decrease in beat-to-beat variability and the FHR tracing can be monitored in the absence of tachycardia or significant decelerations. Narcotics can also produce a sinusoidal heart rate, which has decreased variability and cycles within 15 bpm of the baseline 2–5 times per minute and looks like a sine wave (Figure 3.6). While this is expected in the presence of narcotics, if these have not been given and the pattern persists for > 20 minutes, it can be an ominous finding associated with severe fetal anemia or acidosis. Additional testing, such as scalp stimulation, is required, and if no improvement or response is noted, then delivery may be indicated.

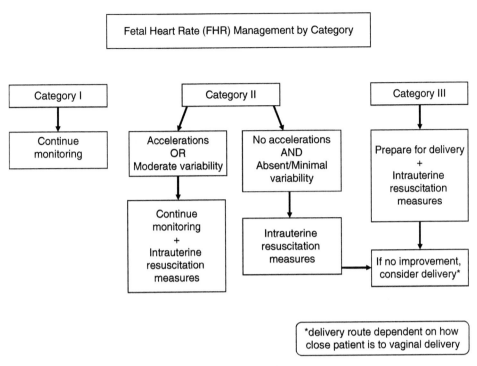

Figure 3.6 Fetal heart rate management by category (adapted from ACOG 2010).

2. **Turn off oxytocin.** If oxytocin is being administered and the variability is decreased, but without evidence of significant decelerations, the oxytocin should be stopped and the fetus monitored. If the decreased variability is due to uterine hyperstimulation, stopping the oxytocin should help to correct this. If uterine hyperstimulation is present in the face of significant decelerations, medications, usually terbutaline, can be given to stop the contractions for a short time.

3. **Administer maternal oxygen.** By administering additional O_2 to the mother by a tight-fitting face mask at 8–10 L/minute, you will increase the O_2 delivery to the fetus and can help to correct any fetal hypoxia.

4. **Change maternal position.** Changing the maternal position may allow for improved oxygenation of the fetus if cord compression is present. If the patient is supine, then moving her to either side is appropriate. If she is on her side already, have her turn to the other side or roll over to a knee–chest position.

5. **Correct maternal hypotension.** If the mother is hypotensive, especially after an epidural or spinal anesthesia, then correct this with a bolus of intravenous crystalloid (lactated Ringer's or normal saline, 1000 mL) or by administering ephedrine 2.5–10 mg IV or IM.

6. **Place an FSE.** If the membranes are intact and the fetus is low enough that the membranes can be ruptured, then rupturing the membranes and placing an FSE will allow for a better assessment of the beat-to-beat variability.

7. **Perform scalp stimulation.** Perform a vaginal exam and stroke the fetal scalp with your fingers. If you see an acceleration of ≥10 bpm after 15 seconds of stimulation, then this is reassuring, and you can continue to monitor the fetus (Elimian *et al.* 1997).

8. **Consider delivery.** If the variability is still minimal to absent after these interventions, and tachycardia or late decelerations are present, then consideration must be given to immediate delivery of the fetus. The route of delivery depends on how far the patient has advanced in labor. If an operative vaginal delivery cannot be safely performed, then a cesarean section may be necessary (see Chapter 9, *Operative Vaginal Delivery*, and Chapter 10, *Cesarean Delivery*).

Fetal Tachycardia

Common reasons for fetal tachycardia, as well as the interventions required, include the following:

Maternal fever. If the mother is febrile, then the source of the fever should be found. Often, in labor, this will be the result of intra-amniotic infection (chorioamnionitis), which is an acute inflammation of the membranes and chorion of the placenta (see Chapter 14). When this is diagnosed, appropriate antibiotics should be started and acetaminophen given to decrease the maternal temperature. Resolution of the fever will usually result in resolution of the tachycardia.

Medications. Terbutaline, given as an intervention for uterine hyperstimulation, and ephedrine, given to correct hypotension from conduction anesthesia, are probably the most common medications that cause fetal tachycardia during labor. If these have been given recently and tachycardia is present, then the fetus may simply be monitored, and as long as significant decelerations are not present, no other intervention is needed.

Fetal distress. If the tachycardia persists without other identifiable causes, such as intra-amniotic infection or medications as mentioned above, or if it is associated with decreased variability or significant decelerations (variable or late), then delivery may be required.

Cardiac arrhythmias. Fetal arrhythmias are an uncommon cause of fetal tachycardia, and often appear on the FHR tracing as intermittent spiking (Figure 3.7). When these are present, they are usually not a problem in labor and no intervention is required if the FHR tracing is otherwise reassuring. If they interfere significantly with the interpretation of the FHR tracing, then a detailed echocardiogram of the fetal heart may be indicated if it has not been done previously, and consideration for delivery by cesarean section if you cannot reliably monitor the fetus in labor.

Variable Decelerations

Because variable decelerations are due to cord compression, the interventions taken to resolve them aim to correct this problem and are indicated when they become recurrent or prolonged in nature. While what follows is a basic algorithm that can be used, note that some of these interventions will occur at the same time. For instance, when you enter the room, you can ask the nurse to turn off the oxytocin, give the patient oxygen by face mask, and cycle the blood pressure cuff while you put on a glove to examine the patient.

1. **Turn off oxytocin.** If oxytocin is being administered then it should be stopped, as the contractions it causes may be compressing the umbilical cord. When there are

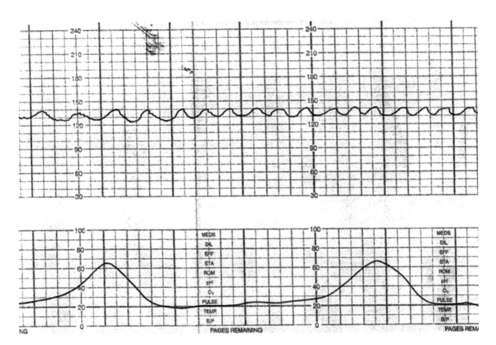

Figure 3.7 Sinusoidal FHR pattern.

significant variable decelerations, especially in the face of uterine tachysystole, this should be your first intervention.

2. **Change maternal position.** Changing the maternal position may allow for improved oxygenation of the fetus if cord compression is present. If the patient is supine, then moving her to either side is appropriate. If she is on her side, then move her to her other side or to a knee–chest position.

3. **Administer maternal oxygen.** By administering additional O_2 to the mother by a tight-fitting face mask at 8–10 L/minute, you will increase the O_2 delivery to the fetus and can help to correct any fetal hypoxia.

4. **Check blood pressure and correct maternal hypotension.** Have the patient's blood pressure cuff cycled to take a reading upon entering the room. If the mother is hypotensive or has demonstrated a recent significant drop in her mean arterial pressure (MAP), especially after an epidural or spinal anesthesia, then correct this with a bolus of intravenous crystalloid (lactated Ringer's or normal saline, 1000 mL) or by administering ephedrine 2.5–10 mg IV or IM. Correcting this is important because, with maternal hypotension, the fetus is less able to tolerate umbilical cord compression with contractions.

5. **Perform vaginal exam.** A vaginal exam will quickly allow you to rule out a prolapsed umbilical cord, which can result in significant variable decelerations due to cord compression. If a prolapsed cord is present, you will usually feel a pulsating section of the umbilical cord ahead of the presenting part of the fetus. This complication requires urgent delivery and is discussed in Chapter 14. The vaginal exam also allows you to determine if the patient's labor is progressing. Sometimes rapid descent of the fetus

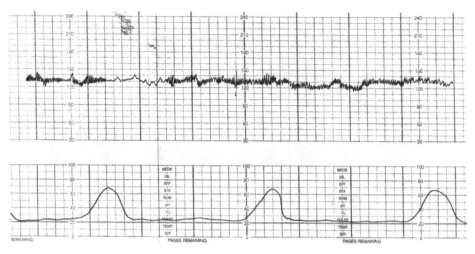

Figure 3.8 Fetal cardiac arrhythmia.

through the birth canal will result in variable decelerations or even a prolonged deceleration.

6. **Place an FSE.** If the membranes are intact and the fetus is low enough that the membranes can be ruptured, then rupturing the membranes and placement of an FSE will allow for a better assessment of the beat-to-beat variability.

7. **Place an IUPC.** Placement of an IUPC will allow you to determine the timing of the contractions and the decelerations more accurately, and can also be used to administer an amnioinfusion.

8. **Give terbutaline.** Administering terbutaline 0.25 mg IV or SQ will decrease contractions for a short time, which will hopefully decrease the cord compression that is causing the variable decelerations. (Note: giving terbutaline IV will result in much quicker results than SQ, i.e., seconds rather than minutes.)

9. **Consider amnioinfusion.** If the decelerations are not repetitive and prolonged and urgent delivery is not required, then an amnioinfusion can be performed, which will provide increased fluid around the fetus and decrease the amount of cord compression that occurs with contractions and stop the decelerations.

10. **Consider delivery if no resolution.** If the FHR tracing continues to show significant, repetitive variable decelerations despite interventions, then delivery will need to be accomplished, especially if a prolonged deceleration or bradycardia develops. If the fetus is low enough in the pelvis and meets criteria for an operative vaginal delivery, this may be done (see Chapter 9). If not, then an urgent cesarean delivery is performed (see Chapter 10).

Late Decelerations

Because late decelerations are the result of uteroplacental insufficiency, interventions are meant to correct this issue. The steps taken are very similar to those for variable decelerations, with some small differences, most notably that an amnioinfusion will not help to improve blood flow to the fetus. As these have been previously discussed and explained, just the interventions are listed below.

1. Turn off oxytocin
2. Change maternal position
3. Administer maternal O_2
4. Check blood pressure and correct maternal hypotension
5. Perform vaginal exam
6. Place an FSE
7. Place an IUPC
8. Give terbutaline if evidence of uterine hyperstimulation
9. Consider delivery if no resolution

Uterine Tachysystole

If uterine tachysystole is present (defined as a persistent pattern of more than five contractions in 10 minutes averaged over 30 minutes) then it is important to monitor and take action to prevent prolonged periods of decreased fetal perfusion. Management is outlined in Figure 3.9.

Prolonged Deceleration or Fetal Bradycardia

When a prolonged deceleration or significant bradycardia develops, immediate intervention is required to resuscitate the fetus. Keep in mind that as you are attempting these actions to resuscitate the baby, you must keep track of how long the deceleration has lasted and make plans for an urgent delivery if the fetus does not recover. The time limits in the algorithm (Figure 3.10) are estimates of when preparation for emergency delivery should be considered and performed.

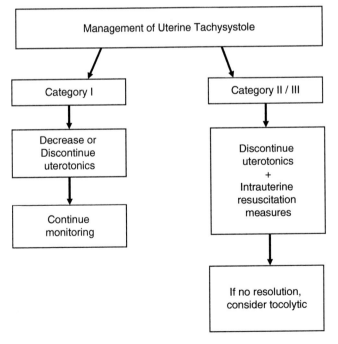

Figure 3.9 Management of uterine tachysystole (adapted from ACOG 2010).

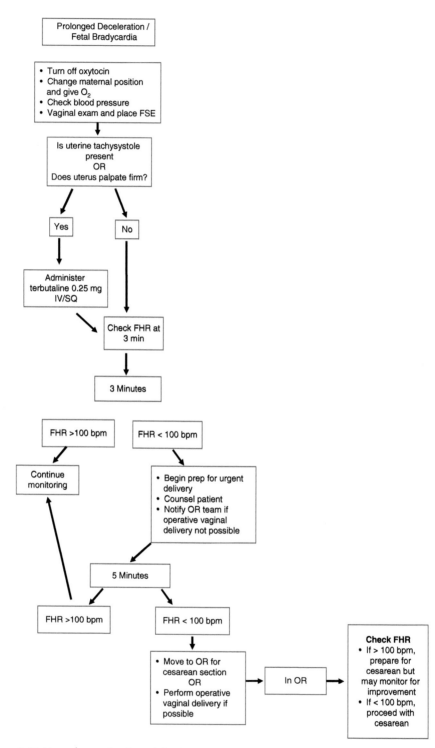

Figure 3.10 Management of prolonged deceleration or fetal bradycardia.

Upon entering the room, ask the nurse to do the following:

- Turn off oxytocin.
- Administer maternal O_2.
- Check blood pressure and correct maternal hypotension.

Put sterile glove on and:

- Perform vaginal exam (rule out a prolapsed umbilical cord).
- Place an FSE.

After vaginal exam:

- **Change maternal position.** Changing the maternal position may allow for improved oxygenation of the fetus if cord compression is present. If the patient is supine, then moving her to either side is appropriate. If she is on her side, then move her to her other side. If this does not resolve the deceleration, then have the patient move to the "knee–chest" position with her head on a pillow at the head of the bed. (This is often difficult or impossible with a dense epidural block, so keep in mind how much motor control your patient actually has.)
- **Place the bed in Trendelenburg.** Most labor and delivery beds have a mechanism by which the head of the bed can be lowered. This is done in an attempt to move the fetus and resolve any compression of the cord that could be causing the deceleration. After this, proceed by following the algorithm in Figure 3.10.

References

ACOG (2009). Intrapartum fetal heart rate monitoring: nomenclature, interpretation, and general management principles. *ACOG Practice Bulletin #106*, July 2009, reaffirmed 2017.

ACOG (2010). Management of intrapartum fetal heart rate tracings. *ACOG Practice Bulletin #116*, November 2010, reaffirmed 2017.

Elimian A, Figueroa R, Tejani N (1997). Intrapartum assessment of fetal well-being: a comparison of scalp stimulation with scalp pH sampling. *Obstet Gynecol* **83**: 373–6.

Kim SY, Khandelwal M, Gaughan JP, Agar MH, Reece EA (2003). Is the intrapartum biophysical profile useful? *Obstet Gynecol* **102**: 471–6.

Macones GA, Hankins GDV, Spong CY, Hauth J, Moore T (2008). The 2008 National Institute of Child Health and Human Development Workshop Report on Electronic Fetal Monitoring: update on definitions, interpretation, and research guidelines. *Obstet Gynecol* **112**: 661–6.

Thacker SB, Stroup DF (2000). Continuous electronic heart rate monitoring for fetal assessment during labor. *Cochrane Database Syst Rev* (2): CD000063.

Management of the First Stage of Labor

Emily Sheikh and Shad Deering

Definition and Normal Duration

As described in Chapter 2, labor is divided into three stages. The first stage begins with regular uterine contractions and cervical change (dilation and effacement), and ends when the cervix is dilated (10 cm) and completely effaced (100%). This stage of labor takes the longest and often requires some intervention from the provider, either to offer analgesia or to augment the progress of labor. The first stage of labor is further divided into latent and active phases. The second stage is the time from completely dilated and effaced to delivery of the neonate, and the third stage involves delivery of the placenta.

Latent Phase

The latent phase of labor begins with regular uterine contractions and cervical dilation and lasts until the cervix is dilated to at least 5–6 cm and almost completely effaced. The length of this stage differs between nulliparous and multiparous patients. In the classic paper on this subject by Friedman, the average lengths of the latent phase of labor were reported as shown in Table 4.1.

These definitions are helpful in determining who needs to be admitted to the hospital, who can be allowed to go home, and who may require labor augmentation, and provide guidance in counseling women as to how long they can expect this part of labor to last. It is important to note that patients who undergo *induction of labor* will not necessarily

Table 4.1 Average length of latent phase of labor

	Normal	Prolonged
Nullipara	6.4 hours (± 5.1 hours)	> 20 hours
Multipara	4.8 hours (± 4.9 hours)	> 14 hours
(Friedman 1978)		

follow the same timeline, as many will require cervical ripening, which is discussed in Chapter 7.

It should also be noted that, historically, the transition from latent to active labor was thought to occur around the time a patient achieved approximately 4 cm dilation with cervical effacement. The Friedman curves, as noted above, are based on this definition. Contemporary studies evaluating normal and prolonged labor curves have demonstrated that the transition to active labor occurs around 5–6 cm dilation with cervical effacement (Zhang *et al.* 2010). This is the point where there is a change in the speed at which cervical change is achieved. Given this new research, the time expected for normal progress in labor has been extended, although the definitions for prolonged latent phase are still based on Friedman's figures.

Active Phase

The active phase of the first stage of labor begins when the cervix is dilated 6 cm and the cervix is almost completely effaced. It is typically much shorter in duration than the latent phase. The average duration of the active phase is expected to be 0.5–0.7 cm/hour in nulliparous women and 0.5–1.3 cm/hour in multiparous women (ACOG 2014). This is important only in that it appears this phase of labor lasts longer than was previously thought, especially in patients undergoing induction of labor. The American College of Obstetricians and Gynecologists (ACOG) has published guidelines on how they define abnormal labor patterns and duration, and these are discussed later in the chapter.

Labor Triage

The triage rooms on labor and delivery are usually where patients are first seen and evaluated and a determination is made as to whether or not they require admission to the hospital. Learning to triage patients efficiently and appropriately is a valuable skill that is essential to managing obstetrical patients.

Triage Decision Analysis

When you see patients on labor and delivery, you will eventually take one of three courses of action. The first is to admit the patient for labor or another indication, the second is to perform further monitoring or workup to ensure the mother and fetus are not in distress, and the third is to discharge the patient to home. A diagram of basic triage decisions is presented in Figure 4.1.

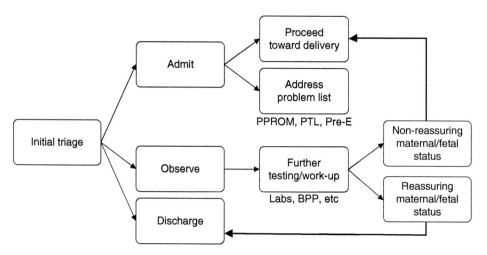

Figure 4.1 Triage pathway.

Determination of Gestational Age

One of the most important tasks you can do on labor and delivery is to determine the patient's gestational age as accurately as possible. This has implications in both the preterm and term fetus with regard to your management. While many patients who present to labor and delivery will have had prenatal care and an accurate due date, you will encounter patients who present late in pregnancy with little or no prenatal care and very unsure dates. Knowing how to correctly date a pregnancy will also assist you in deciding on the most accurate gestational age, and help determine what interventions might be necessary. A simple way to determine the patient's gestational age is by the following algorithm.

1. Ask the patient what the first day of her last menstrual period (LMP) was, and use this to calculate an initial estimated date of delivery (EDD). Historically, Naegele's rule (see below), or a pregnancy wheel have been used to then determine the EDD. There are now calculators, both online and available for your smartphone, which can be used. The ACOG website and phone/tablet application both offer such calculators. These calculators are also particularly useful when calculating EDD for patients who have become pregnant using assisted reproductive technologies (ART), e.g., intrauterine insemination or in vitro fertilization. Naegele's rule:

$$EDD = LMP + 7 \text{ days} + 9 \text{ months}$$

If the patient has a history of irregular menses, then this method is not considered accurate. This is an indication for a first-trimester ultrasound to establish her EDD.

2. Ask the patient if she had an ultrasound early in her pregnancy. If she did, then compare the EDD from the ultrasound with that based on her LMP and determine how different they are. In general, the following rules apply:

   • If the ultrasound was performed in the *first* trimester, the dates should be changed to match the ultrasound if they are different by > 5 days (before 9 weeks EGA) or > 7 days (between 9 weeks and 13^{+6} weeks).

Table 4.2 Adjustment of gestational age based on LMP to match ultrasound

Gestational age by LMP (weeks)	Difference between ultrasound and LMP that justifies changing EDD
$\leq 8^{+6}$ weeks	> 5 days
$9^{+0} - 15^{+6}$ weeks	> 7 days
$16^{+0} - 21^{+6}$ weeks	> 10 days
$22^{+0} - 27^{+6}$ weeks	> 14 days
$\geq 28^{+0}$ weeks	> 21 days

EDD, estimated date of delivery LMP, last menstrual period (ACOG 2017a)

- If the ultrasound was performed in the *early second* trimester, the dates should be changed to match the ultrasound if they are different by > 7 days (between 14 weeks and 15^{+6} weeks EGA) or > 10 days (between 16 weeks to 21^{+6} weeks).
- If the ultrasound was performed in the *late second* trimester, the dates should be changed to match the ultrasound if they are different by > 10 days (between 21 weeks and 27^{+6} weeks EGA).
- If the ultrasound was performed in the *third* trimester, the dates should be changed to match the ultrasound if they are different by > 21 days.
- If there are no ultrasound examinations, but the patient has a sure LMP, use this to determine the EDD.
- If the patient has irregular menses and has not had an ultrasound, perform an ultrasound and use the EDD from this.

These recommendations are summarized in Table 4.2. The important thing to remember is that, once the dates are set by a first-trimester ultrasound, they are not changed based on later ultrasounds. The most accurate dating possible is a sonogram between 6 and 12 weeks that measures the *crown–rump length* of the fetus.

Common Presenting Complaints

While patients will present with a wide variety of complaints, what follows are some of the more common presenting complaints that patients have when they come for evaluation.

Decreased Fetal Movement

Many patients, especially near term, will present with a complaint of decreased fetal movement. This may be either a subjective decrease in overall (global) movement, or they may not have been able to get their "kick counts" (10 kicks/movements in an hour at least once a day) as they are instructed to check for. While a pregnant woman may begin feeling fetal movement between 18 and 20 weeks estimated gestational age (EGA), the movements often do not become consistent until later in development. Starting around 28 weeks, she should count fetal movements until she either reaches 10 movements or an hour passes. If she does not feel 10 movements, then this is considered decreased fetal movement, and she should be asked to present for evaluation. When this occurs, the following actions should be taken:

1. After establishing the patient's gestational age, ask the four basic questions:
   a. Are you having any **BLEEDING?**
   b. Are you having any **CONTRACTIONS?** (include time of onset/frequency/intensity)
   c. Do you feel like you broke your **WATER?** (include time/color of fluid)
   d. When was the last time you felt your baby **MOVING?** (this fourth question is slightly modified, as the patient's presenting complaint is decreased movement)

   If the patient answers yes to any of the first three questions, then these issues must also be addressed during her time in triage and on labor and delivery. After asking these questions, proceed to steps 2 and 3.
2. Obtain a fetal non-stress test (NST) by placing external fetal heart monitor and tocometer (see Chapter 2).
3. Perform an abdominal ultrasound to determine the amniotic fluid index (AFI), fetal presentation, and placental location (see Chapter 2).

Interventions

- If the patient has a reactive NST and a normal AFI, and is not in labor, she may be reassured that her fetus demonstrates no evidence of distress and then discharged to home to follow up with her regular provider.
- If the patient has a non-reactive fetal heart rate (FHR) tracing, then she should not be discharged until additional evaluation is done. In general, a biophysical profile (BPP) should be performed at this point. This exam is discussed in detail in Chapter 2.
- If the patient has an AFI of less than 5 or an MVP of less than 2, then this is classified as oligohydramnios (see Chapter 14). In a term patient, induction or augmentation of labor is usually undertaken. It is also important to note that oligohydramnios may result from spontaneous rupture of membranes with a slow leak that the patient did not notice. Because of this, when oligohydramnios is present, you should perform an examination to rule out ruptured membranes, which is discussed later in this section.

Rule Out Labor at Term (≥ 37 weeks)

This is probably the most common reason that women come to labor and delivery. It is not uncommon for a woman, especially a primigravida, to be evaluated multiple times before she actually goes into active labor and is admitted. The following steps are taken to rule out *term* labor:*

1. After establishing the patient's gestational age, ask the four basic questions:
   a. Are you having any **BLEEDING?**
   b. Are you having any **CONTRACTIONS?** (include time of onset/frequency/intensity)
   c. Do you feel like you broke your **WATER?** (include time/color of fluid)
   d. Are you feeling regular fetal **MOVEMENTS?**

4. Obtain a fetal non-stress test (NST) by placing external fetal heart monitor and tocometer (See Chapter 2).
5. Perform an abdominal ultrasound to determine the amniotic fluid index (AFI), fetal presentation, and placentation (see Chapter 2).

---

* A patient with complaint of *preterm* labor requires a different evaluation, which is discussed in Chapter 14.

6. Perform a sterile digital cervical examination (or a sterile speculum examination if there is a possibility of ruptured membranes).

Considerations

The two key things to evaluate when a patient presents for evaluation of possible term labor are fetal status and the presence or absence of cervical change. In general, only the patient with a reassuring FHR tracing who is not in labor will be discharged, while all others will be at least kept for observation.

It is important to realize that the actual cervical dilation or effacement that physicians use to determine if a patient is in labor and requires admission to labor and delivery may vary significantly. It is dependent both on the patient's parity and on other factors, such as the amount of pain she is experiencing, whether or not she has a history of rapid labor, and how far away she lives. Some general guidelines for labor triage are as follows:

- If the patient does not have regular contractions (at least every 5–7 minutes) and is < 3 cm dilated, she may be discharged to home with labor precautions. These precautions should include instructions to call back or return if she feels that her membranes rupture, if she experiences significant vaginal bleeding, or if the contractions become more frequent and painful. If the patient has significant pain, but is not in labor, she may be given medications for the pain to go home with, assuming the fetal status is reassuring. You should also ensure she has a plan for follow-up, as well (see Chapter 8).
- If the patient has regular contractions (at least every 5–7 minutes) and is 2–3 cm dilated, she may be offered the option of walking for 1–2 hours and then having her cervix checked again to determine if she is progressing in labor. If the patient makes cervical change when rechecked, she may be admitted.
- Also, if the patient has a history of rapid labor, is in significant pain, or lives more than 30 minutes from the hospital, it is reasonable to have her walk even if she is only 1–2 cm dilated. If the patient has regular contractions and is > 4 cm dilated, she will usually be admitted to labor and delivery.

Remember that these are just guidelines, and there will be circumstances where patients will be kept for observation or given pain medication for latent labor and monitored to see if they progress in labor.

Rule Out Ruptured Membranes

Many women will call labor and delivery and report that they have experienced a large "gush" of fluid. Regardless of the gestational age, the patient should be advised to come in to labor and delivery for evaluation.

1. After establishing the patient's gestational age, ask the four basic questions and perform an NST (see Chapter 2):
   a. Are you having any **BLEEDING?**
   b. Are you having any **CONTRACTIONS?** (include time of onset/frequency/intensity)
   c. What time do you feel like you broke your **WATER?** (include color of fluid and if she is continuing to leak fluid)
   d. Are you feeling regular fetal **MOVEMENTS?**

2. After asking these questions, perform a sterile speculum examination and observe the cervical os.

There are four different parameters you will observe for during your exam. First, look for evidence of **POOLING** of amniotic fluid in the vagina as well as for fluid coming from the os as the patient bears down with a **VALSALVA** maneuver. Obtain a small amount of fluid from the posterior vaginal fornix or lateral sidewall with a sterile cotton swab and smear this on a slide. Allow the slide to dry and then look for evidence of a **FERNING** pattern. (Ferning will often not appear until the slide is *completely* dry.) Also, place some of the vaginal secretions collected with the swab on **NITRAZINE** paper to see if the color changes because of an increased vaginal pH, which is seen with amniotic fluid – this will usually turn nitrazine paper blue. If the patient is preterm, other specimens/swabs may need to be collected during this exam (see Chapter 14).

False-positive results may occur for the following reasons:

- Nitrazine: contamination with blood, semen, alkaline antiseptics, or bacterial vaginosis (Mercer 2003).
- Ferning: cervical mucus may demonstrate some degree of ferning.

False-negative results may occur in the following situations:

- Nitrazine/ferning: prolonged leakage of a small amount of fluid, or minimal fluid present in the vagina.

3. Perform an abdominal ultrasound to determine the amniotic fluid index (AFI), fetal presentation, and placentation (see Chapter 2).

If the patient has a good history for ruptured membranes, i.e., a large gush of fluid with continuing leakage, but the tests above are negative, or are inconclusive, further evaluation is required. If the amniotic fluid volume is normal (AFI between 5 and 25 at term – see Chapter 2), then ruptured membranes is very unlikely. There are now proprietary tests that can be performed to rule out rupture of membranes. They work by detecting proteins found only in amniotic fluid, e.g. alpha-macroglobulin-1 (PAMG-1). These test kits are usually reserved for cases where rupture is more difficult to determine, as they can be expensive.

In rare circumstances (e.g., preterm or pre-viable rupture of membranes) an ultrasound-guided amniocentesis with instillation of indigo carmine (1 mL in 9 mL of sterile saline) may be done with observation for passage of blue fluid from the vagina. However, this procedure is not generally performed unless there is a very high index of suspicion for ruptured membranes in a preterm patient.

Interventions

- If the patient is at *term* and found to have ruptured membranes, you may perform a digital examination to determine how dilated the cervix is if you could not see this on the speculum examination. If you could see the cervix well, then perform an abdominal ultrasound quickly to confirm that the fetus is in a vertex position and admit the patient to labor and delivery.
- If, however, the patient is *preterm*, less than 34 weeks, please refer to the section on preterm premature rupture of membranes (PPROM) in Chapter 14 for a discussion of how to proceed with these patients.

There has been a debate for some time regarding whether or not the term patient with ruptured membranes who is not in labor should undergo labor induction or just conservative monitoring, as the majority of term patients will enter labor spontaneously within 24 hours of rupture of membranes. There are now multiple studies, however, that have demonstrated a significant decrease in the risk of both maternal infection (intra-amniotic infection and endometritis postpartum) and neonatal NICU admissions and overall morbidity with induction of labor (Middleton *et al.* 2017). These studies also did not demonstrate an increase in the risk of cesarean section with induction compared to conservative management. Because of these recommendations, especially in patients who are known to have a positive culture for group B streptococcus, admission and induction of labor is recommended (see *Group B Streptococcus Prophylaxis*, later in this chapter).

Make a note in the chart and admission history and physical of the time at which the patient believes the membranes ruptured, as well as the color of the fluid (see *Management of Meconium*, later in this chapter).

Rule out Preeclampsia

Patients may be referred to labor and delivery for evaluation of possible preeclampsia after 20 weeks' gestation. Or they may call with complaints of worsening edema, a severe headache, right upper quadrant (RUQ) pain, or visual disturbances. This is not an uncommon reason to see a patient after a clinic visit where the patient is found to have new-onset hypertension. In these cases, the initial approach should be the same, beginning with the standard four questions about bleeding, contractions, ROM, and fetal movement, obtaining an NST, and performing an abdominal ultrasound. In addition to these, you should inquire about symptoms that may be associated with preeclampsia. These questions include the following:

a. Are you having any swelling? Edema is common in preeclampsia but will often be in the upper extremities and the face rather than just in the lower extremities, which may occur with normal pregnancy. (Note that edema is NOT part of the diagnostic criteria for preeclampsia, but should increase your suspicion.)
b. Are you having any headaches? Severe headaches may be a sign of severe preeclampsia and CNS irritation and should be noted.
c. Are you experiencing any RUQ pain? Another possible component of severe preeclampsia is severe RUQ pain from liver involvement or an expanding liver hematoma.
d. Have you noticed any changes in your vision, e.g., flashing lights? Scotomata is another sign of CNS irritation and possible severe preeclampsia.

After asking these questions, you should send some basic laboratory tests. These tests include:

- Urinalysis (for evidence of proteinuria) with a urine protein/creatinine ratio
- CBC (to assess for hemoconcentration and/or thrombocytopenia)
- Chemistries/electrolytes (with particular attention to the creatinine)
- Uric acid
- AST/ALT
- LDH

During the time you are waiting for these results, the fetus should be placed on the monitor to obtain an NST and the patient should have serial blood pressure readings taken.

Table 4.3 Diagnostic criteria for preeclampsia and preeclampsia with severe features

Preeclampsia

- BP ≥ 140 systolic or ≥ 90 mmHg diastolic on two occasions at least 4 hours apart (at least 20 weeks EGA without history of hypertension) OR ≥ 160 systolic or ≥ 110 diastolic at a single encounter

AND

- ≥ 300 mg urine total protein/24-hour urine collection OR protein/creatinine ratio ≥ 0.3 (preferably a catheterized specimen without the presence of blood)

Severe features*

- Systolic > 160 or diastolic > 110 on two occasions at least 4 hours apart
- Platelet count < 100,000
- Impaired liver function (LFTs 2× normal) or severe RUQ or epigastric pain
- Renal insufficiency (serum creatinine > 1.1 mg/dL or 2× patient's baseline)
- Pulmonary edema
- New-onset cerebral or visual disturbances

* In the absence of documented proteinuria, symptoms of severe features and new-onset hypertension also meets criteria for preeclampsia.

Interventions

Please refer to Chapter 14 for a thorough discussion of the diagnosis of preeclampsia, including risk factors, laboratory results, and management. See Table 4.3 for diagnostic criteria for *preeclampsia* and *preeclampsia with severe features*. Diagnosis of preeclampsia requires the presence of both hypertension and proteinuria (unless there are severe features present, in which case it can be diagnosed without proteinuria). The terminology and differentiation of "mild" versus "severe" preeclampsia nomenclature is no longer used. It should also be emphasized that patients with persistent severe-range blood pressure readings (systolic > 160 or diastolic > 110) require prompt attention and treatment.

Management of the Latent Phase

The latent phase of labor begins with regular uterine contractions and cervical change and ends when the cervix is 5–6 cm dilated and almost completely effaced. While many patients will not be admitted until they are in active labor, patients may present with ruptured membranes or be admitted for delivery for other indications while in the latent phase. If the patient progresses in labor and enters the active phase, then no intervention is required. Latent labor can last for many hours, and may require intervention if prolonged, or if there is a medical indication to expedite delivery.

Prolonged Latent Phase

A prolonged latent phase of labor is defined as > 20 hours in nulliparous patients and > 14 hours in multiparous patients. An unfavorable cervix (see Chapter 7) at the onset of labor is a risk factor for prolonged latent phase. Women with a prolonged latent phase are at increased risk for postpartum hemorrhage, cesarean delivery, and neonatal admission to the NICU (Cheng *et al.* 2009). For the patient who has a prolonged latent phase, then consideration must be given to how best to augment labor. Options for treatment include the following:

Therapeutic rest. This involves administering narcotics to the patient and is discussed in the next section.

Amniotomy. If the patient is a candidate for artificial rupture of membranes (AROM), then this intervention may be performed. It has been shown to decrease the duration of the first stage of labor and is more effective when used in conjunction with oxytocin augmentation (Macones *et al.* 2012). See Chapter 2 for details on the indications, contraindications, and steps of performing an amniotomy.

Labor augmentation. The latent phase may be augmented with one of two methods. First, if the cervix is unfavorable, then cervical ripening may be attempted (see Chapter 7). Oxytocin augmentation of labor may also be used with either a favorable or an unfavorable cervix, though greater success is achieved after cervical ripening. Success rates (i.e., getting patients to transition from latent to active labor) of more than 70% of women have been reported with the use of oxytocin (Rouse *et al.* 2011, Kawakita *et al.* 2016).

You will probably notice that cesarean delivery is not listed as a treatment option for a prolonged latent phase of labor. This is because there is no increase in perinatal mortality associated with a protracted latent phase as long as the fetal status remains reassuring (ACOG 2014). This recommendation is specific to those patients presenting in spontaneous latent labor. For those undergoing *induction of labor* for medical indications, prolonged latent phase may be an indication for cesarean delivery. In general, a cesarean section in the latent phase should be reserved for fetal distress or other indications, such as presentation in labor with a breech fetus or for a repeat cesarean delivery for those not wanting a trial of labor after cesarean (TOLAC), or for those who are not candidates for such.

Pain Control

When a patient presents with regular uterine contractions and you determine that she is in the latent phase of labor, pain is often a significant concern. In the nulliparous patient experiencing labor for the first time, early labor can be extremely uncomfortable. Also, when a patient is admitted for labor induction and is in the latent phase, contractions from oxytocin or other induction agents can be very painful as well. When you talk with patients about options for pain management, make sure to explain that you want to support their desires, which may be to avoid pain medication, and be sensitive to their requests. Options for pain control for patients who desire this during the latent phase of labor include narcotics and epidural anesthesia.

Narcotics

A good rule of thumb when administering narcotics during labor is to ask yourself: what are the chances of the patient delivering within 2 hours? If a significant amount of the narcotic is present in the fetal system at the time of delivery, then the infant can be significantly depressed and require resuscitation. This complication, fortunately, rarely occurs with the specific formulations of narcotics that are given in latent labor.

Administration of narcotics for therapeutic rest for the patient in pain during latent labor is a reasonable option in many cases, and you can reassure the woman that the medication will not stop labor. One study reported that after therapeutic rest, more than 60% of women will transition into active labor (Mackeen *et al.* 2014). Because of the effects on the FHR tracing, which include decreased variability, narcotics should only be administered after obtaining reassuring fetal testing, usually in the form of a reactive non-stress test. If the patient is only in latent labor and fetal testing is reassuring, then the patient can be discharged to home with PO medication for pain if she has not demonstrated cervical change. If, however, PO pain medication has not been successful, or the woman is extremely uncomfortable, she can be given IV medication and monitored on labor and delivery to ensure it is effective. (See Chapter 8, *Obstetric Analgesia and Anesthesia*, for doses of narcotics used for therapeutic rest.)

Epidural

This is not the first choice for latent labor, since it restricts a patient's ability to walk and move. Whether or not early epidural prolongs the latent phase of labor remains controversial. A Cochrane review demonstrated that there were no significant increases in time to delivery (13 minutes), and no differences in risk of cesarean delivery between those with and without epidural (Anim-Somuah *et al.* 2011). However, there are cases in which this is a reasonable thing to pursue during latent labor. ACOG does not recommend that a woman be required to achieve a certain degree of cervical dilation before an epidural is administered, and clarifies that patient comfort is an important consideration (ACOG 2017b). Some indications for an epidural in the latent phase of labor include the following:

- Induction for intrauterine fetal demise (IUFD)
- Inability to control pain with adequate doses of IV/IM narcotics
- Maternal cardiac or CNS conditions for which pain may cause maternal or fetal compromise

Non-Narcotic Pain Control

Historically, nitrous oxide (N_2O) gas administration was used to help patients cope with labor pain. While the use of N_2O had fallen out of favor (in the United States) for many years, it appears to be becoming more common in some hospitals and birth centers. N_2O is delivered as a mixture of 50% N_2O and 50% oxygen. It is self-administered by the patient, and is considered a safe, effective alternative to IV narcotics or intrathecal anesthesia (ACOG 2017b). Benefits to using N_2O include freedom of movement, patient-controlled pain relief, and no need for additional monitoring (ACOG 2017b). Check with your institution to see if this is offered as an option and what is in the specific protocol.

Fetal Distress

Whenever a patient is evaluated for labor at the hospital, you must evaluate the FHR tracing. If a patient is in the latent phase of labor and there is fetal distress, the first thing to do is determine the etiology and correct it if possible. See Chapter 3, *Intrapartum Fetal Heart Rate Monitoring*, for non-reassuring testing. If you cannot correct the underlying cause, or a non-reassuring FHR tracing persists despite appropriate interventions, the standard of care for a timely delivery is a cesarean section.

Management of the Active Phase

The active phase of labor begins when the cervix is dilated 6 cm and almost completely effaced and ends when the cervix is completely dilated (no cervix is palpable around the fetal vertex). In contrast to the latent phase of labor, a woman in the active phase is expected to make cervical change every 1–2 hours. If she does not, then she may have either a protraction or an arrest disorder, and the labor may require augmentation in an attempt to accomplish a vaginal delivery.

Protraction and Arrest Disorders

The overall incidence of protraction and arrest disorders in the first stage of labor is around 8–12% (Ramus 2017). A protraction disorder simply implies that the patient has continued to make cervical change, just at a much slower rate than anticipated, while an arrest disorder means she has ceased to make progress at all.

Protraction Disorders

A nulliparous patient has a protracted active phase of labor when she fails to dilate at least 1 cm/hour, or a multiparous patient if she dilates less than 1.2–1.5 cm/hour. These rates are two standard deviations below what is normally expected. When this occurs, there are two interventions that may be attempted. These are amniotomy (see Chapter 2) and oxytocin augmentation (see Chapter 7). If a patient has a protracted active phase of labor, you should also consider the placement of an intrauterine pressure catheter (IUPC) to better assess the adequacy of the patient's contractions, once the membranes are ruptured.

Arrest Disorders

A patient is diagnosed with arrest of dilation when she has demonstrated no cervical change for at least 4 hours with adequate uterine contractions. Adequate uterine contractions are measured with an IUPC and defined as > 200 Montevideo units (a measure of the area-under-the-curve on the tocometer – see Chapter 2). If the patient meets these criteria, then a cesarean section may be recommended. Part of the reasoning behind performing a cesarean section for an arrest of dilation is that the absence of any change over this time period may imply that either the fetus is too large or the patient's pelvis too small to permit a vaginal delivery, or the fetus may be positioned in a way that does not allow passage (e.g., asynclitism – which refers to the fetal head being tilted to the side such that it is not in line with the birth canal). An algorithm for the management of the active phase of labor is shown in Figure 4.2.

For the indications, contraindications, and standard dose regimens for oxytocin augmentation of labor, please refer to Chapter 7, *Induction and Augmentation of Labor*.

Pain Control

Options for pain control during the active phase of labor are similar to those available during latent labor. The difference is that intravenous narcotics should not be administered if you believe the patient may deliver within the next 2 hours. For this reason, narcotics are rarely given after a patient reaches approximately 6 cm, and some form of conduction anesthesia (epidural or spinal) is generally the recommended option at this time (see Chapter 8, *Obstetric Analgesia and Anesthesia*).

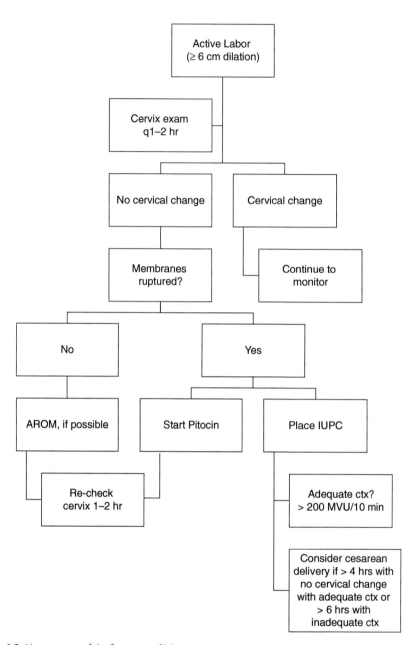

Figure 4.2 Management of the first stage of labor.

Fetal Distress

Similar to the latent phase, if fetal distress occurs, you must attempt to determine the reason and correct it if possible (see Chapter 3, *Intrapartum Fetal Heart Rate Monitoring*). If you cannot accomplish this in a timely fashion, then you must perform a cesarean delivery, as an operative vaginal delivery is not possible during the first stage of labor.

Management of Meconium

Meconium passage prior to birth occurs in approximately 8–18% of all term births (Lee *et al.* 2011, Lindenskov *et al.* 2015). If a patient is noted to have meconium-stained fluids in the latent phase of labor, this implies that she has ruptured membranes and will therefore be admitted to labor and delivery. More often, this complication is not seen until the active phase of labor, which is when most patients will spontaneously rupture their membranes.

When noting meconium passage in the chart, you should write both the time it was noted and whether it appeared thin, thick, or particulate. Given that unique neonatal resuscitation strategies are used when meconium is present, it is also very important to notify your pediatrician or baby care team of its presence and the timing, to provide a description (thin, thick, particulate, etc.) of the meconium, and to ensure they are present for the delivery. Neonatal aspiration of meconium-stained amniotic fluids can lead to meconium aspiration syndrome, which is characterized by neonatal respiratory distress and oxygen requirement, and can lead to pulmonary hypertension, with significant morbidity and mortality. With improved neonatal resuscitation strategies, the incidence of meconium aspiration syndrome has decreased from 22% to 0.2% over the past several decades, with improvement in neonatal outcomes as well (Lindenskov *et al.* 2015).

While there is some controversy regarding the use of an amnioinfusion when meconium is present during labor in the absence of variable decelerations (which is another common indication for amnioinfusion), there are several trials that have demonstrated a reduction in the rate of meconium aspiration syndrome and fetal distress when an amnioinfusion is performed for patients found to have meconium-stained amniotic fluid, as well as a trend toward reduced perinatal mortality (Hofmeyr *et al.* 2014). The current recommendation from ACOG, however, is to consider an amnioinfusion when there are variable decelerations present, regardless of the presence or absence of meconium (ACOG 2006, reaffirmed 2016).

Group B Streptococcus Prophylaxis

Group B streptococcus (GBS), or *Streptococcus agalactiae,* is an encapsulated Gram-positive organism that is the most common pathogenic bacterium found in newborns. These bacteria can colonize as many as 33% of pregnant women, and because of this, it is important to administer antibiotics during labor to prevent the occurrence of early neonatal sepsis from this organism (Kwatra *et al.* 2014).

Historically, patients were risk-stratified and treated based on risk factors for GBS (such as gestational age < 37 weeks, ruptured membranes for > 18 hours, or a previously affected baby). Contemporary standard of care is to screen all patients for the presence of GBS in the urogenital tract. The Centers for Disease Control and Prevention (CDC) have published clear guidelines for GBS screening and prophylaxis (Verani *et al.* 2010). These recommendations include the screening of all pregnant patients between 35 and 37 weeks' gestation and the treatment of all patients during labor who have positive cultures. See Figure 4.3 for an algorithm for term patients and Figure 4.4 for preterm patients.

Ideally, a patient should receive at least a 4-hour course of prophylactic antibiotics prior to delivery (Berardi *et al.* 2011). At times, this may mean waiting to rupture a patient's membranes, or not augmenting labor as aggressively as you might in a GBS-negative

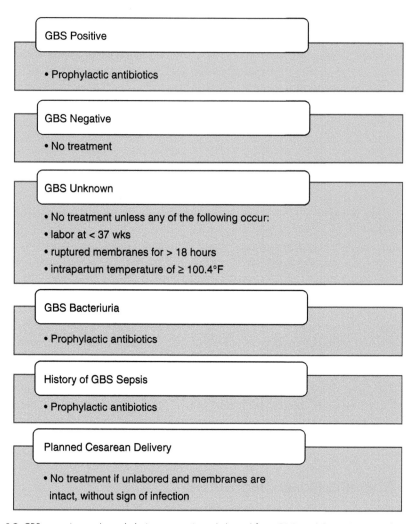

Figure 4.3 GBS screening and prophylaxis: term patients (adapted from CDC guidelines: Verani *et al.* 2010).

patient, especially a multiparous patient who presents in active labor that you expect to deliver quickly.

Penicillin (PCN) is the first-line treatment for GBS prophylaxis. Ampicillin can also be used, and it confers a broader spectrum of coverage – though there is concern for antibiotic resistance. Given that many patients report PCN allergy, alternative treatments, based on CDC guidelines, can be found in Figure 4.5. It should be noted that although 10% of patients report PCN allergy, studies show that 90% of those patients do not have any clinically identifiable allergy, e.g., presence of IgE to PCN (Raja *et al.* 2009). Some institutions offer PCN allergy testing, which could limit the morbidity and risk factors associated with alternative antibiotic regimens in some patients.

According to CDC guidelines, positive GBS culture in a previous pregnancy is not an indication for antibiotic prophylaxis during the current pregnancy unless the previous child

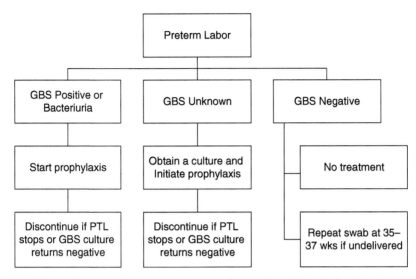

Figure 4.4 GBS screening and prophylaxis: preterm patients (adapted from CDC guidelines: Verani *et al.* 2010). PTL, preterm labor.

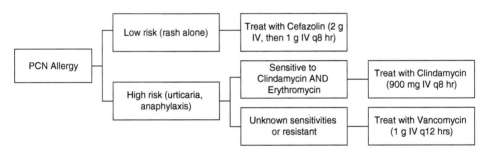

Figure 4.5 GBS prophylaxis for penicillin (PCN)-allergic patients (adapted from CDC guidelines: Verani *et al.* 2010).

was noted to have GBS-positive cultures, as well. Also, if a patient has demonstrated GBS in her urine during pregnancy, she should receive antibiotic prophylaxis during labor, and screening between 35 and 37 weeks is not necessary. Of note, patients who have a planned cesarean delivery, and who do not labor or have ruptured membranes prior to the procedure, do not require GBS prophylaxis regardless of the GBS culture results.

It is important to note that antibiotic treatment does not reduce the incidence of late-onset GBS infections, which are those that occur between 7 and 89 days of life (Verani *et al.* 2010). Several vaccine prototypes have been developed and are in or nearing clinical trials (Kobayashi *et al.* 2016). In the near future, these may become available, and could reduce or obviate the need for patients to receive antibiotic prophylaxis during labor. The added benefit of such a vaccine is that the conferred immunity could also protect against late-onset neonatal sepsis (Kobayashi *et al.* 2016).

References

ACOG (2006). Amnioinfusion does not prevent meconium aspiration syndrome. *ACOG Committee Opinion #346*, October 2006, reaffirmed 2018.

ACOG (2014). Safe prevention of the primary cesarean delivery. *ACOG Obstetric Care Consensus #1*, March 2014, reaffirmed 2016.

ACOG (2017a). Methods for estimating the due date. *ACOG Committee Opinion #700*, May 2017.

ACOG (2017b). Obstetric analgesia and anesthesia. *ACOG Practice Bulletin #117*, April 2017.

Anim-Somuah M, Smyth RM, Jones L (2011). Epidural versus non-epidural or no analgesia in labour. *Cochrane Database Syst Rev* (12): CD000331.

Berardi A, Rossi C, Biasini A, *et al.* (2011). Efficacy of intrapartum chemoprophylaxis less than 4 hours duration. *J Matern Fetal Neonatal Med* 24: 619–25.

Cheng YW, Delaney SS, Hopkins LM, Caughey AB (2009). The association between the length of first stage of labor, mode of delivery, and perinatal outcomes in women undergoing induction of labor. *Am J Obstet Gynecol* 201: 477.e1–7.

Friedman EA (1978). *Labor: Clinical Evaluation and Management*, 2nd edn. New York: Appleton-Century-Crofts.

Hofmeyr GJ, Xu H, Eke AC (2014). Amnioinfusion for meconium-stained liquor in labour. *Cochrane Database Syst Rev* (1): CD000014.

Kawakita T, Reddy UM, Iqbal SN, *et al.* (2016). Duration of oxytocin and rupture of the membranes before diagnosing a failed induction of labor. *Obstet Gynecol* 128: 373–80.

Kobayashi M, Vekemans J, Baker CJ, *et al.* (2016). Group B streptococcus vaccine development: present status and future considerations, with emphasis on perspectives for low and middle income countries. *F1000Res* 5: 2355.

Kwatra G, Adrian PV, Shiri T, *et al.* (2014). Serotype-specific acquisition and loss of group

B streptococcus recto-vaginal colonization in late pregnancy. *PloS one* 9 (6): e98778.

Lee KA, Mi Lee S, Jin Yang H, *et al.* (2011). The frequency of meconium-stained amniotic fluid increases as a function of the duration of labor. *J Matern Fetal Neonatal Med* 24: 880–5.

Lindenskov PH, Castellheim A, Saugstad O, Mollnes TE (2015). Meconium aspiration syndrome: possible pathophysiological mechanisms and future potential therapies. *Neonatology* 107: 225–30.

Mackeen AD, Fhenel E, Berghella V, Klein T (2014). Morphine sleep in pregnancy. *Am J Perinatol* 31: 85–90.

Macones GA, Cahill A, Stamilio DM, Odibo AO (2012). The efficacy of early amniotomy in nulliparous labor induction: a randomized controlled trial. *Am J Obstet Gynecol* 207: 403. e1–5.

Mercer BM (2003). Preterm premature rupture of the membranes. *Obstet Gynecol* 101: 178–93.

Middleton P, Shepherd E, Flenady V, McBain RD, Crowther CA (2017). Planned early birth versus expectant management (waiting) for prelabour rupture of membranes at term (37 weeks or more). *Cochrane Database Syst Rev* 1: CD005302.

Raja AS, Lindsell CJ, Bernstein JA, Codispoti CD, Moellman JJ (2009). The use of penicillin skin testing to assess the prevalence of penicillin allergy in an emergency department setting. *Ann Emerg Med* 54: 72–7.

Ramus RM (2017). Abnormal labor. *Medscape.* https://emedicine.medscape.com/article/273053 (accessed May 2018).

Rouse DJ, Weiner SJ, Bloom SL, *et al.* (2011). Failed labor induction: toward an objective diagnosis. *Obstet Gynecol* 117: 267–72.

Verani JR, McGee L, Schrag SJ (2010). Prevention of perinatal group B streptococcal disease: revised guidelines from CDC, 2010. *MMWR Recomm Rep* 59 (RR-10): 1–36.

Zhang JJ, Landy HJ, Branch DW, *et al.* (2010). Contemporary patterns of spontaneous labor with normal neonatal outcomes. *Obstet Gynecol* 116: 1281–7.

Management of the Second Stage of Labor

Kelsey J. Simpson and Shad Deering

Definition

The second stage of labor begins when the woman's cervix is completely dilated and completely effaced (usually reported as "complete/complete" or "C/C" in the chart). It is during this stage that the patient will push to deliver, and it ends with the delivery of the baby.

Normal Duration

The normal duration of the second stage of labor is dependent on parity and epidural usage. When patients have an epidural, the duration of second stage for nulliparous women is approximately 70 minutes, compared to 25 minutes for multiparous patients. Without an epidural, these times are shorter, at approximately 35 and 15 minutes respectively (Zhang *et al.* 2010).

Multiple additional factors can also affect the length of the second stage of labor, including fetal size, occiput position, maternal body mass index (BMI), and station at which complete dilation occurs. ACOG recommends that the second stage should be allowed to progress without operative intervention as long as the fetal heart rate (FHR) tracing remains reassuring and the fetus demonstrates some descent during pushing until the patient meets criteria for dystocia, which is defined later in this chapter. If fetal distress develops during this stage, then an operative intervention – forceps, vacuum extraction, or cesarean section – is indicated (ACOG 2014).

Routine Management

Fetal Monitoring

While pushing, the FHR is usually monitored in a continuous fashion, with attention to any decelerations and their timing related to contractions. If the patient has been using intermittent monitoring during labor or desires this while pushing, then the FHR must be recorded every 15 minutes after a contraction in a low-risk patient. High-risk patients (e.g., suspected fetal growth restriction, preeclampsia, or type 1 diabetes) are not candidates for intermittent fetal monitoring (ACOG 2009).

If you have difficulty monitoring the fetus with external monitors, which often need to be adjusted inferiorly during pushing as the baby descends, then you may place a fetal scalp electrode (FSE) in order to better assess fetal status (see Chapter 2, *Common Examinations and Procedures*).

Anesthesia Support

Most commonly, if a patient desired an epidural for pain relief, it will already be in place by the time she enters the second stage of labor. An epidural is generally not administered this late in labor. However, if a patient is able to sit for placement, it may be possible to have either a spinal or even an epidural placed for analgesia. The advantage of the spinal in this situation is in its rapid onset of analgesia. A combined spinal/epidural technique, discussed in Chapter 8, may also be of benefit, as it provides rapid pain relief with the spinal component but also allows for additional boluses through the epidural catheter, which is left in place if needed. In a multiparous patient with a history of rapid deliveries, it may be impossible to place either a spinal or an epidural prior to delivery. Whether or not conduction anesthesia (i.e., spinal or epidural) may be administered at this stage is dependent on the clinical situation as well as the individual anesthesia provider. Before calling to discuss with your anesthesia provider, it is prudent to perform a cervical examination so that you know exactly what the fetal station and cervical dilation are, so you can communicate this to the provider.

Narcotics should generally not be used during the second stage of labor, as delivery will likely occur soon enough that the fetus could be affected. If any narcotics have been given within 2 hours of delivery, then you should notify the pediatrician and have naloxone hydrochloride (0.1 mg/kg) drawn up in case there is significant neonatal depression. See Table 5.1 for doses based on fetal weight.

A pudendal nerve block is another option during the second stage of labor. It is performed by inserting a needle through the vagina and injecting the pudendal nerves with a local anesthetic. When performed correctly, this technique provides anesthesia that is adequate for operative vaginal delivery. This technique is discussed in detail in Chapter 8.

Table 5.1 Doses of naloxone hydrochloride

Fetal weight (g)	Dose (mL of 0.4 mg/mL concentration)
4000	1.0 mL
3000	0.75 mL
2000	0.5 mL

Pediatric Consultation

There are certain situations where it is prudent to have a pediatrician attend a delivery. In general, whenever you anticipate there is some risk that the fetus will require immediate attention and possibly resuscitation, you should contact a pediatrician to discuss the situation. Some of these situations include the following:

- Cesarean section
- Meconium
- Forceps or vacuum delivery
- Breech vaginal delivery
- Umbilical cord prolapse
- Delivery after significant hemorrhage (placental abruption/vasa previa)
- Intra-amniotic infection
- Maternal history of substance abuse
- Recent administration of narcotics or the use of general anesthesia
- Multiple pregnancy
- Fetal distress/non-reassuring fetal heart rate tracing
- Preterm delivery (< 37 weeks)
- Known/suspected fetal anomaly

By keeping these situations in mind, you will be able to call the pediatricians prior to delivery, and you will have time to brief them so they can be prepared and present at delivery. This will also help reassure the parents should the baby require immediate resuscitation after delivery.

Perineal Care

As one of the risks of any vaginal delivery is lacerations, it is important to use both proper technique during delivery and also any interventions that can decrease this risk. A recent meta-analysis of over 1500 women, looking at third- and fourth-degree perineal lacerations, found that starting perineal massage at 36 weeks gestational age significantly reduced lacerations. Additionally, the application of a warm compress during the second stage of labor reduced rates compared to a hands-off approach (Aasheim *et al.* 2017). Another recent study showed that the incidence of significant lacerations could be reduced by more than 50% by the use of perineal massage beginning around 36 weeks, warm compress use during labor, avoiding midline episiotomy and using a mediolateral approach if an episiotomy was indicated, and supporting the perineum and controlling the head at delivery (Fausett *et al.* 2017).

Pushing

Much is written in the lay press about how and when to push during labor. While there is some science involved in the process, much of this phase is an art, especially in teaching and coaching the patient in pushing, and there is much you can learn from experienced delivery nurses, midwives, and other providers.

Pushing Position and Coaching

In general, whatever position the patient desires to assume that still allows you to adequately monitor the fetus is acceptable. Some women will feel more comfortable on their back while others will want to push on their side or use a "squatting bar" to support themselves while they bear down. When patients begin pushing, especially nulliparous patients or those with a dense epidural, it is sometimes helpful to place your fingers into the vagina and push posteriorly to assist them in knowing where to push. This will also allow you to determine if they are pushing effectively, as you will feel the fetal head applying pressure to your fingers when the woman bears down in the correct manner. Once the patient understands where to push you do not need to keep your fingers in place as you may cause lacerations in edematous tissue.

When coaching, or explaining pushing to patients, many physicians and nurses will have the patient take a deep breath as the contraction begins to build (which can be seen on the monitor if you are using either external or internal monitors) and then hold her breath and bear down in a similar manner to having a bowel movement while the coach (partner, nurse, birthing assistant, or physician) counts to 10. At this point, the patient exhales and quickly takes another deep breath and bears down again while the coach counts. Usually, patients will do three sets of pushes with each contraction. Again, this is something of an art rather than a science, and women may want to push differently. Some providers will not have the patient hold her breath, and rather use an "open glottis" technique. A recent meta-analysis of 21 randomized trials concluded that there is no clear difference in the length of pushing when women follow their own instincts versus directed pushing with Valsalva maneuver (Lemos *et al.* 2017). Remember that your goal in this process is to help patients push effectively while doing your best to respect their desires for the delivery.

When to Begin Pushing

While this may sound like a simple decision, you will find a lot of different opinions on this topic. Once they patient is completely dilated, if she feels the urge to push, then you should have her begin. If, however, she is completely dilated but does not feel the need to push, then you have some options to consider, and there have been several recent studies that have examined whether pushing as soon as they are completely dilated or if either waiting for a specified amount of time or until they feel the urge to push (which is called "laboring down") is best for mother and baby.

Two different studies have randomized patients with epidurals to either immediate pushing or waiting for up to 2 hours or when the head was visible at the introitus (Fraser *et al.* 2000, Hansen *et al.* 2002). Both of these showed that the group that delayed pushing had an overall longer total second stage but shorter time spent actually pushing. In the Hansen study, the difference in actual pushing time was 110 minutes with immediate pushing versus only 68 minutes with delayed pushing. It is also important to note that there was no increase in the risk of significant lacerations or complications, and that neonatal outcomes were the same between the groups.

Based on the available literature and evidence, at this time ACOG recommends that in the absence of indications for expeditious delivery women may be offered a period of rest of 1–2 hours at the onset of the second stage (ACOG 2017b).

Spontaneous Vaginal Delivery

The majority of deliveries are uncomplicated. What follows is a description of how to perform an uncomplicated vaginal delivery, as well as notes for different times when complications may occur. Delivery of a breech presentation is discussed separately in Chapter 14.

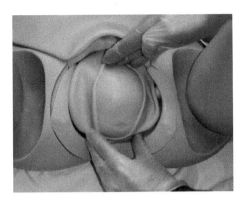

Figure 5.1 Hand position at the time of vaginal delivery, supporting the perineum.

Delivery of the Head

As the mother bears down with contractions, the fetal head will cause the perineum to bulge. When this occurs, place one hand at the inferior vaginal opening (Figure 5.1). The other hand is placed on the anterior portion of the fetal head. The goal is to protect the perineum by applying slight pressure with the posterior hand while at the same time controlling the head to prevent a significant anterior tear.

> **Episiotomy.** If an episiotomy is required, it will almost always be just prior to delivery of the fetal head. An episiotomy is an incision made in the perineum during delivery to provide additional room for the fetus to deliver. A 2015 review of hospital discharge data reported that episiotomies are performed in approximately 12% of deliveries (Friedman *et al.* 2015). It is not, however, a procedure that should be performed as a standard part of every delivery, as there may be significant short- and long-term morbidity to the mother. Types of episiotomies, indications, repair techniques, and complications are discussed in detail in Chapter 11.

Allow the head to deliver, and then have the mother stop pushing and pant. (Some women, especially those without an epidural, may not be able to stop pushing, and you will simply proceed with the delivery.) After the head delivers, it will restitute/turn to one side or the other.

Next, palpate the fetal neck to determine if there is a nuchal cord present. Nuchal cords occur in approximately 5% of all deliveries (Dhar *et al.* 1995). If one is present, then reduce it by pulling it gently over the fetal head. If it is too tight to allow this, you can attempt to deliver with it in place. If this is not possible, then as a last resort, place two Kelly clamps on the cord and cut in between with scissors.

The presence or absence of a nuchal cord as well as the manner in which it is reduced should be included in the delivery summary. Also, be careful not to accidentally cut the baby when you have a tight nuchal cord and you are "surgically reducing" it with clamps and scissors.

Delivery of the Shoulders

Place your hands on the fetal head with the fingers pointing toward the nose and have the mother begin to push again (Figure 5.2). As you apply gentle downward traction to deliver

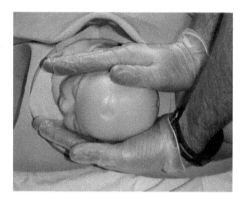

Figure 5.2 Hand position for shoulder delivery.

the anterior shoulder, you will see it appear at the introitus. If it does not come with relative ease, then you have a shoulder dystocia and must take immediate action to free the shoulder which is stuck behind the pubic symphysis (see the section in Chapter 14 on *Shoulder Dystocia*).

After the anterior shoulder appears at the introitus, change the direction of traction upward, and the posterior shoulder will deliver. (If you have cut an episiotomy, or are concerned about a perineal laceration, you or your assistant can attempt to support the perineum with a hand.)

Delivery of the Body and Clamping of the Cord

After the shoulders have delivered, the rest of the baby will almost always rapidly deliver. The most important thing to remember here is to not drop the child, as they are quite slippery when they come out! You can use your arms and body to cradle the child if needed and stay close to the perineum. (Do *anything* but drop a baby!)

ACOG now recommends delaying umbilical cord clamping for 30–60 seconds in vigorous infants, with benefits for both preterm and term infants without increasing maternal morbidity (ACOG 2017a). A 2012 Cochrane review looking at preterm infants found that delayed cord clamping was associated with fewer transfusions and lower incidence of intraventricular hemorrhage and necrotizing enterocolitis, with no significant difference in the rates of phototherapy (Rabe *et al.* 2012). A Cochrane review from 2013 looking at term infants found that delayed cord clamping increased hemoglobin concentration at birth, as well as iron stores (McDonald *et al.* 2013).

Upon delivery, the newborn infant may be placed on the maternal abdomen to allow for skin-to-skin contact while placental transfusion occurs. Normal newborn care should be initiated with stimulation and drying of the infant. If the baby is born with meconium and is vigorous, delayed cord clamping can still be performed. It is important, however, to keep in mind the situations in which delayed cord clamping is contraindicated (Table 5.2).

Once 30–60 seconds have elapsed, take two clamps and clamp the umbilical cord. Exactly where you do this is not terribly important, as another plastic clamp will be placed by the delivery room nurse and the cord trimmed to the appropriate length. In general, doubly clamping and cutting the cord around 30–40 cm (12–16 inches) from the umbilical

Table 5.2 Contraindications to delayed cord clamping

Maternal	Hemorrhage
	Hemodynamic instability
	Abnormal placentation (placenta previa, abruption)
Fetal	Need for immediate resuscitation
	Placental circulation no longer intact (abruption, placenta previa, cord avulsion)

cord insertion is adequate. (If the delivery has been uncomplicated, some fathers may want to cut the cord. This is something you can discuss with the parents prior to delivery. If you allow them to do this, make sure that you clearly show them where to cut and keep all fetal extremities and other parts away from the scissors.)

After the cord is cut, the infant may remain on the mother's abdomen if it has good color, respirations, and no evidence of distress. If additional resuscitation is needed, then the newborn is given to the labor and delivery nurse and taken over to the warmer.

At this point, the second stage of labor is over and the third stage begins.

Potential Second-Stage Complications

Meconium

In 2015, the American Academy of Pediatrics and the American Heart Association updated their guidelines on delivery of infants with meconium-stained amniotic fluid. Infants with meconium-stained fluid should no longer routinely receive intrapartum suction on the perineum, regardless of whether or not they are vigorous. The resuscitation should follow the same guidelines as those with clear fluid (ACOG 2017c).

Fetal Distress

During pushing, it is not uncommon to have FHR decelerations. Early decelerations, caused by compression of the fetal head during contractions, are not associated with fetal distress and may be watched and the patient reassured. Variable decelerations, however, may become more severe with pushing and must be monitored closely. Between pushes, the fetus should recover from these decelerations back to a normal baseline. When moderate to severe variable decelerations are present with pushing, having the patient push with every other contraction will sometimes allow the fetus enough time to recover between pushes to allow for a vaginal delivery. Late decelerations may occur intermittently, but if they become repetitive, then some action should be taken (see Chapter 3, *Intrapartum Fetal Heart Rate Monitoring*).

If normal conservative interventions are not able to correct fetal distress during the second stage of labor, then a decision must be made as to what the best route of delivery will be. If the fetus is at an appropriate station (+2 or lower) and meets the criteria listed in Chapter 9, *Operative Vaginal Delivery*, then either forceps or a vacuum device may be used to facilitate the delivery.

If, on the other hand, the fetus is not close enough to delivery to perform an operative delivery, then a cesarean section must be performed. The speed at which this is accomplished should depend on the degree of fetal distress. If there is a prolonged deceleration or fetal bradycardia, then an urgent cesarean is indicated. If this is the case, the following steps need to be taken and personnel mobilized in a rapid fashion:

1. Quickly counsel the patient on the need for an urgent cesarean delivery and explain the indications.
2. Call for additional assistance (resident/staff) as appropriate.
3. Inform the charge nurse you are calling for an urgent cesarean section.
4. Alert the anesthesia provider.
5. Unhook the patient's bed from the wall and any monitor cords and make sure any attached intravenous lines are secured.
6. Call the OR technician to the OR.
7. Call the NICU/pediatrics and alert them to the situation.
8. Ask for antibiotics in the OR.

For specifics regarding the procedure, see Chapter 10, *Cesarean Delivery.*

Labor Dystocia

Dystocia is defined as difficult labor. In the second stage of labor, dystocia may result from any of the following:

Cephalopelvic disproportion. This simply means that the fetus is too large or in a position such that it will not fit through the maternal pelvis. Unfortunately, this is not a diagnosis that can often be predicted, given the difficulty of accurately determining fetal weight prior to birth as well as our limited ability to clinically judge which women have an adequate pelvis for childbirth. While there are specific cases when a cesarean section for fetal macrosomia is indicated, in general, prophylactic cesarean delivery for a fetus that is "too large" has not been shown to be a reasonable or cost-effective intervention (Herbst 2005).

Malpresentation. Approximately 5% of fetuses will remain in a persistent occiput posterior or occiput transverse position during the second stage of labor (Vitner *et al.* 2015). These patients tend to have a longer second stage of labor and are at increased risk of intervention.

Epidural use. Current evidence demonstrates that that epidural analgesia prolongs the second stage by an average of 13.66 minutes. However, there are no negative effects on the fetus or neonate (Anim-Somuah *et al.* 2011).

Uterine hypocontractility. There are times when, even in the second stage of labor, uterine contractions may space out to the point where adequate progress is not made. In this situation, it is reasonable to begin oxytocin in order to help labor along.

Interventions that can be used if the patient is not making good progress with pushing efforts and the FHR tracing is reassuring include the following:

- Delayed pushing (discussed earlier in this chapter)
- Decreasing the epidural infusion rate if there is a very dense block, in order to allow the patient to push more effectively
- Changing maternal pushing position
- Administering oxytocin if uterine contractions are not frequent enough

Table 5.3 Definitions of second-stage dystocia (arrest of descent)

	Epidural	No epidural
Nulliparous	4 hours	3 hours
Multiparous	3 hours	2 hours

(Spong *et al.* 2012)

In 2012, the Eunice Kennedy Shriver National Institute of Child Health and Human Development, the Society for Maternal–Fetal Medicine, and ACOG convened a workshop to discuss concepts to prevent the first cesarean section by clarifying how long the second stage of labor could last without negatively impacting fetal outcomes (Spong *et al.* 2012). During this workshop, the criteria for second-stage arrest (called arrest of descent) were defined as shown in Table 5.3.

When patients do not progress well during the second stage of labor and meet the criteria for dystocia listed in Table 5.3, then there are several options that may be considered. These are:

Continued observation. If a patient has been making steady progress during pushing and the FHR tracing has remained reassuring, then the time limits set in Table 5.3 are not absolute indications for operative intervention. Interventions mentioned previously, such as decreasing the epidural rate, changing the maternal position, or administering oxytocin may be attempted, with continued close monitoring of the fetal status.

Operative vaginal delivery. If the fetus is felt to be an appropriate candidate for operative vaginal delivery and has met the criteria listed in Table 5.3, then this option may be discussed with the patient. If the patient has not exceeded these time limits, but has become exhausted from pushing, then operative intervention may also be offered (see Chapter 9, *Operative Vaginal Delivery*).

Cesarean delivery. If the fetus is not felt to be a candidate for operative vaginal delivery, and continued observation is not desired by the patient or there is evidence of fetal distress, then a cesarean delivery may be offered to the patient.

References

Aasheim V, Nilsen ABV, Reinar LM, Lukasse M (2017). Perineal techniques during the second stage of labour for reducing perineal trauma. *Cochrane Database Syst Rev* (6): CD006672.

ACOG (2009). Intrapartum fetal heart rate monitoring: nomenclature, interpretation, and general management principles. *ACOG Practice Bulletin #106*, July 2009, reaffirmed 2017.

ACOG (2014). Safe prevention of the primary cesarean delivery. *ACOG Obstetric Care Consensus #1*, March 2014, reaffirmed 2016.

ACOG (2017a). Delayed umbilical cord clamping after birth. *ACOG Committee Opinion #684*, January 2017.

ACOG (2017b). Approaches to limit intervention during labor and birth. *ACOG Committee Opinion #687*, February 2017.

ACOG (2017c). Delivery of a newborn with meconium-stained amniotic fluid. *ACOG Committee Opinion #689*, March 2017.

Anim-Somuah M, Smyth RM, Jones L (2011). Epidural versus non-epidural or no analgesia in labour. *Cochrane Database Syst Rev* (12): CD000331.

Dhar KK, Ray SN, Dhall GI (1995). Significance of nuchal cord. *J Indian Med Assoc* **93**: 451–3.

Fausett M, Staat B, Crosiar J, Deering S (2017). SAFE PASSAGES implementation reduces perineal trauma. *Am J Obstet Gynecol* **216** (1 Suppl.): S39.

Fraser WD, Marcoux S, Krauss I, *et al.* (2000). Multicenter, randomized, controlled trial of delayed pushing for nulliparous women in the second stage of labor with continuous epidural analgesia. *Am J Obstet Gynecol* **182**: 1165–72.

Friedman A, Ananth C, Prendergast E, D'Alton M, Wright J (2015). Variation in and factors associated with use of episiotomy. *JAMA* **313**: 197–9.

Hansen SL, Clark SL, Foster JC (2002). Active pushing versus passive fetal descent in the second stage of labor: a randomized controlled trial. *Obstet Gynecol* **99**: 29–34.

Lemos A, Amorium MM, Dornelas de Andrade A, *et al.* (2017). Pushing/bearing down methods for the second stage of labour. *Cochrane Database Syst Rev* (3): CD009124.

McDonald SJ, Middleton P, Dowswell T, Morris PS (2013). Effect of timing of umbilical cord clamping of term infants on maternal and neonatal outcomes. *Cochrane Database Syst Rev* (7): CD004074.

Rabe H, Diaz-Rossello JL, Duley L, Dowswell T (2012). Effect of timing of umbilical cord clamping and other strategies to influence placental transfusion at preterm birth on maternal and infant outcomes. *Cochrane Database Syst Rev* (8): CD003248.

Herbst MA (2005). Treatment of suspected fetal macrosomia: a cost-effectiveness analysis. *Am J Obstet Gynecol* **193**: 1035–9.

Spong CY, Berghella V, Wenstrom KD, Mercer BM, Saade GR (2012). Preventing the first cesarean delivery: summary of a joint Eunice Kennedy Shriver National Institute of Child Health and Human Development, Society for Maternal–Fetal Medicine, and American College of Obstetricians and Gynecologist Workshop. *Obstet Gynecol* **120**: 1181–93.

Vitner D, Paltieli Y, Haberman S, *et al.* (2015). Prospective multicenter study of ultrasound-based measurements of fetal head station and position throughout labor. *Ultrasound Obstet Gynecol* **465**: 611–15.

Zhang J, Landy HJ, Branch DW, *et al.* (2010). Contemporary patterns of spontaneous labor with normal neonatal outcomes. *Obstet Gynecol* **116**: 1281–7.

Management of the Third Stage of Labor

Kelsey J. Simpson and Shad Deering

Definition

The third stage of labor begins after the delivery of the fetus and ends when the placenta and membranes have been removed. While this may seem anticlimactic compared to the actual delivery of the baby, you must remember to be vigilant, as significant complications, including catastrophic hemorrhage, can occur either before or after the placenta delivers. In fact, at times a large amount of blood may build up behind the placenta and surprise you as the placenta delivers.

Normal Duration

The average length of the third stage is 5–6 minutes, with 90% of placentas delivered by 15 minutes and 97% within 30 minutes of birth. If the placenta has not been delivered within 30 minutes, the third stage of labor is considered prolonged, and it may be necessary to manually remove the placenta (Combs and Laros 1991, Dombrowski *et al.* 1995).

Routine Management

After the baby is delivered, the cord clamped and cut, and the infant given to the mother or pediatrician, the removal of the placenta may be managed in either an active or a passive manner. Passive management generally means simply awaiting the spontaneous delivery of the placenta, while active management involves early cord clamping, the use of uterotonics (such as oxytocin), and gentle traction on the umbilical cord. Active management is recommended, as it significantly decreases the risk of postpartum hemorrhage – by more than 60% – and also lowers the chance of a blood transfusion and the need for uterotonic agents within the first 24 hours (Begley *et al.* 2015).

One recent development has been the recommendation by the American College of Obstetricians and Gynecologists for delayed cord clamping in both term and preterm infants (ACOG 2017a). This has slightly changed the general practice of the third stage, which now includes the following steps (each of which is discussed in the following sections):

1. Delay cord clamping for 30–60 seconds (if no contraindications exist)
2. Administration of oxytocin after cord clamping
3. Gentle traction on the umbilical cord and delivery of the placenta
4. Inspection of the placenta
5. Evaluation of uterine tone and vaginal/cervical lacerations

Delayed Cord Clamping

It is now recommended that, if possible, cord clamping be delayed for 30–60 seconds after delivery in both preterm and term infants (ACOG 2017a). Delayed cord clamping has not been shown to increase the risk of postpartum hemorrhage. The evidence for this is discussed in more detail in Chapter 5.

In situations where delayed cord clamping cannot be performed (maternal instability, need for immediate fetal resuscitation: see Table 5.2), another option is umbilical cord milking. Several studies suggest that this achieves increased placental transfusion in a rapid time frame with similar benefit to delayed cord clamping; however, there is currently insufficient evidence to support or refute the practice (ACOG 2017a).

Administration of Oxytocin

This is a major component of third-stage management. A Cochrane review showed that oxytocin administration resulted in a significant reduction of postpartum hemorrhage of nearly 50% (Westhoff *et al.* 2013). Additionally, another publication compared controlled cord traction with a hands-off approach and found that controlled cord traction significantly decreased the need for manual removal of the placenta, mean blood loss, and the incidence of hemorrhage, and decreased the duration of the third stage of labor by 3 minutes (Du *et al.* 2014).

A standard routine for oxytocin after delivery is 10–40 units in 500 mL of lactated Ringer's (LR) or normal saline (NS) at 10 mL/minute, per your hospital's protocol. There have been studies that have evaluated whether or not it makes a difference if the oxytocin is given before or after delivery of the placenta, and there appears to be no significant difference in blood loss with either method at this time – so make sure to check what your institution's protocol calls for (Prendiville *et al.* 2000, Jackson *et al.* 2001).

Delivery of the Placenta

After delivery of the infant, when the cord has been clamped and cut and the infant given to either the mother or a nurse, place a sterile towel on the maternal abdomen and keep one hand on the uterus, applying mild pressure in the suprapubic region (Figure 6.1).

This is done to assess uterine tone and monitor for evidence of atony. With the other hand, apply gentle downward traction on the cord. It is imperative that you do not apply

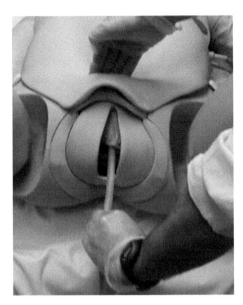

Figure 6.1 Delivery of the placenta by gentle traction on the cord, with one hand on the maternal abdomen to prevent uterine inversion.

excessive force on the cord, as it is possible to both avulse the cord, which results in bleeding and the need to manually extract the uterus, and to cause a uterine inversion, which is an emergency and associated with severe hemorrhage. The following are signs that the placenta is separating from the uterus:

1. The uterus will become more firm.
2. A sudden gush of blood will occur.
3. The umbilical cord will descend or lengthen.

As these occur, you can have the mother gently bear down to assist with delivery of the placenta. As the placenta delivers, take care not to leave the membranes behind, as they can cause problems with bleeding later. In order to prevent this, you can either take ring forceps and gently tease out any that remain attached or twist the placenta in either a clockwise or counterclockwise direction to ensure they are removed. Once the placenta and membranes are out, ask the nurse to start the oxytocin infusion, if it is not already running, and inspect the placenta.

Inspection of the Placenta

Upon inspection of the placenta, you should make a note of the following things:

1. **How many vessels are in the cord?** Normal is three, two arteries and one vein. If there are only two vessels, then you should alert the pediatricians to this fact, as it can be associated with other congenital anomalies.
2. **Is the cord insertion normal?** The umbilical cord usually inserts into the center of the placenta. Two common variations are a marginal insertion, where the cord inserts into the edge of the placenta, which occurs in 7% of term deliveries; and a velamentous

insertion, where the umbilical vessels separate in the membranes away from the placenta (Benirschke and Kaufmann 2000).

3. **Is the placenta intact?** This is important in preventing hemorrhage from retained placenta. If there is a large area that appears to be missing, an ultrasound may be performed to look for any retained portion of the placenta or membranes, and manual exploration of the uterus is done.

Evaluation of Uterine Tone and Vaginal/Cervical Lacerations

After the placenta is delivered, it is important to use your abdominal hand to assess uterine tone, because poor tone, known as uterine atony, is the most common reason for a postpartum hemorrhage. With uterine massage, the uterus should become firm and bleeding decrease. If this does not happen, then you will need to take additional steps to improve uterine tone: these are discussed in Chapter 14, in the section on postpartum hemorrhage.

At the same time you are performing uterine massage to assess/improve uterine tone, inspect the vagina and cervix for any lacerations that may have occurred during delivery. This includes both spontaneous lacerations and one caused by an episiotomy. You should also evaluate the cervix, because significant lacerations of the cervix can result in significant blood loss as well. To do this, you will need to use a light source and place your hand on the posterior wall of the vagina to push inferiorly, sometimes using a ring forceps to grasp the cervix, and visualize it to see if there is any significant bleeding. If there is active bleeding from lacerations, then you will need to repair them. These techniques are discussed in detail in Chapter 11, *Lacerations and Episiotomies*.

Potential Third-Stage Complications

Retained Placenta

If the placenta has not delivered within approximately 30 minutes, it is considered to be retained and manual removal is generally indicated. (Also, if there is significant bleeding prior to the placenta delivering, then manual removal may be required to enable the uterus to contract.) This complication occurs in approximately 0.5–3% of vaginal deliveries (Weeks and Mirembe 2002).

If the patient requires manual removal of the placenta, first ensure that she has adequate anesthesia. If the epidural is functioning, this will almost always suffice. If not, then it may be necessary to administer IV narcotics, such as fentanyl, to allow you to perform the exam. If pain control is an issue or the patient is becoming unstable, then contact your anesthesia provider early in the process, rather than later, to assist.

After the patient is comfortable, use one hand to grasp the uterine fundus abdominally, and then place the other hand into the uterus through the vagina. Once your hand is inside the uterus, find the edge of the placenta and then create a cleavage plane between the uterine wall and the placenta with your fingers. Continue to extend this plane until you have separated the placenta from the uterine wall, and then grasp the placenta in your hand and gently remove it through the vagina. Any trailing membranes are grasped with ring forceps in the same manner as with spontaneous delivery of the placenta. If there is any question that there may be retained membranes or part of the placenta still in the uterus, take a sponge and insert it with your hand back into the uterus and wipe the uterine cavity to remove any remaining debris. (Make sure you do not leave a sponge in the uterus, as it can cause continued bleeding and become a nidus for infection.)

If you have any question about whether or not you have removed all of the placenta, an abdominal ultrasound can quickly be done to determine if there is any remaining placental tissue in the uterus, which will often show up as a hyperechoic (bright) area rather than a thin endometrial stripe. One study found that the ultrasound appearance of retained placental tissue was variable, and the examination was most reassuring if there was a thin endometrial stripe and no hyperechoic areas: the negative predictive value (i.e., there is no retained placental tissue) when this is seen is 87% (Carlan *et al.* 1997). Another study reported that, when the uterus appeared empty on ultrasound, 17 of 18 patients did not have any pathologic evidence of placental tissue after dilation and curettage (Shen *et al.* 2003).

If you are unable to completely remove the placenta at this point, you may use a banjo curette in order to attempt to remove any remaining placental tissue. Doing this under ultrasound guidance may be helpful in locating any retained tissue as well. To perform this procedure, take the following steps:

1. Ensure adequate anesthesia (may use epidural if this is in place, or IV narcotics).
2. Notify anesthesia support, as you may need the patient to go to the OR for help with this.
3. Counsel the patient on the procedure.
4. Grasp the anterior cervix with a ring forceps.
5. Gently insert the banjo curette into the uterus and perform a curettage (have an assistant monitor with an abdominal sonogram if available).
6. Be prepared for additional bleeding.
7. Monitor urine output closely after the procedure.
8. Consider sending a CBC 4–6 hours after the procedure if there was significant blood loss.

Some physicians will place patients on prophylactic antibiotics for 24 hours after manual removal of the placenta. There are no data to support or refute this practice at this time, and the decision is left up to the preference of the provider, but it is common at most institutions (Chongsomchai *et al.* 2014).

Avulsion of Umbilical Cord

If the umbilical cord detaches while you are applying gentle traction, then it is important to proceed quickly to perform a manual removal of the placenta to prevent a significant hemorrhage. Exactly what constitutes "gentle traction" is something that you will learn by doing deliveries, and it is important to err on the side of less traction at first. This complication seems to occur more often with very preterm deliveries, when the placenta does not separate as easily as after a term delivery, and extra care should be taken in these cases. The procedure for manual removal is the same as described under *Routine Management*, above.

Postpartum Hemorrhage

This complication occurs in approximately 4–6% of deliveries and is caused by uterine atony in 80% or more of cases (ACOG 2017b). It is a significant problem that can rapidly cause a patient to become hemodynamically unstable, and it requires quick intervention to correct. A thorough discussion of this problem is found in Chapter 14, *Common Obstetric Complications and Emergencies*.

Uterine Inversion

This complication occurs in approximately 1 in 2500 deliveries (ACOG 2017b). It is often associated with an abnormally implanted placenta, such as a placenta accreta, increta, or percreta, although excessive traction on the umbilical cord has also been implicated. When this occurs it is an obstetric emergency and must be dealt with quickly to avoid significant maternal morbidity and mortality. This complication is discussed in detail in Chapter 14.

References

ACOG (2017a). Delayed umbilical cord clamping after birth. *ACOG Committee Opinion* #684, January 2017.

ACOG (2017b). Postpartum hemorrhage. *ACOG Practice Bulletin* #183, October 2017.

Begley CM, Gyte GM, Devane D, McGuire W, Weeks A (2015). Active versus expectant management for women in the third stage of labour. *Cochrane Database Syst Rev* (3): CD007412.

Benirschke K, Kaufmann P (2000). *Pathology of the Human Placenta*, 4th edn. New York: Springer-Verlag.

Carlan SJ, Scott WT, Pollack R, Harris K (1997). Appearance of the uterus by ultrasound immediately after placental delivery with pathologic correlation. *J Clin Ultrasound* 25: 301–8.

Chongsomchai C, Lumbiganon P, Laopaiboon M (2014). Prophylactic antibiotics for manual removal of retained placenta in vaginal birth. *Cochrane Database Syst Rev* (10): CD004904.

Combs CA, Laros RK (1991). Prolonged third stage of labor: morbidity and risk factors. *Obstet Gynecol* 77: 863–7.

Dombrowski MP, Bottoms SF, Saleh AA, Hurd WW, Romero R (1995). Third stage of labor: analysis of duration and clinical practice. *Am J Obstet Gynecol* 172: 1279–84.

Du Y, Ye M, Zheng F (2014). Active management of the third stage of labor with and without controlled cord traction: a systematic review and meta-analysis of randomized controlled trials. *Acta Obstet Gynecol Scand* 93: 626–33.

Jackson KW, Allbert JR, Schemmer GK, et al. (2001). A randomized controlled trial comparing oxytocin administration before and after placental delivery in the prevention of postpartum hemorrhage. *Am J Obstet Gynecol* 185: 873–7.

Prendiville WJ, Elbourne D, McDonald S (2000). Active versus expectant management in the third stage of labor. *Cochrane Database Syst Rev* (3): CD000007.

Shen O, Rabinowitz R, Eisenberg VH, Samueloff A (2003). Transabdominal sonography before uterine exploration as a predictor of retained placental fragments. *J Ultrasound Med* 22: 561–4.

Weeks AD, Mirembe FM (2002). The retained placenta: new insights into an old problem. *Eur J Obstet Gynecol and Reprod Biology* 102: 109–10.

Westhoff G, Cotter AM, Tolosa JE (2013). Prophylactic oxytocin for the third stage of labour to prevent postpartum haemorrhage. *Cochrane Database Syst Rev* (10): CD001808.

Induction and Augmentation of Labor

Irina U. Tunnage and Shad Deering

Introduction

Making a decision to influence labor is central to managing patients on labor and delivery. It is a common practice in obstetrics, but one that can cause fetal distress and increase a mother's chance of requiring a cesarean delivery. The decision must, therefore, be handled carefully. In general, labor may be induced or augmented. The difference is that with induction the patient has not yet begun to labor and demonstrate cervical change, and with augmentation the labor is simply being assisted.

Induction of Labor

Labor induction is a commonplace occurrence in modern obstetric practice. From 1990 to 1998, the rate of labor induction in the United States increased from 9.5% to 22% of all births (Martin *et al.* 2009). As induction has become much more common, it is imperative for providers to understand both the indications and the potential complications that can occur.

Indications for Induction

A decision to induce labor must take into consideration both the maternal and fetal conditions. When contemplating induction, you must be able to clearly state in the medical record why you are intervening. This is important because there has been a long-held belief that labor induction increases the risk of cesarean section. However, a meta-analysis carried out in 2015 concluded that **when stratifying groups of women appropriately, induction of labor does not increase the risk of cesarean section** (Little and Caughey 2015). Induction of labor is indicated when the benefits of delivery, to either the mother or the fetus, outweigh the risks of prolonging the pregnancy. Some commonly accepted indications for induction of labor are:

- Intra-amniotic infection
- Fetal demise
- Pregnancy-induced hypertension
- Preeclampsia/eclampsia
- Post-term pregnancy (usually defined as > 42 weeks*)
- Premature rupture of membranes (at > 34 weeks)
- Fetal compromise (e.g., FGR, oligohydramnios, isoimmunization)
- Maternal medical conditions (e.g., diabetes, chronic hypertension, renal disease)
- History of rapid labors (when the patient lives a significant distance from the hospital)
- Elective (> 39 weeks)

Contraindications to Induction

The following are contraindications to labor induction:

1. **Fetal**

    a. Evidence of significant fetal compromise, i.e., an ominous fetal heart rate (FHR) tracing or biophysical profile (BPP) of 4 or less (if this is the case, immediate delivery, not induction, is required)
    b. Malpresentation (e.g., transverse lie, incomplete breech)
    c. Placenta previa or vasa previa
    d. Fetal anomalies that would not allow passage of the fetal head (such as severe hydrocephalus)
    e. Umbilical cord prolapse

2. **Maternal**

    a. Inadequate pelvis (determined by clinical pelvimetry to be too small for vaginal delivery)
    b. Active genital herpes infection
    c. Medical conditions that make labor dangerous for the mother

3. **Uterine**

    a. Previous uterine incision (classical, "T," or "J"; see Chapter 10)
    b. Prior myomectomy with entrance into the uterine cavity

The baseline risk of uterine rupture for patients with a previous low transverse cesarean section who have spontaneous labor is only 0.5% (Lydon-Rochelle *et al.* 2001). For patients who undergo induction of labor with oxytocin the risk is approximately 1%, and as high as 2% with prostaglandins (ACOG 2009). These risks do not appear to increase with induction with an unfavorable cervix. Given the current evidence, it is recommended that misoprostol

---

* A post-term pregnancy is defined as one lasting 42 weeks or more (ACOG 2014b). However, there is a good deal of literature, including a meta-analysis of 19 trials of routine care versus selective induction after 41 weeks, that has demonstrated that induction of labor at 41 weeks does not result in an increase in the cesarean section rate, and may even lower the perinatal mortality rate (Hannah *et al.* 1992, Crowley 2000).

(a prostaglandin) not be used for induction or augmentation of labor in patients with a previous cesarean section.

Even though the risk of uterine rupture is higher for patients with a prior cesarean section, the American College of Obstetricians and Gynecologists (ACOG) states that "induction of labor for maternal or fetal indications remains an option for women undergoing a trial of labor after cesarean" (ACOG 2010a). It is important, however, that the potentially increased risk of uterine rupture associated with any induction should be discussed with the patient and documented in the patient's medical record. Additionally, in these patients the indication for induction must be clearly stated in the chart.

Timing of Induction

When labor induction is undertaken for either logistic reasons or electively, and not for fetal or maternal disease states, then ACOG recommends that either fetal lung maturity be documented by amniocentesis or one of the following criteria be met (ACOG 2009):

- Fetal heart tones documented for at least 30 weeks by Doppler.
- It has been at least 36 weeks since the patient had a positive urine or serum pregnancy test.
- Ultrasound examination prior to 20 weeks supports a gestational age of at least 39 weeks.

Other things that must be considered prior to induction of labor include an assessment of the following:

1. **Gestational age** (as mentioned above).
2. **Fetal size.** Induction of labor for presumed macrosomia has not been shown to decrease the risk of shoulder dystocia, but in certain situations a cesarean section may be offered for an extremely macrosomic fetus (see Chapter 10, *Cesarean Delivery*).
3. **Fetal presentation.** Induction should not be performed if the fetus is breech or transverse. In this situation, an external cephalic version may be attempted if appropriate (see Chapter 2, *Common Examinations and Procedures*).
4. **Clinical pelvimetry.** An assessment of the patient's pelvis should be performed, and induction of labor may not be recommended if the patient has a significantly contracted pelvis. This is uncommon and rarely used as a reason not to attempt induction.
5. **Cervical examination.** Examination of the cervix will help you to determine what method to use for induction, as well as allow you to counsel the patient on the anticipated success rate (see Bishop score, below).

Methods of Induction

After the decision has been made to proceed with induction of labor, then attention is turned to how to proceed. The method of induction will depend on the cervical examination and whether or not cervical ripening is felt to be needed prior to the administration of oxytocin.

Cervical Ripening

When the cervix is not prepared for regular labor, it is often referred to as "unfavorable." The goal of cervical ripening is to make the cervix more "favorable" for labor and thus increase the chances of having a vaginal delivery. One method used to grade the cervix in

Table 7.1 Calculation of Bishop score

	Bishop score			
	0	1	2	3
Dilation (cm)	Closed (0)	1–2	3–4	5+
Effacement (%)	0–30	40–50	60–70	80+
Station	−3	−2	−1, 0	+1 or more
Cervix	Firm	Medium	Soft	—
Position	Posterior	Mid-position	Anterior	—

Station is on a +3 to −3 scale. "Position" refers to the position of the cervix in the vagina. "Cervix" refers to the consistency of the cervix on exam.

terms of how "favorable" it is at the beginning of an induction is the Bishop score, which grades cervical dilation, effacement, station of the fetal vertex, consistency of the cervix, and the position of the cervix. It can range from 0 to 13. With a Bishop score of ≥ 8, induction of labor will usually be successful, or at least as successful as normal spontaneous labor, and oxytocin is often started without cervical ripening in these cases (Bishop 1964). See Table 7.1 for how to calculate the score.

It is also important to note that success rates are dependent on parity as well. Multiparous patients with a Bishop score > 5 are much more likely to have a successful induction than nulliparous patients with the same score (Mhaske *et al.* 2015).

When it comes to deciding which agent to use, much of this is based on individual preference. It is important, however, to understand how each method works, the potential complications, and what the fetal monitoring requirements are for the different medications.

Medications Available for Cervical Ripening

Prostaglandin E2. This is also called dinoprostone (see Appendix A, *Medication Database*, for additional information). It can be applied either as a gel, or as a vaginal insert which is called Cervidil. The price for a single application of this is approximately $160. A general protocol for the insertion of either is as follows:

- Confirm patient's EDD.
- Confirm fetus is vertex by ultrasound.
- Review the FHR tracing.
- Insert either gel (intravaginal or intracervical) or vaginal insert.
- Have the patient remain recumbent for 30 minutes after placement.

If dinoprostone gel is inserted, monitor FHR for 2 hours. If the FHR remains reassuring and there is no change in uterine activity, you can discontinue monitoring.

If Cervidil is placed, continuously monitor FHR while it is in place, until 15 minutes after it is removed.

It is recommended that oxytocin not be started for at least 6–12 hours after these medications are used.

Prostaglandin E1. Misoprostol, or Cytotec, is a synthetic prostaglandin E1 that is marketed for prevention of peptic ulcers. It is inexpensive but is not used in patients who have had a previous cesarean section because of an increased risk of uterine rupture (ACOG 2010a). It has been shown in several studies to be as good as or better than prostaglandin E2, but should be used in doses of 25 mcg q3–6 hours to minimize the occurrence of uterine tachysystole and fetal distress. If the patient is contracting more than three times in 10 minutes when it is time for subsequent doses, then the next dose is usually not placed in an attempt to avoid uterine tachysystole. The procedure is the same as for prostaglandin E2, but the patient must be continuously monitored after this is used. In post-term pregnancies, dosing and route of administration of Cytotec has recently been studied, finding that oral administration is more effective than vaginal administration. An oral dose of 100 mcg (vs. 25 mcg or 50 mcg vaginally) for labor induction decreases time to delivery and has shown better neonatal and maternal outcomes in post-term pregnancies (Rezaie *et al.* 2016). Oxytocin should not be started until at least 4 hours after the last dose of misoprostol.

As with all interventions, there are pros and cons to each. It is helpful to look at them when deciding between prostaglandin choices:

Dinoprostone. When used as an insert (Cervidil), it is left in place for 12–24 hours, which can be considered for overnight cervical ripening. It is also useful for women who are already contracting but who still would benefit from cervical ripening, because the insert allows for easy removal in the event of uterine tachysystole. The downside, as previously mentioned, is the cost.

Misoprotol. In contrast, the cost of misoprostol is only about $2 per dose. This drug can be used q3–6 h. The downside of this administration is that it is a dissolvable pill, and therefore it cannot be removed once administered if uterine tachysystole occurs.

Other Methods for Cervical Ripening

Foley balloon. Using this method, a Foley catheter, often with a 30 mL balloon instead of the smaller 10 mL balloon, is inserted into the cervical os and then inflated. It can be placed either during a speculum exam, using ring forceps to place the catheter (although you must be careful where you grasp the catheter, as you can make a hole in the balloon doing this), or during a digital vaginal exam. If it is difficult to place through the cervix, then it is possible to place a urologic sound through the catheter to assist in the placement. The catheter is then taped to the patient's leg and oxytocin is often started. It is not necessary to place a weight on the end of the catheter. The use of oxytocin at the same time as Foley bulb administration has been shown to decrease the time that the Foley bulb is in place, but has no effect on time to delivery (Fitzpatrick *et al.* 2012). This procedure has been shown to be as effective as misoprostol and prostaglandin (ACOG 2009).

Hygroscopic cervical dilators. These may be placed into the cervical os in the same manner as a Foley catheter balloon. They are generally very safe, although rare cases of anaphylaxis have been reported after their insertion. These work by slowly expanding in the cervix, and may be used concurrently with oxytocin.

Membrane stripping. This involves performing a vigorous cervical exam and rotating the examining finger 360 degrees once your finger is through the internal os in an attempt to separate the membranes from the lower uterine segment. This will increase the level of prostaglandins present, which is important for the stimulation of labor. This is generally not performed until 38 or 39 weeks' gestation. It will result in approximately two-thirds of patients going into spontaneous labor within the next 48 hours, and reduces the incidence of induction with other methods (ACOG 2009).

Complications of Induction

The major complications associated with labor induction are related to the risk of uterine tachysystole and uterine rupture. With the use of any of the prostaglandins or oxytocin, uterine tachysystole may occur and lead to fetal distress. The relative potential for this complication to occur is the reason for the different monitoring requirements for oxytocin versus the various prostaglandins. This complication is discussed in detail later in this chapter.

An unlikely, but potentially catastrophic complication of labor induction is uterine rupture, where a full-thickness defect in the uterine wall can result in massive hemorrhage and a compromised fetus. This is fortunately a rare occurrence (Table 7.2) but because prostaglandins have been associated with an increased risk of uterine rupture in patients with a previous cesarean delivery, they are not used in that population. This complication is discussed in detail in Chapter 14.

Table 7.2 Incidence of uterine rupture in patients who have had a previous cesarean delivery

	Risk of uterine rupture
Spontaneous labor	0.52%
Induced without prostaglandins	0.77%
Induced with prostaglandins	2.24%

(ACOG 2010a)

Augmentation of Labor

Augmentation of labor refers to interventions to stimulate uterine contractions when the woman's spontaneous contractions have not resulted in labor progress within a reasonable time period.

Indications for Augmentation

If a patient has a labor protraction disorder, then augmentation of labor is indicated if the fetal status is reassuring. In the latent phase, labor is historically defined as prolonged when it exceeds 20 hours in nulliparous women, and 14 hours in multiparous women (ACOG 2014a). In the active phase of labor, nulliparous patients should dilate at least 1 cm/hour and multiparous patients around 1.5 cm/hour. If they are not continuing to progress on serial cervical examinations, then it is reasonable to consider augmentation.

Contraindications to Augmentation

Contraindications to labor augmentation are essentially the same as the contraindications to labor induction. One additional note is that if a fetus demonstrates an intolerance to contractions with spontaneous labor, and has a non-reassuring FHR tracing, then labor cannot be augmented at that time as it will likely worsen the fetal condition by causing additional stress and decreased uterine perfusion with more frequent and intense contractions.

Methods of Augmentation

When labor augmentation is considered, there are generally two options, medications and amniotomy.

Medications Available

In general, oxytocin is almost always the medication utilized for labor augmentation, although rarely, with a very unfavorable cervix, misoprostol is utilized at the same doses as previously discussed.

Oxytocin (Pitocin)

Pitocin is a synthetic version of the natural hormone oxytocin. When given intravenously, it will stimulate uterine contractions by acting on oxytocin receptors in the myometrium (see Appendix A, *Medication Database*, for additional information on this).

Preparation

Oxytocin is diluted in a lactated Ringer's (LR) solution, usually with 10–20 units of oxytocin per 1000 mL of LR. This will result in a concentration of either 10 mU/mL or 20 mU/mL.

Dosage

Oxytocin for labor augmentation is given IV, and the dosage varies. It is always started slowly, and then titrated up to achieve adequate contractions. (Note: When external tocometry is used to record contractions, only the duration and timing and not the actual strength of the contraction is measured. When an intrauterine pressure catheter (IUPC) is used, then the pressure of each contraction can be measured. This is important when attempting to define "adequate" contractions.)

Oxytocin is usually given in either a "low-dose" or "high-dose" protocol. There are many studies which have demonstrated that the high-dose protocols result in a shorter duration of labor and fewer cesarean deliveries for dystocia, but an increased incidence of uterine tachysystole. In general, the high-dose protocols are not used in patients with a prior cesarean delivery. Also, most institutions have a written protocol for what regimens are acceptable, so check with your unit and ask to see this. Some common protocols are listed in Table 7.3.

While there is no maximum dose established for oxytocin, most institutions do not run infusions at more than 40 mU/min. At high doses for long periods of time, there is a risk of water intoxication, which is discussed later in this chapter.

Please refer to Appendix B, *Sample Notes and Orders*, to see an example of how to write orders for each of these oxytocin protocols.

Table 7.3 Oxytocin dosing protocols for augmentation of labor

	Starting dose	Maximum dose	Dose increase	Interval
High dose	6 mU/min	42 mU/min	6 mU/min*	15–40 min
Low dose	1–2 mU/min	20–40 mU/min	1–2 mU/min	15–40 min

* The dosage increase of 6 mU/min in the high-dose protocol should be changed to 3 mU/min if significant uterine tachysystole occurs.

Contraindications

- Same as for induction of labor
- Allergy to oxytocin

Fetal Monitoring

Continuous fetal monitoring is recommended while oxytocin is given.

Complications

There are several potential complications with IV oxytocin administration. Some common problems are as follows:

Acute hypotension. If the IV pump used to administer the dilute oxytocin malfunctions, an accidental bolus can cause sudden maternal hypotension. The treatment for this is to immediately discontinue the infusion and correct the hypotension as needed.

Water intoxication. When oxytocin is administered in doses of ≥ 20 mU/minute, it exerts a powerful antidiuretic action. This is because oxytocin is similar in its molecular structure to vasopressin. If additional IV fluids are given to patients on high doses of oxytocin (for things such as maternal hypotension or prior to an epidural being placed), then water intoxication may develop – which can lead to convulsions, coma, and even death. Monitoring fluid intake is a must when patients are receiving high doses of oxytocin for a long period of time.

Uterine tachysystole. Even at normal doses given for labor augmentation, uterine tachysystole and resulting fetal distress secondary to decreased perfusion may develop. The mechanism is simple: with each contraction the blood flow to the fetus decreases, and if contractions are too strong, too frequent, or too long in duration, the fetus cannot tolerate the decrease in perfusion.

Uterine tachysystole is defined as a persistent pattern of more than five contractions in 10 minutes averaged over 30 minutes (ACOG 2010b).

In the presence of uterine tachysystole, the intervention depends on the fetal response. If the fetus is tolerating the increased uterine activity, then the dose of oxytocin can simply be decreased to correct it. If, however, the fetus is demonstrating distress in the form of variable or late decelerations, or even worse, bradycardia, then the oxytocin must be stopped and immediate interventions made, which often include the administration of terbutaline to cause the uterine muscle to relax and improve perfusion. See Chapter 3, *Intrapartum Fetal Heart Rate Monitoring*, for a protocol for intervention.

Uterine rupture. While this is a rare event, and almost always occurs in women with a previous uterine scar, the use of oxytocin can increase the risk of this happening. This complication is discussed in detail in Chapter 14, *Common Obstetric Complications and Emergencies*.

Amniotomy

This involves the artificial rupture of the amniotic membranes (see Chapter 2). It is often used when the latent phase of labor is prolonged or there are inadequate contractions during the active phase. Performing this prior to starting oxytocin is a reasonable intervention, and it also allows you to place an IUPC to determine the strength of the patient's contractions or a fetal scalp electrode (FSE) if you need to monitor the FHR tracing more closely. It has been shown that amniotomy during the active phase of labor will shorten the duration of labor and can decrease the need for oxytocin augmentation. In a trial of amniotomy combined with early oxytocin infusion, compared with amniotomy alone, the induction-to-delivery interval was shorter with amniotomy alone than with amniotomy combined with oxytocin (ACOG 2014a).

References

ACOG (2009). Induction of labor. *ACOG Practice Bulletin #107*, August 2009, reaffirmed 2016.

ACOG (2010a). Vaginal birth after previous cesarean delivery. *ACOG Practice Bulletin #115*, August 2010, reaffirmed 2017.

ACOG (2010b). Management of intrapartum fetal heart rate tracings. *ACOG Practice Bulletin #116*, November 2010, reaffirmed 2017.

ACOG (2014a). Safe prevention of the primary cesarean delivery. *ACOG Obstetric Care Consensus #1*, March 2014, reaffirmed 2016.

ACOG (2014b). Management of late-term and postterm pregnancies. *ACOG Practice Bulletin #146*, August 2014, reaffirmed 2016.

Bishop EH (1964). Pelvic scoring for elective induction. *Obstet Gynecol* **24**: 266–8.

Crowley P (2000). Interventions for preventing or improving the outcome of delivery at or beyond term. *Cochrane Database Syst Rev* (2): CD000170.

Fitzpatrick CB, Grotegut CA, Bishop TS, et al. (2012). Cervical ripening with Foley balloon plus fixed versus incremental low-dose oxytocin: a randomized controlled trial. *J Matern Fetal Neonatal Med* **25**: 1006–10.

Hannah ME, Hannah WJ, Hellmann J, et al. (1992). Induction of labor as compared with serial antenatal monitoring in post-term pregnancy: a randomized controlled trial. The Canadian Multicenter Post-term Pregnancy Trial Group. *N Engl J Med* **326**: 1587–92.

Little SE, Caughey AB (2015). Induction of labor and cesarean: what is the true relationship? *Clin J Obstet Gynecol* **58**: 269–81.

Lydon-Rochelle M, Holt VL, Easterling TR, Martin DP (2001). Risk of uterine rupture during labor among women with a prior cesarean delivery. *N Engl J Med* **345**: 3–8.

Martin JA, Hamilton BE, Sutton PD, et al. (2009). Births: final data for 2006. *Natl Vital Stat Rep* **57**: 1–102.

Mhaske N, Agarwal R, Wadhwa RD, Basannar DR (2015). Study of the risk factors for cesarean delivery in induced labors at term. *J Obstet Gynecol India* **65**: 236–40.

Rezaie M, Farhadifar F, Sadegh SM, Nayebi M (2016). Comparison of vaginal and oral doses of misoprostol for labour induction in post-term pregnancies. *J Clin Diagn Res* **10**: QC08–11.

Obstetric Analgesia and Anesthesia

Elise Diamond and Shad Deering

Principles of Pain Relief During Labor

Whereas in the past many women gave birth under heavy sedation and barely remembered the experience, in modern obstetrics the objective now is to provide adequate relief from the pain of childbirth while allowing the woman to fully participate in her delivery. Providing adequate pain control during labor is one of the most important functions of the obstetrician, and maternal request is considered to be sufficient medical indication for pain relief when a patient has been determined to be in labor.

When counseling patients about options for anesthesia during labor, it is important to know what services are available at your particular facility. Also, if support is available for epidural/spinal anesthesia, make sure you check with the anesthesiologist on call before you promise a laboring patient that she will receive her pain relief "right away." This is important in that the anesthesiologist often is responsible for many patients (including those undergoing cesarean section or even postpartum tubal ligations) and may not be immediately available for this non-emergency procedure.

Some women will also request to go through labor without the assistance of analgesia. If this is the patient's desire, make it clear to her that you will fully support her decision and that, if she should change her mind, you will make whatever you can available to her, depending on where she is in labor.

A common question that many women ask regarding all types of analgesia is "Is this safe for my baby?" After reading this chapter, you will be able to confidently answer this question and speak about specific medications and techniques available, which will go a long way toward reassuring the patient.

Oral Intake During Labor and Delivery

In general, most anesthesia providers agree that oral intake of a moderate amount of "clear liquids" during labor is acceptable. These can include but are not limited to juice (without particulates), water, transparent jello, frozen pops, clear tea, or black coffee. The volume of liquid is less important than the presence of particulate matter. One study even showed that oral intake of carbohydrates during labor shortened the second stage of labor without adversely affecting maternal or neonatal outcomes (Rahmani *et al.* 2012).

If a scheduled cesarean delivery is planned or a postpartum tubal ligation is anticipated, the patient should ideally be kept NPO for 6–8 hours prior to the procedure. Before surgical procedures (cesarean section or postpartum tubal ligation) an H_2 blocker, non-particulate antacids, or metoclopramide can be administered for aspiration prevention.

Anesthesia Consultation

When evaluating a patient on labor and delivery, it is important to determine if she has any significant anesthetic risk factors for which an anesthesiologist should see her early in labor in case any emergencies arise. Some situations in which this would be appropriate are listed in Table 8.1.

By notifying the anesthesia provider of these patients so they can be seen early in their labor and a plan made for analgesia, you can avoid many complications should an emergency occur. Early and ongoing conversations between anesthesia teams and obstetric teams are critical for the best outcomes.

Options for Pain Relief During Latent Labor

During latent labor, narcotics are often used to make the patient more comfortable. If the patient does not meet criteria for admission to labor and delivery, then narcotics can be given to relieve the pain of contractions. This is sometimes referred to as therapeutic rest. It is extremely important to ensure that fetal testing, usually in the form of a reactive non-stress test (NST), is reassuring prior to giving a patient any of these medications. If the patient is admitted to the hospital but has not yet entered active labor, either intravenous or intramuscular narcotics, or a combination of both, may be used for pain control in latent labor as well.

Medications utilized for analgesia during latent labor are usually opioid agonists/ antagonists, and mainly work by sedating the patient (Olofsson *et al.* 1996). Benzodiazepines, on the other hand, are not recommended during labor because they can cause significant neonatal depression, hypotonia, and problems with neonatal temperature regulation.

It is important to realize that, unlike conduction anesthesia (epidural or spinal techniques; discussed later in this chapter), all parenteral medications can cross the placenta and

Table 8.1 Conditions requiring anesthesiology consultation

- Morbid obesity (BMI of 50 or higher)
- Severe preeclampsia or HELLP syndrome
- Known coagulopathy or thrombocytopenia
- Use of anticoagulant medications
- Previous history of anesthetic complications (malignant hyperthermia)
- Previous difficult or failed neuraxial block
- History of neck or spine trauma or surgery (including rod placement or vertebral fusion)
- Severe scoliosis
- Dwarfism
- Significant maternal cardiac disease (valvular disease, implanted pacemaker, WPW, history of SVT)
- Significant pulmonary disease (obstructive sleep apnea, pulmonary hypertension, anticipated difficult airway)
- Significant neurologic disease (AV malformation, aneurysm, intracranial mass, Chiari malformation)
- Significant renal or liver disease
- Placenta previa or accreta
- History of multiple abdominal operations
- Spinal cord lesion above T6 (at risk for autonomic hyperreflexia)
- Myasthenia gravis
- Neurofibromatosis
- Sickle cell anemia
- Planned concurrent abdominal procedure along with cesarean delivery

have some effect on the fetus and the fetal heart rate (FHR) tracing (Hawkins 2000). In fact, some opioid drugs, such as meperidine, are not recommended in the peripartum period. This is because the active metabolite of meperidine, normeperidine, has a prolonged half-life of up to 72 hours in the neonate and its effects cannot be antagonized by naloxone. When choosing to give narcotics during labor, you must take into account how quickly the medication will provide some pain relief to the patient, how long it is until you anticipate the patient will deliver, whether the drug has pure agonist or has mixed agonist/antagonist effects, and what the half-life of the medication and its metabolites is in the neonate. A good rule of thumb is to not give parenteral narcotics after the patient is 4–5 cm dilated. While narcotics can be given after this, they should not be given if you expect the patient to deliver within 2–3 hours of the dose, because of the increased risk of neonatal respiratory depression.

An additional aspect of care to consider when using opioids is any possible effects on breastfeeding. Intravenous opioids can cause drowsiness in neonates that can interfere with suckling, and additional lactation support may be needed. Overall, however, studies have shown no difference in duration of breastfeeding or in continued breastfeeding at 12 months (Wilson *et al.* 2010).

Despite these possible complications, and the specific ones listed with each agent in the next section, the American College of Obstetricians and Gynecologists (ACOG) recognizes the role of parenteral opioids in peripartum analgesia as having several unique benefits. These include being widely available, being able to be administered without skilled support personnel, supporting patient autonomy as an alternative choice to neuraxial analgesia, use for therapeutic rest in the early first stage of labor, and administration to patients who may have contraindications to neuraxial analgesia.

In the past, there had been a suggestion in the literature about whether placement of an epidural early in labor increases the cesarean section rate, especially in nulliparous patients. It is now generally recognized that it does not increase the rate of cesarean delivery, and ACOG recommends that neuraxial analgesia should not be withheld for that concern and can be given at any time rather than waiting for any predetermined amount of cervical dilation (ACOG 2017).

It is a reasonable strategy to attempt to utilize parenteral narcotics during the latent phase of labor in an attempt to make the patient more comfortable, and then an epidural when she enters the active phase. If you cannot adequately control the pain with IV/IM narcotics until the patient enters active labor, then you can discuss the risks and benefits of an epidural and proceed with that course of action.

Note: Because all narcotics can cause maternal nausea/vomiting, an antiemetic, most often promethazine 12.5–25 mg IV, can be given along with the narcotic. This not only decreases the nausea, but also provides additional sedation.

Narcotics

Indications
- Relief of pain during the first stage of labor
- Therapeutic rest for patients in latent labor
- Need for additional analgesia when repairing vaginal lacerations

Contraindications
- Known allergy to specific medication
- Imminent delivery (i.e., within approx. 2 hours)

Procedure
- IV and/or IM administration as per medication specification
- Monitor FHR (external or internal monitors)
- Monitor maternal vital signs and watch for respiratory depression

Complications
- Maternal respiratory depression
- Fetal respiratory depression
- Decreased FHR variability
- Sinusoidal FHR pattern
- Nausea/vomiting
- Pruritis
- Loss of gag reflex (with inability to protect airway)

There are many options available, and Table 8.2 provides a comparison of some of the most common medications with regard to their dosage, onset and duration of action, and neonatal and maternal half-life.

Table 8.2 Narcotics for pain relief during labor and delivery

Butorphanol	A synthetic opioid agonist/antagonist with rapid onset of both analgesia and sedation	
	Dosage	1–2 mg IV or IM. May be repeated every 4 hours as needed
	Onset of action	5–10 minutes (IV)
		30–60 minutes (IM)
	Neonatal half-life	The neonatal half-life is unknown, but is similar to that of nalbuphine in adults
	Maternal half-life	2–5 hours (duration of action: 4–6 hours)
	Notes	This medication has been reported to increase blood pressure and should be avoided in patients with chronic hypertension or preeclampsia. It may also produce a temporary sinusoidal fetal heart rate pattern.
Fentanyl	A synthetic opioid with rapid onset of action but short duration	
	Dosage	50–100 mcg IV every hour as needed. Alternatively administered as a PCA (loading dose of 50 mcg, followed by 10–25 mcg every 10–12 minutes)
	Onset of action	2–4 minutes
	Neonatal half-life	5.3 hours
	Maternal half-life	3 hours (duration of action: 30–60 minutes)
	Notes	This medication is a rapidly acting narcotic that is also cleared relatively quickly. It may, however, require an anesthesiologist to administer, depending on the monitoring requirements of your hospital.
Morphine sulfate	A systemic opioid with a long half-life, which is very sedating	
	Dosage	Typical doses are 2–5 mg IV or 5–10 mg IM every 4 hours as needed
	Onset of action	5–10 minutes (IV)
		30–40 minutes (IM)
	Neonatal half-life	7 hours
	Maternal half-life	2 hours (duration of action: 1–3 hours)
	Notes	This medication is often used for therapeutic rest and less commonly for patients actually in labor. It is very sedating and often gives patients excellent pain relief for several hours.

Table 8.2 (cont.)

Nalbuphine	A synthetic opioid agonist/antagonist with rapid onset of both analgesia and sedation	
	Dosage	10 mg IV and/or IM. May be repeated every 3 hours. May be co-administered as a 10 mg IV dose with a 10 mg IM dose for immediate as well as delayed pain relief in latent labor
	Onset of action	2–3 minutes (IV)
		15 minutes (IM)
	Neonatal half-life	4.1 hours
	Maternal half-life	2–5 hours (duration of action: 2–4 hours)
	Notes	This medication may produce a transient sinusoidal fetal heart rate pattern.
Remifentanil	A synthetic opioid with an ultra-short half-life that allows for easy titration with PCA and has been shown to provide better pain relief than other opioids during labor in this manner	
	Dosage	0.15–0.5 mcg/kg every 2 minutes via PCA
	Onset of action	20–90 seconds
	Neonatal half-life	Unknown (likely similar to maternal half-life)
	Maternal half-life	9–10 minutes (duration of action: 3–4 minutes)
	Notes	This medication may produce a transient sinusoidal fetal heart rate pattern.

(Adapted from ACOG 2017)

Options for Pain Relief During Active Labor

During active labor, intravenous or intramuscular narcotics can still be administered. However, care must be taken not to administer too many repeat doses, especially intramuscularly with the delayed release and effect, and not to give them too close to delivery, as they can cause significant neonatal depression – as previously discussed. When active labor starts and the contraction pain becomes more intense, many women request either an epidural or spinal anesthesia.

There has been significant debate about what effect an epidural has on the length of labor, the incidence of operative vaginal delivery, the risk of cesarean section, and how it may affect breastfeeding.

With regards to the timing of an epidural, "early" placement (prior to 4 cm dilation) is not contraindicated, and indeed in certain patients with high-risk pregnancies and a significant possibility of requiring emergency cesarean delivery (twins, known difficult airway, significant pulmonary or cardiac disease, etc.) an earlier epidural may in fact be preferable to allow easy titration should emergency operative delivery be indicated. Many studies have evaluated the effect of epidural anesthesia on labor duration and delivery. High-quality studies and Cochrane reviews have demonstrated that the initiation of epidural analgesia at any stage of labor does **not** increase the risk of cesarean delivery (Wong *et al.* 2005, Anim-Somuah *et al.* 2011, Jones *et al.* 2012, Sng *et al.* 2014). Patient satisfaction and neonatal outcomes are significantly better with an epidural when compared with parenteral narcotic analgesia (Halpern *et al.* 1998).

Neuraxial anesthesia during labor has also not been shown to decrease the success of breastfeeding, and a negligible concentration of opioid enters the maternal plasma (Montgomery and Hale 2012). Fears related to breastfeeding should not deter women from receiving an epidural if they desire one during labor (Halpern *et al.* 1999).

Indications and contraindications for both epidural and spinal anesthesia, as well as the technique and potential complications, are detailed below.

Other options for pain relief during active labor include pudendal nerve block and inhaled nitrous oxide.

Epidural Anesthesia

Indications
- Anesthesia during labor
- Multiple gestation
- Maternal cardiac, pulmonary, or neurologic disease

Contraindications
- Patient refusal/inability to remain still for the procedure
- Infection at site of needle placement
- Intra-amniotic infection*
- Coagulopathy (platelets $< 80 \times 10^9$/L, DIC, hemophilia, etc.)**
- Increased intracranial pressure from mass lesions
- Maternal hypovolemia

Procedure
A needle is inserted into the epidural space through the ligamentum flavum in the region of L2–5 and a small catheter is then threaded into this space.

---

* Intra-amniotic infection is listed as a contraindication to epidural/spinal anesthesia in anesthesia texts, but this is usually only in cases where the patient appears septic and the risk of bacteremia is felt to be high (Norris 2000). Antibiotics should be started as soon as intra-amniotic infection is diagnosed and the case discussed with the anesthesiologist on call if an epidural is desired.

** There is no known safe lower limit for platelet count. Generally epidural or spinal anesthesia is acceptable when platelet count is $\geq$ 80,000 according to ACOG. In some cases it may be acceptable at even lower levels, depending on the comfort level of the anesthesiologist. Even though this evidence exists, if an anesthesiologist does not feel comfortable with the patient's platelet count and the risk of an epidural hematoma, they may still decline to place it.

Potential Complications

- Postdural puncture headache (0.7%)
- Failure to provide adequate pain relief (10%)
- Maternal hypotension (up to 10%)
- Maternal fever (30% will experience a fever of 37.5 °C or higher)
- Epidural hematoma (1 in 250,000)
- Fetal heart rate decelerations
- Pruritus

(Beilin *et al.* 1998, Segal 2010, Chestnut *et al.* 2014)

Spinal Anesthesia

Indications

- Anesthesia during labor
- Cesarean section

Contraindications

- Patient refusal/inability to remain still and cooperate
- Infection at site of needle placement
- Intra-amniotic infection
- Coagulopathy (platelets $< 80 \times 10^9$/L, DIC, hemophilia, etc.)
- Increased intracranial pressure
- Maternal hypovolemia

Procedure

A spinal needle is inserted through the arachnoid and dura, and opioids and/or local anesthetics are injected intrathecally.

Potential Complications

- Postdural puncture "spinal" headache (1–3%)
- Maternal hypotension (10%)
- Fetal heart rate decelerations
- Pruritis
- Failure to provide adequate pain relief (or the effect wears off prior to delivery or conclusion of cesarean section)

(Chestnut *et al.* 2014)

Combined Spinal/Epidural

This technique is helpful as it provides rapid onset of analgesia from the spinal component, combined with the ability to continue providing pain relief with the epidural catheter that is placed during the procedure. It is also effective in providing postoperative pain control after cesarean section with the epidural component. One reported side effect has been a small increased risk of fetal bradycardia and even emergency cesarean delivery in 1.5% of cases in one study (Gambling *et al.* 1998). This is independent of maternal hypotension and is postulated to be due to elevated uterine tone and speed of pain relief, which is more common with combined spinal/epidural analgesia than with epidural analgesia. Despite this, outcomes such as rates of cesarean delivery, low Apgar score, or neonatal acidemia did not differ between the two types in one study (Abrao *et al.* 2009).

Pudendal Nerve Block

The pudendal nerve includes fibers from S2–4 and innervates the vagina, vulva, and perineum. It also has motor fibers going to the pelvic floor and perineum. Descent of the fetal vertex in the second stage of labor can result in significant pain through the stretching of the pelvic floor. By performing an anesthetic block of this nerve, pain relief for the second stage of labor, and even an operative vaginal delivery, can be obtained.

Indications
- Second stage anesthesia
- Operative vaginal delivery
- Augmentation of an epidural that did not cover the sacral nerves
- Obstetric laceration repair

Contraindications
- Allergy to local anesthetic agent to be used

Procedure

A pudendal nerve block kit comes with a needle guide that is inserted into the vagina and directed just posterior to the ischial spines. When injecting the patient's left pudendal nerve, place the needle guide with your left hand, and when injecting the right side, use your right hand to place the needle guide. The needle is then inserted through the needle guide and into the vaginal mucosa until it touches the sacrospinous ligament. At this time, advance the needle approximately 1 cm through the sacrospinous ligament medial and posterior to the ischial spine. Prior to injecting approximately 10 mL of 1% lidocaine or 1% mepivacaine on each side, you must aspirate to ensure you are not directly injecting the pudendal vessels, which are in close proximity to the nerves.

Potential Complications
- Systemic lidocaine toxicity with convulsions may occur with intravascular injection
- Hematoma formation
- Infection (very rare)
- Maternal fever (30% will experience a fever of 37.5 °C or higher)

(Segal 2010)

Nitrous Oxide

This is a self-administered inhaled anesthetic that has been used for decades for anesthesia in other specialties and has a long track record of safety. It has a mild analgesic and amnestic effect but does not eliminate pain; rather the benefit is in the dissociative effect it creates. The nitrous oxide (N_2O) is absorbed by the lungs and is then exhaled. It is not metabolized by the body. Recent formulations have a decreased amount of nitrous oxide, allowing the patient to remain aware and participate in her care but also to experience relief from labor pain. A skilled provider is not required to administer nitrous oxide. The relief provided by nitrous oxide is not as effective as that from epidural analgesia, but it does have benefits – including allowing continued mobility during labor. Additional benefits include rapid onset of anesthesia (1–2 minutes) and short duration of effect (1–2 minutes). Not all hospitals are providing this form of anesthesia yet but the number is increasing (Rosen 2002, Likis *et al.* 2014).

Indications
- Second stage anesthesia
- Operative vaginal delivery
- Augmentation of an epidural that did not cover the sacral nerves
- Obstetric laceration repair
- External cephalic version

Contraindications
- A patient's inability to hold her own face mask
- Patients who are acutely intoxicated or have impaired consciousness
- Patients who have received intravenous opioids in the last 2 hours
- Patients with pernicious anemia or documented B_{12} deficiency (patients taking B_{12} as a nutritional supplement without a deficiency are not contraindicated from this therapy)
- Potential for trapped gas (pneumothorax, intraocular surgery, middle ear surgery, bowel obstruction)

Procedure
The current formulation has a 50%–50% blend of nitrous oxide and oxygen. Measures are in place on the device to decrease ambient levels of nitrous oxide. These include a demand valve that only releases the gas when the patient inhales from the mask, as well as a scavenging apparatus that removes exhaled nitrous oxide. The patient must exhale directly into the mask for the scavenger to adequately remove the exhaled nitrous oxide, and the patient should be coached in this technique.

Potential Complications
Maternal adverse effects can include nausea/vomiting, lightheadedness, or drowsiness. Additionally the nitrous oxide does transmit through the placenta, but the effect on the neonate is negligible as it is rapidly eliminated by neonatal respiration.

Anesthesia Options for Procedures

Cesarean Delivery
In preparing for a cesarean delivery, either an epidural or a spinal anesthesia is normally placed. An epidural takes longer to achieve an adequate level of anesthesia than a spinal, but is less likely to cause maternal hypotension. If a patient has been laboring and has a functioning epidural in place, additional medication may be administered through the

catheter to obtain a surgical anesthesia level. In cases where the delivery is more urgent and there is not time for conduction anesthesia, emergency cesarean delivery under general anesthesia may be the best option. Adequate general anesthesia can typically be achieved within 2 minutes (5 minutes if including a 3-minute preoxygenation period). The decision to administer general anesthesia should not be taken lightly, as the risk of maternal complications is much higher than with either a spinal or an epidural.

Operative Vaginal Delivery

Often, when time comes to consider an operative delivery, the patient will have already received either a spinal or an epidural, which should provide sufficient analgesia. If the epidural is not adequate, then it may be re-dosed by the anesthesia provider as long as there is no pressing fetal distress. If the patient does not have any anesthesia and an operative delivery is required, then some form of pain relief is usually necessary. This is one instance where a vacuum device is advantageous over forceps. The vacuum needs only to be placed on the fetal vertex and does not cause as much maternal discomfort as the placement of forceps. Even in this case, though, anesthesia is usually required. Options for anesthesia with an operative delivery include:

Epidural. This is rarely chosen at the time a decision is made for an operative delivery, because of the relatively long time it takes to place and then take effect.

Spinal. This may be performed relatively rapidly, and the onset of pain relief is also very quick. However, if there is evidence of fetal compromise or distress, then there is usually not time for this method. It does, however, provide excellent analgesia when forceps are to be used.

Pudendal block. This can be performed in patients without any other anesthesia, or in those in whom an epidural/spinal is not providing adequate relief to allow for an operative delivery. It can be performed rapidly in the presence of fetal distress, and when placed properly, provides excellent pain relief for either a vacuum or forceps delivery. See the previous section for instructions on how to perform the procedure and potential complications.

Perineal infiltration. This method involves local infiltration of the perineal area with a local anesthetic. It is not generally adequate for a forceps delivery, but may provide some relief if an episiotomy must be made during an operative delivery.

Repair of Vaginal Lacerations

For most first- and second-degree lacerations, injections of local anesthetic are usually sufficient to complete the repair with adequate pain relief for the mother. Typically, 1% lidocaine is used for this purpose. It is drawn up into a 5–10 mL syringe and injected into and around the area to be sutured using a small, usually 21–23 gauge needle. If the patient has a working epidural or pudendal block, then these are almost always adequate as well. If the epidural is not adequate, it can be re-dosed by the anesthesiologist for the repair. The maximum doses of commonly used local anesthetics are shown in Table 8.3.

For third- and fourth-degree lacerations, greater visualization is required as well as more time for the repair. If the patient does not have a working regional anesthetic, then IV narcotics and local anesthetics may be required. Some common narcotics used for this include morphine sulfate, and fentanyl, all of which have been previously described. In those

Table 8.3 Maximum doses of local anesthetics

Local anesthetic	Without epinephrine	With epinephrine
Lidocaine	5 mg/kg	7 mg/kg
Bupivacaine	3 mg/kg	3 mg/kg
Ropivacaine	2 mg/kg	2 mg/kg

(Adapted from ACOG 2017)

cases where adequate analgesia cannot be obtained with these measures and the patient is hemodynamically stable, you can consult your anesthesiologist regarding regional anesthesia.

Postpartum Tubal Ligation

Patients should be kept NPO for 6–8 hours prior to planned postpartum tubal ligation. Anesthesia for tubal ligation can be done with a previously placed epidural catheter left in place for this purpose, or under spinal anesthesia. Alternatively, this can be done under general anesthesia. However, general anesthesia is not recommended, as patients are still considered physiologically pregnant until 6 weeks postpartum, and the incidence of failed intubation is much higher than in the non-pregnant population.

Obstetric Emergencies

When the situation arises and urgent delivery is required, the choice of anesthesia must ensure the ability to rapidly deliver the fetus while making sure the mother remains stable. The type of anesthesia depends on both the fetal status and the proposed route of delivery.

If the fetus meets criteria for an operative vaginal delivery, then analgesia needs to be adequate for the procedure. If the patient has a functioning epidural or spinal anesthesia, then this is usually adequate. If she does not, then a pudendal block may be attempted. In general, vacuum devices require less analgesia than do forceps, which should be taken into account depending on the situation.

If labor has not progressed to the point where an operative vaginal delivery is possible, and fetal distress is present, then a cesarean delivery is performed. If the patient has a functioning epidural, this can usually be used to administer additional medications and achieve an adequate level of analgesia for cesarean section. This does, however, depend on the degree of fetal distress. If severe distress exists, such as a profound bradycardia without recovery, then you may not have time to wait the 10–15 minutes it takes to augment an epidural or place a spinal anesthetic. In this case, a general anesthetic is required. This should not be undertaken lightly, as the risk of complications with general anesthesia is significantly higher than with conduction anesthesia. In fact, in pregnancy the risk of maternal death from general anesthesia is 16.7 times greater than with regional anesthesia, and the incidence of failed intubation is much higher than in the non-pregnant population (Samsoon and Young 1987, Hawkins *et al.* 1997, Barnardo and Jenkins 2000, Quinn *et al.* 2013, Kinsella 2015).

Making a decision about what type of anesthesia to use is sometimes difficult, and the decision should be made in conjunction with the anesthesiologist as you inform them of exactly what level of distress is present and how quickly you need to effect delivery. They will tell you how long it will take for either conduction or general anesthesia to achieve an adequate surgical level. An anesthesiologist will usually recommend general anesthesia if delivery must occur in less than 5–10 minutes.

In rare, extreme emergencies, a cesarean section can be started with local anesthesia while the patient is being intubated or the spinal/epidural anesthesia is becoming adequate. Conditions where this may be necessary include a failed (or contraindicated) regional anesthesia with an inaccessible airway, failed intubation with significant fetal distress, an inadequate regional anesthesia, or no trained personnel available for other types of anesthesia (Norris 2000). A large syringe is filled with local anesthetic and injected subcutaneously where the incision will be made (usually 200–300 mL of 0.5% lidocaine with epinephrine). The incision is then made and successive layers injected as needed until the peritoneal cavity is entered. (You must take into account the maximum doses of local anesthetic that can be used, which are listed in Table 8.3.) By this time, the anesthesiologist should have the patient asleep, or additional intravenous medications can be given after the baby is delivered. Fortunately, this is a very rare occurrence.

Postpartum

In the postpartum patient, the most common emergency requiring anesthesia is postpartum hemorrhage. It is often necessary to make the patient more comfortable in order to manually explore the uterus or repair lacerations that are causing the bleeding. If the bleeding is secondary to uterine inversion, then anesthetic consultation is urgently needed to facilitate replacement of the uterus.

Anesthetic options for postpartum hemorrhage, which usually involves manually exploring the uterus, include the following:

- For manual uterine exploration (retained placenta/uterine atony):
    - Bolus through an existing epidural catheter
    - Intravenous opioids (fentanyl, morphine)
    - Inhalational nitrous oxide (50% N_2O + 50% O_2)
    - General anesthesia

- For vaginal/cervical lacerations:
    - Infiltration with local anesthetic
    - Bolus through an existing epidural catheter
    - Intravenous opioids (fentanyl, morphine)
    - Inhalational nitrous oxide (50% N_2O + 50% O_2)
    - Pudendal nerve block

- For uterine inversion:
    - Intravenous opioids (fentanyl, morphine)
    - Inhalational nitrous oxide (50% N_2O + 50% O_2)
    - General anesthesia

Postpartum Pain Management

Planning for postpartum pain control should begin prior to delivery. If a patient receives a cesarean section, injection of an opioid along with the spinal anesthesia can provide effective postpartum pain relief for 12–24 hours (Goodman *et al.* 2005). This does have the side effects of increased pruritus, nausea, and possible respiratory depression. Antihistamines or a mixed agonist/antagonist drug such as nalbuphine can provide relief from pruritus. A local anesthetic may also be given at the time of cesarean delivery by irrigation and infiltration of the wound, which is easy to perform and reduces postoperative opioid consumption (Bamigboye and Hofmeyr 2009). If injection of neuraxial opioid is not possible, or if general anesthesia is used for cesarean section, postoperative pain control can be achieved with a patient-controlled analgesia (PCA) with fentanyl or hydromorphone (Dilaudid), or if skilled anesthetic personnel are present, a transversus abdominis plane (TAP) block can be performed, usually under ultrasound guidance. A TAP block with ropivacaine at the time of cesarean section has been shown to decrease postoperative narcotic requirements by 70% (McDonnell *et al.* 2008).

NSAIDs

Intravenous NSAID preparations such as ketorolac (Toradol) may be used postoperatively as long as the patient does not have any contraindications to NSAID use or concerns for bleeding. Oral formulations of NSAIDs are commonly used for postpartum pain management. Previous recommendations were to not use NSAIDs in patients with hypertension, but recent data show that this is not a concern even in patients with preeclampsia (Viteri *et al.* 2017).

Acetaminophen

Intravenous acetaminophen (paracetamol) can be given, but oral formulations have been shown to have similar efficacy, and the IV formulation is more expensive (Alhashemi *et al.* 2006, McDonnell *et al.* 2008). Care should be taken in patients with underlying liver disease, including preeclampsia or HELLP syndrome. Acetaminophen can be used in combination with oral or parenteral NSAIDs or opioids.

Oral Opioids

Oral opioids can be used in patients with significant vaginal lacerations or after cesarean section, but their use should be limited given the recent epidemic of opioid abuse in the United States. It is important not to prescribe too many pills at the time of discharge, as overprescribing can lead to leftover medication being used when not needed or even misused. A recent multicenter study of opioid prescriptions and use after cesarean section showed that patients only used about half of what was given to them (20 of 40 Percocet) at the time of discharge (Bateman *et al.* 2017). Given this, limiting initial prescriptions to no more than 30 tablets is a reasonable place to start, although it is important to check with your institution's guidelines as well.

Additionally, the FDA recently issued a strengthened "warning" against codeine or tramadol in breastfeeding mothers because of the risk of serious adverse reactions in breastfed infants, including excess sleepiness, difficulty breastfeeding, or serious breathing problems that could result in death (FDA 2017).

References

Abrao KC, Francisco RP, Miyadahira S, Cicarelli DD, Zugaib M (2009). Elevation of uterine basal tone and fetal heart rate abnormalities after labor analgesia: a randomized controlled trial. *Obstet Gynecol* **113**: 41–7.

ACOG (2017). Obstetric analgesia and anesthesia. ACOG Practice Bulletin #177, April 2017. *Obstet Gynecol* **129**: e73–89.

Alhashemi JA, Alotaibi QA, Mashaat MS, *et al.* (2006). Intravenous acetaminophen vs oral ibuprofen in combination with morphine PCIA after cesarean delivery. *Can J Anaesth* **53**: 1200–6.

Anim-Somuah M, Smyth RM, Jones L (2011). Epidural versus non-epidural or no analgesia in labour. *Cochrane Database Syst Rev* (12): CD000331.

Bamigboye AA, Hofmeyr GJ (2009). Local anaesthetic wound infiltration and abdominal nerves block during cesarean section for postoperative pain relief. *Cochrane Database of Systematic Reviews* (3): CD006954.

Barnardo PD, Jenkins JG (2000). Failed tracheal intubation in obstetrics: a 6-year review in the UK region. *Anaesthesia* **55**: 690–4.

Bateman B, Cole N, Maeda A, *et al.* (2017). Patterns of opioid prescription and use after cesarean delivery. *Obstet Gynecol* **130**: 29–35.

Beilin Y, Zahn J, Bernstein HH, *et al.* (1998). Treatment of incomplete analgesia after placement of an epidural catheter and administration of local anesthesia for women in labor. *Anesthesiology* **88**: 1502–6.

Chestnut DH, Wong CA, Tsen LC, *et al.* (eds.) (2014). *Chestnut's Obstetric Anesthesia: Principles and Practice*, 5th edn. Philadelphia, PA: Elsevier Saunders 2014.

FDA (2017). *FDA Drug Safety Communication: FDA restricts use of prescription codeine pain and cough medicines and tramadol pain medicines in children; recommends against use in breastfeeding women.* Silver Spring, MD: Food and Drug Administration.

Gambling DR, Sharma SK, Ramin SM, *et al.* (1998). A randomized study of combined spinal–epidural analgesia versus intravenous meperidine during labor: impact on cesarean delivery rate. *Anesthesiology* **89**: 1336–44.

Goodman SR, Drachenberg AM, Johnson SA, *et al.* (2005). Decreased postpartum use of oral pain medication after a single dose of epidural morphine. *Reg Anesth Pain Med* **30**: 134–9.

Halpern SH, Leighton BL, Ohisson A, *et al.* (1998). Effect of epidural vs parental opioid analgesia on the progress of labor: a meta-analysis. *JAMA* **280**: 2105–2110.

Halpern SH, Levine T, Wilson DB, *et al.* (1999). Effect of labor analgesia on breastfeeding success. *Birth* **26**: 83–8.

Hawkins JL (2000). Obstetric anesthesia and analgesia. In Mitchell JL (ed.), *Precis: Obstetrics*, 2nd edn. Washington, DC: ACOG.

Hawkins JL, Koonin LM, Palmer SK, Gibbs CP (1997). Anesthesia-related deaths during obstetric delivery in the United States 1979–1990. *Anesthesiology* **86**: 277–84.

Jones L, Othman M, Dowswell T, *et al.* (2012). Pain management for women in labour: an overview of systematic reviews. *Cochrane Database Syst Rev* (3): CD009234.

Kinsella SM, Winton AL, Mushambi MC, *et al.* (2015). Failed tracheal intubation during obstetric general anesthesia: a literature review. *Int J Obstet Anesth* **24**: 356–74.

Likis FE, Andrews JC, Collins MR, *et al.* (2014). Nitrous oxide for the management of labor pain: a systematic review. *Anesth Analg* **118**: 153–67.

McDonnell JG, Curley G, Carney J, *et al.* (2008). The analgesic efficacy of transversus abdominis plane block after cesarean delivery: a randomized controlled trial. *Anesthesia* **106**: 186–91.

Montgomery A, Hale TW; Academy of Breastfeeding Medicine (2012). ABM clinical protocol #15: analgesia and anesthesia for the breastfeeding mother, revised 2012. *Breastfeed Med* **7**: 547–53.

Norris MC (ed.) (2000). *Handbook of Obstetric Anesthesia*. Philadelphia, PA: Lippincott, Williams & Wilkins, pp. 147, 437.

Olofsson C, Ekblom A, Ekman-Ordeberg G, Hjelm A, Irestedt L (1996). Lack of analgesic effect of systemically administered morphine or pethidine on labour pain. *Br J Obstet Gynaecol* **103**: 968–72.

Quinn AC, Milne D, Columb M, Gorton H, Knight M (2013). Failed tracheal intubation in obstetric anaesthesia: 2 year national case-control study in the UK. *Br J Anaesth* **110**: 74–80.

Rahmani R, Khakbazan Z, Yavari P, Granmayeh M, Yavari L (2012). Effect of oral carbohydrate intake on labor progress: randomized controlled trial. *Iranian Journal of Public Health* **41**: 59–66.

Rosen MA (2002). Nitrous oxide for relief of labor pain: a systematic review. *Am J Obstet Gynecol* **186** (5 Suppl. Nature): S110–26.

Samsoon GL, Young JR (1987). Difficult tracheal intubation: a retrospective study. *Anaesthesia* **42**: 487–90.

Segal S (2010). Labor epidural analgesia and maternal fever. *Anesth Analg* **111**: 1467–75.

Sng BL, Leong WL, Zeng Y, *et al.* (2014). Early versus late initiation of epidural analgesia for labour. *Cochrane Database Syst Rev* (10): CD007238.

Viteri OA, England JA, Alrais MA, *et al.* (2017). Association of nonsteroidal anti-inflammatory drugs and postpartum hypertension in women with preeclampsia with severe features. *Obstet Gynecol* **130**: 830–5.

Wilson MJ, MacArthur C, Cooper GM, *et al.* (2010). Epidural analgesia and breastfeeding: a randomized controlled trial of epidural techniques with and without fentanyl and a non-epidural comparison group. COMET Study Group UK. *Anaesthesia* **65**: 145–53.

Wong CA, Scavone BM, Peaceman AM, *et al.* The risk of cesarean delivery with neuraxial analgesia given early versus late in labor. *N Engl J Med* 2005; **352**: 655–65.

Operative Vaginal Delivery

Morgan Light and Shad Deering

Indications for Operative Vaginal Delivery

The most recent ACOG Practice Bulletin on the subject states that only 3.30% of all deliveries in 2013 were operative vaginal deliveries (ACOG 2015). This being said, in the right hands, these procedures can allow you to deliver a fetus safely and rapidly, and acquiring these skills is an essential part of any obstetric provider's training. Indications for an operative vaginal delivery, according to ACOG, include:

- Presumed or imminent fetal compromise (example – severe variable decelerations or repetitive late decelerations with pushing)
- Maternal indication for shortened/passive second stage (example – severe maternal cardiac disease or CNS disease)
- Prolonged second stage of labor (see Chapter 5 for definitions, as they differ for nulliparous/multiparous patients)
- Aftercoming head of a vaginal breech delivery

Essential Criteria

If the patient meets one of the common indications for an operative delivery, you will need to consider the essential criteria that must be met prior to performing an operative delivery. These include the following:

- Size of the baby (EFW, either from sonogram or estimated by Leopold's maneuvers)
- Leading part of the fetal skull at +2 station or lower

- Adequate pelvis
- Adequate pain control
- Cervix completely dilated
- Known fetal head position
- Ruptured membranes
- Willingness to abandon the procedure (if you are unable to place the instrument, or if there is no descent with appropriate traction, you must always be willing to stop and proceed to cesarean section)

Acronym: **SLAACKR-W**

Size of baby. The first parameter you must consider is whether or not you believe the fetus is small enough to be delivered vaginally. This is why performing Leopold's maneuvers at the time of admission is important in establishing an estimated fetal weight (EFW). If you feel that the fetus is large (> 4000 grams), then, although you may attempt the delivery if you feel the pelvis is adequate (i.e. large enough to allow passage of the fetus), there is a higher chance of a shoulder dystocia or no fetal descent with traction and you must be prepared for these complications and willing to abandon the attempt.

Leading part of the fetal skull at +2 station or lower. If the fetus is not at least at +2 station, then you are performing a mid-forceps delivery, which is rarely used, and only when it is felt that the fetus can be more rapidly delivered by this method than by cesarean. A mid-forceps delivery also requires a provider who has been trained and is comfortable with the procedure, as the risks to the mother and fetus are increased over low or outlet forceps deliveries.

Adequate pelvis. If you determine that the patient has a contracted pelvis on clinical pelvimetry, then performing an operative delivery is contraindicated. Regardless of how much traction you apply, if the space is too small, the baby still won't fit. (Clinical pelvimetry is described in Chapter 2.)

Adequate pain control. In general, some form of anesthesia (epidural or spinal) is required to perform a forceps delivery. The pressure from the application of forceps can be very uncomfortable. With a vacuum device, less anesthesia is needed for the application, which is one reason this device is often used when a patient does not have an epidural. If the patient does not have neuraxial anesthesia, or if anesthesia is not adequate, then a pudendal nerve block may be attempted. (See Chapter 8 for a discussion of these options.)

Cervix completely dilated. Unless the cervix is completely dilated, an operative vaginal delivery should not be attempted. If any part of the cervix is caught in the forceps or vacuum device then significant cervical lacerations and hemorrhage can occur.

Known fetal head position. In order to appropriately and safely apply either forceps or a vacuum device, it is imperative that you know the baby's head's position (i.e., OA, OP, LOA, etc.). This can be very difficult after a patient has been pushing for several hours and developed caput, which is why is it important that you check the fetal head position on every labor exam and document it in the record. An ultrasound, either transabdominal or translabial, may also be performed at bedside to aid in determining position.

Ruptured membranes. You cannot place the instruments with the membranes still intact. If the membranes are still intact, which is unlikely when the cervix is completely dilated

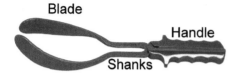

Figure 9.1 Parts of a forceps.

and effaced, then perform an artificial rupture of membranes (AROM) prior to placement of the instrument.

Contraindications to Operative Vaginal Delivery

Just as important as knowing the indications and prerequisites for performing an operative vaginal delivery is understanding the conditions when you should not attempt it. These situations include:

- General contraindications:
  - Fetus is known or strongly suspected to have a bone demineralization condition (osteogenesis imperfecta)
  - Fetus is known or strongly suspected to have a bleeding disorder (hemophilia, von Willebrand's, etc.)
  - Fetal head is not engaged
  - Fetal head position is not known

- Specific contraindications for vacuum:
  - Preterm status (< 34 weeks' gestation) (risk of fetal intraventricular hemorrhage)*
  - Face presentation

Forceps Delivery

There are multiple texts written on this subject, and some of these are listed in the reference section for this chapter, as there is too much to cover completely in this brief text. This section describes the types of forceps to choose for different deliveries, and provides basic instructions on how to apply them in the occiput anterior (OA) position and the checks to perform before applying traction. In order to really learn this, you must get a pair in your hands and practice. This is something that can be done on labor and delivery in any free minutes you have.

The parts of a forceps (Figure 9.1) are:

Blades. The blades of the forceps are applied to the fetal head. There are several variations, which can be seen in Figure 9.2(a–e).

Shanks. The shanks connect the handles of the forceps to the blades. Depending on the type of forceps, these may be overlapping or parallel.

Handles. The handles also vary according to the type of forceps. They usually incorporate different locking mechanisms.

---

* The fact that vacuum devices should not be used with a preterm fetus is one of the reasons why it is important to learn how to use forceps.

Types of Forceps and Indications

Simpson forceps (Figure 9.2a). These are a classic instrument with parallel shanks to allow the blades to fit around any molding that occurs with labor. They are typically used in nulliparous patients when the fetus has a significant amount of molding present.

Elliot forceps (Figure 9.2b). The Elliot forceps are similar in appearance to Simpson forceps, but the shanks are overlapping and not parallel. They are used for delivery of a fetus with minimal molding, usually in multiparous patients.

Keilland forceps (Figure 9.2c). These are the forceps of choice for rotation of the fetal head (i.e. from OP to OA), especially when the rotation is > 45 degrees. The reason for this is the absence of a significant pelvic curve, which makes rotation easier through a smaller arc of movement. After rotation, the infant can be delivered with these forceps, although the angle of traction will be different than with the classic instruments such as Simpson or Elliot forceps.

Piper forceps (Figure 9.2d). These forceps are used to deliver the aftercoming head of a breech presentation during vaginal delivery. They are applied after the arms of the fetus are delivered and used to prevent the fetal neck from being hyperextended during delivery.

Luikart modification (Figure 9.2e). This modification is often seen with Simpson forceps (making them Simpson–Luikart forceps) and is notable for the solid blades rather than the fenestrated ones on the classic Simpsons. The advantage of this modification is that vaginal tissue is less likely to be caught in the fenestrations during application, and this may decrease the incidence of vaginal lacerations.

(a)

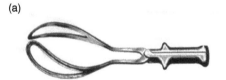

Figure 9.2a Simpson forceps.

(b)

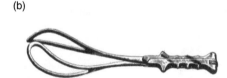

Figure 9.2b Elliot forceps.

(c)

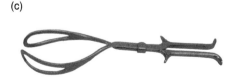

Figure 9.2c Keilland forceps.

(d)

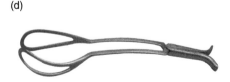

Figure 9.2d Piper forceps.

(e)

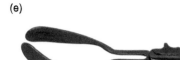

Figure 9.2e Simpson–Luikart forceps.

After you have gone through the acronym **SLAACKR**, you are ready to apply the forceps. When placing forceps, the steps are as follows:

1. Counsel and verbally consent the patient (patients should be counseled for the potential of an operative delivery at the time of admission).
2. Choose appropriate forceps (see above).
3. Check forceps to ensure they match and articulate (sometimes after sterilization they are not packaged together correctly). The handles usually have numbers stamped on them that should match.
4. Empty the bladder (or remove the Foley catheter).
5. Remove intrauterine pressure catheter (IUPC) if present.
6. Remove fetal scalp electrode (FSE) if it interferes with placement (which it often will) and replace external monitor.
7. Confirm fetal head position.
8. Begin application between contractions.
9. Check placement with three checks (see below).
10. Apply traction with next contraction.
11. Monitor the fetal heart rate between pushes.

Application of Forceps

When the fetus is in the occiput anterior (OA) position, the left blade is applied first. (Note that the LEFT blade refers to the blade that will be on the fetus's LEFT and not yours.) If the fetus is rotated to either side, then the posterior blade is placed first, as it will act as a splint when the anterior blade is placed (Hale 2001). In the OA position, the left blade is held in the right hand, with the left hand holding the handle. The blade of the forceps is held vertically and inserted into the vagina, with the right hand between the vaginal sidewall and the blade. The right hand then guides the blade into place with gentle pressure as the left hand guides the handle through a wide arc in a counterclockwise fashion (Figures 9.3, 9.4.) The left hand does **not** force the forceps into place, but guides it. Grasping the handle with only the thumb and two fingers will help to avoid any temptation to use the left hand too aggressively and apply excessive pressure. Once applied, have an assistant hold the handle in position as you prepare to place the next blade. The right blade is then grasped in the left hand and applied in the same manner, but the arc is in a clockwise direction (Figure 9.5).

After both blades are placed and the handles are articulated, or put together, you will perform three checks. If placement is not adequate, the handles may be disarticulated and small adjustments made. If the handles do not articulate, attempt placement again. If the forceps are not able to be articulated, the forceps delivery cannot be attempted.

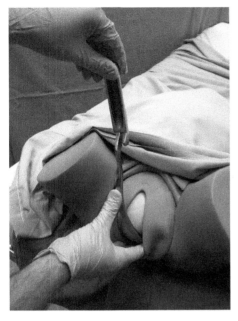

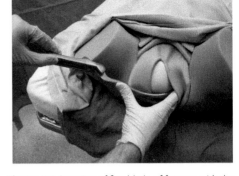

Figure 9.4 Insertion of first blade of forceps, with the left hand guiding the handle through a counterclockwise arc.

Figure 9.3 Application of first blade of forceps.

Figure 9.5 Application of second blade of forceps.

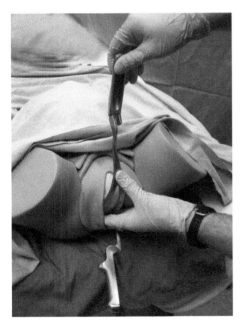

Checking Placement of Forceps

1. Ensure the sagittal suture is centered between the blades and running perpendicular to the plane of the shanks.
2. Be able to place no more than one finger between the fenestrations of each blade and the fetal skull. The amount of the fenestration felt on both sides should be equal.
3. The posterior fontanelle should be midway between the sides of the blades and only one finger breadth above the shanks.

(Hale 2001)

Applying Traction

When applying traction, it is important to apply it in the appropriate direction. This is often referred to as "axis traction," as you are attempting to apply force in the plane of least resistance and help guide the fetal head under the pubic symphysis. The dominant hand is used to grasp the handles of the forceps and the other hand is placed on the shanks to push down in a vertical manner, which is called the Pajot maneuver (Hale 2001). This will guide a fetus in the OA position under the pubic symphysis. At times, an instrument called a Bill handle is attached to the handle of the forceps, which will accomplish the same axis traction (Figure 9.6). The direction of traction is generally slightly different (less downward traction) for a fetus in the OP position, as the Pajot maneuver can cause hyperextension when the occiput is posterior.

The amount of traction applied should be the least possible to accomplish descent of the fetal head. Traction is applied in a steady manner, gradually increasing in intensity as needed, during a contraction with maternal pushing, and then gradually relaxed after the contraction ends.

An episiotomy does not have to be cut just because forceps are placed. If there is significant resistance from the soft tissues, then it can be performed either between pushes or as the perineum is being distended by the fetal head. If an episiotomy is performed, care must be taken not to cut the infant, and it is extremely important to support the perineum as the infant delivers to try and avoid extension of the incision into the anal sphincter and rectum.

As the fetal head descends and distends the perineum, the forceps handles are elevated with the dominant hand. The other hand, or an assistant, supports the perineum. (The handles should not be elevated more than 45 degrees above a horizontal plane, to protect against sulcus lacerations.) The blades are then removed by reversing the movements used to apply them, with the right blade first. Make sure to use the same arc motion with removal. After the forceps are removed, delivery of the shoulders and body should proceed in the normal manner.

After the delivery, it is important to examine the vagina, including the sidewalls, for lacerations, and to look for extension of lacerations or an episiotomy into the anal sphincter or rectum.

Note: If the fetal head does not descend with appropriate traction, then you can reassess head position, because traction from the OP position is different from the OA position. The most important thing to remember is that, if a fetus does not descend with appropriate traction generated by the arms and shoulders, then there is probably a good reason. It takes

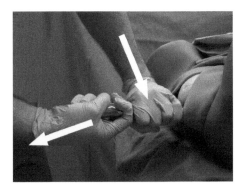

Figure 9.6 Axis traction.

practice to understand exactly how much traction to apply, but never make the mistake of applying too much.

Vacuum Delivery

Use of the vacuum device can result in similar complications to forceps. After determining that an operative vaginal delivery is indicated, and going through your acronym SLAACKR-W, consider whether you can use a vacuum (i.e., gestational age at least 34 weeks, no known bleeding disorders, and no need for rotation). General reasons for choosing a vacuum device over forceps are more experience with vacuum devices and less need for pain control for placement.

Application and Traction

After counseling the patient and confirming fetal head position, empty the patient's bladder. Then place the vacuum device so that it covers the midline of the vertex. Make sure that it does not overlap either the anterior or posterior fontanelle, and that there is no vaginal tissue trapped in between the vacuum and the fetal scalp.

When the patient experiences a contraction, have your assistant bring the pressure up to an appropriate level, which should not generally exceed 500–600 mmHg or 0.6–0.8 kg/cm^2 (it is important to make sure and review the instructions for the vacuum device that your institution uses so that you will know the appropriate pressure). Using a Kiwi vacuum device, you may bring the pressure up yourself (500–600 mmHg is the "green zone"). After you have done this, apply traction with each push in the appropriate axis (see the forceps section, above, for a description of this). It is important to avoid a rocking or jerking motion and instead to use gentle and steady traction.

There is debate about what to do between pushes and whether it is necessary to release the vacuum seal between pushes in order to decrease rates of cephalohematoma. One randomized trial has examined the rates of cephalohematoma by comparing two groups. One group was randomized to continuous vacuum application during and between contractions; in the other, the vacuum seal was released between contractions. Incidence of cephalohematoma was similar between the two groups (Bofill *et al.* 1997a). The biggest risk factor for development of cephalohematoma is the duration of vacuum application, with one trial reporting a 28% incidence in neonates when application time exceeded 5 minutes (Bofill *et al.* 1997b). Given all of the data, the most recent ACOG Practice Bulletin on operative vaginal delivery states that releasing vacuum pressure between contractions does not appear to reduce the incidence of fetal scalp injury or improve other outcomes such as time to delivery, method success, maternal lacerations, or other neonatal outcomes (ACOG 2015).

If the vacuum seal breaks and it "pops off" three separate times, it is generally wise to abandon the procedure. Be sure to read the package insert included with vacuum devices at your institution for recommended number of allowed "pop-offs," as some instruments will specify two times as an indication to abandon the procedure. Also, when this happens, recheck the fetal head position, because pop-offs will occur more often when the fetus is in the OP position.

Sequential Use of Vacuum and Forceps

With the increased use of vacuum devices, which are not as successful as forceps in completing delivery, there are times where one instrument is used after the initial one has failed. One study reported on the maternal and neonatal morbidity of over 3700 combined vacuum/forceps deliveries with an equal number of deliveries by forceps alone and vacuum alone, as well as an additional 11,000 spontaneous vaginal deliveries (Gardella *et al.* 2001). This study found that the risk of intracranial hemorrhage was significantly increased, by 3.9-fold, when both devices were utilized during delivery. There was also an increased risk of facial nerve injury, neonatal seizures, and postpartum hemorrhage when both instruments were used compared to only one instrument. A more recent study also examined outcomes of 1360 nulliparous women undergoing operative vaginal delivery (Murphy *et al.* 2011). Sequential use of instruments was associated with increased anal sphincter tears and low umbilical artery pH when compared with patients undergoing operative vaginal delivery with a single instrument.

Given the above data demonstrating increased rates of neonatal complications, ACOG states that the available evidence weighs against routine use of sequential vacuum and forceps (ACOG 2015). Extreme care should be taken, both in the choice of the first instrument to use and in making a decision to apply a second instrument should the first one fail.

Potential Complications of Operative Vaginal Delivery

There are potential complications involved in the use of both forceps and vacuum devices. It is imperative that you are knowledgeable regarding both maternal and fetal complications so that you can adequately counsel patients, do your best to avoid them, and recognize them should they occur.

The overall rates of serious complications such as neonatal encephalopathy and neonatal death from intracranial hemorrhage are similar to those of neonates delivered by cesarean section in the second stage of labor. The risk of intracranial hemorrhage with operative vaginal deliveries (both vacuum and forceps) is also similar when compared with spontaneous vaginal delivery (Gardella *et al.* 2001).

Forceps

1. Maternal complications:
   a. Cervical lacerations

  b. Vaginal sidewall lacerations
  c. Third/fourth-degree lacerations (involvement of the anal sphincter/rectum)
  d. Vaginal hematoma
  e. Postpartum hemorrhage

2. Fetal complications:

  a. Cephalohematoma
  b. Neonatal abducens (6th nerve) injury: 2.4% of forceps deliveries (Gailbraith 1994)
  c. Facial nerve palsy: 0.8–7.5 cases per 1000 births, 8.8 per 1000 forceps deliveries (Duval and Daniel 2009)
  d. Facial marks (these usually resolve within the first few days of life)
  e. Neonatal jaundice
  f. Skull fractures

Vacuum

1. Maternal complications:

  a. Vaginal lacerations: these tend to occur less often than with forceps, although if any vaginal tissue is caught between the vacuum device and the fetal head, this can cause significant hemorrhage afterwards. Any operative delivery, especially those that involve an episiotomy, can result in third/fourth-degree lacerations, although vacuum deliveries are less likely than forceps to cause this (see Chapter 11)
  b. Cervical lacerations
  c. Postpartum hemorrhage

2. Fetal complications:

  a. Scalp lacerations (especially if a twisting movement, or "cookie-cutter" motion is used to attempt to rotate the infant)
  b. Cephalohematoma: rates vary depending on the source, ranging from 11% up to 28% when applied for more than 5 minutes
  c. Subgaleal hematoma: bleeding between cranial periosteum and epicranial aponeurosis
  d. Retinal hemorrhages
  e. Neonatal jaundice

Long-term Infant Outcomes with Operative Vaginal Delivery

There have been two long-term studies of the cognitive development of children delivered by forceps or vacuum extractor. These both found no difference when compared to infants delivered spontaneously (Ngan *et al.* 1990, Wesley *et al.* 1993). The forceps study included nearly 1200 children delivered via forceps and the vacuum study nearly 300 vacuum deliveries. No differences were seen in scholastic performance, speech, or neurologic abnormality. These facts are important to know when counseling patients, as they are often nervous when you discuss these interventions with them.

References

ACOG (2015). Operative vaginal delivery. *ACOG Practice Bulletin #154*, November 2015.

Bofill JA, Rust OA, Schorr SJ, *et al.* (1997a). A randomized trial of two vacuum extraction techniques. *Obstet Gynecol* **89**: 758–62.

Bofill JA, Rust OA, Devidas M, *et al.* (1997b). Neonatal cephalohematoma from vacuum extraction. *J Reprod Med* **42**: 565–9.

Duval M, Daniel S (2009). Facial nerve palsy in neonates secondary to forceps use. *Arch Otolaryngol Head Neck Surg* **135**: 634–6.

Gailbraith RS (1994). Incidence of neonatal sixth nerve palsy in relation to mode of delivery. *Am J Obstet Gynecol* **170**: 1158–9.

Gardella C, Taylor M, Benedetti T, Hitti J, Critchlow C (2001). The effect of sequential use of vacuum and forceps for assisted vaginal delivery on neonatal and maternal outcomes. *Am J Obstet Gynecol* **185**: 896–902.

Hale RW (ed.) (2001). *Dennen's Forceps Deliveries*, 4th edn. Washington, DC: American College of Obstetricians and Gynecologists.

Murphy DJ, Macleod M, Bahl R, Strachan B (2011). A cohort study of maternal and neonatal morbidity in relation to use of sequential instruments at operative vaginal delivery. *Eur J Obstet Gynecol Reprod Biol* **156**: 41–5.

Ngan HY, Miu P, Ko L, Ma HK (1990). Long-term neurological sequelae following vacuum extractor delivery. *Aust N Z J Obstet Gynaecol* **30**: 111–14.

Wesley BD, Van den Berg BJ, Reece EA (1993). The effect of forceps delivery on cognitive development. *Am J Obstet Gynecol* **169**: 1091–5.

Chapter 1

Cesarean Delivery

Meghan Yamasaki and Shad Deering

Introduction

Cesarean deliveries are now a routine part of any obstetric practice. The current cesarean rate in the United States is approximately 32% (Martin *et al.* 2017). Of these operations, the majority are repeat cesarean sections. Once a patient has had a cesarean, for any reason, she may choose to have a repeat cesarean delivery with subsequent pregnancies. While attempting to have a vaginal birth after cesarean section (VBAC) is a reasonable option for many women, they must be given the option of a repeat cesarean delivery as there are risks involved in a VBAC. This topic is discussed in detail later in this chapter.

Indications for Cesarean Section

As with nearly everything in obstetrics, there are both maternal and fetal indications for performing a cesarean delivery. Currently, over 85% of cesarean sections performed in the United States are done for one of the following four reasons:

1. Prior cesarean delivery
2. Labor dystocia (arrest of dilation/arrest of descent)
3. Fetal distress
4. Fetal malpresentation (e.g., breech presentation, transverse fetal lie)

(Cunningham *et al.* 2014)

Chapters 4 and 5 contain extensive discussions of exactly when a cesarean delivery is indicated for labor dystocia, as well as what level of fetal distress may require an immediate cesarean section.

Other, less common indications for cesarean delivery can be categorized as either maternal or fetal. Some of these include the following:

Maternal:

1. Placenta previa or vasa previa
2. Placental abruption
3. CNS lesions that make labor contraindicated
4. Active genital HSV infection during labor
5. HIV infection with a detectable viral load (> 1000 copies)*

Fetal:

1. Umbilical cord prolapse
2. Significant hydrocephalus that makes vaginal delivery impossible
3. Fetal macrosomia**
4. Other fetal conditions that preclude vaginal delivery
5. Triplet pregnancy or higher-order multiple gestations
6. Fetal bleeding disorder

Preoperative Evaluation

Prior to beginning a cesarean section, the following steps should be taken:

1. Anesthesia evaluation, to determine type of anesthesia required. This will most often be some form of conduction anesthesia: see Chapter 8.
2. Baseline laboratory testing to include a measurement of hemoglobin, hematocrit, platelets, and an antibody screen.

---

* This recommendation depends on the patient's antepartum treatment as well as on her viral load at the time of delivery (ACOG 2016a).

** Presumed fetal macrosomia is rarely an indication for a primary cesarean section without labor. This is because ultrasound estimation of fetal weight is not very accurate at term. ACOG does, however, recommend offering a prophylactic cesarean section if the estimated fetal weight is > 5000 grams in a non-diabetic patient or > 4500 grams in a patient with diabetes, in an effort to prevent shoulder dystocia (ACOG 2016b).

3. Order antibiotic prophylaxis. This usually consists of ampicillin, an extended-spectrum penicillin, or cephalosporin. Azithromycin may also be used concurrently in certain situations. Please see below for further details.

Anesthesia

Most commonly, either spinal or epidural anesthesia is used to perform a cesarean section. In emergency cases, or when a spinal or epidural is contraindicated (such as patients with thrombocytopenia or a coagulopathy), it may be necessary to administer general anesthesia.

Essential Anatomy

Most cesarean sections will be straightforward in terms of anatomy, but a thorough knowledge of female pelvic anatomy is essential for when complications occur. You must know every layer of tissue that you incise and understand the potential problems that can occur at each step of the operation. Always remember that if there are abdominal adhesions or you are having difficulty repairing the uterine incision, restore normal anatomy first. This will prevent accidental damage of other structures and ensure an appropriate repair. Both written descriptions and diagrams are provided, to help you identify important structures during the operation.

A. Abdominal Wall

When beginning the operation, you will make a sharp incision in the skin with a scalpel. After getting through the skin, you will encounter the following layers in this order:

1. Subcutaneous tissue
   a. Camper's fascia (fatty tissue)
   b. Scarpa's fascia (thick, fibrous tissue)

2. Fascia (musculoaponeurotic layer)
   a. Rectus sheath (formed by the aponeuroses of the external and internal oblique and transversalis muscles)

3. Transversalis fascia
4. Peritoneum

B. Blood Vessels

In general, during an uncomplicated cesarean delivery, you should not encounter or damage any significant blood vessels. However, some large vessels that you may see and should be aware of include the following:

1. **Abdominal wall vessels.** The femoral artery supplies branches to the superficial layers of the abdominal wall, and the external iliac artery gives rise to the inferior epigastric artery. Specifically, some important vessels are the following:
   - Branches of femoral artery:
     - Superficial epigastric artery. This vessel is lateral to the rectus muscle and runs over the external oblique muscle.
     - Superficial circumflex artery. Runs laterally, inferior to the iliac ligament up toward the iliac crest.

- Superficial external pudendal artery. This vessel runs in a medial direction just above the inguinal ligament.

- Branches of external iliac artery:

   - Inferior epigastric artery. This vessel runs superiorly on the posterior and lateral portion of the rectus abdominal muscles. It is not incised with a transverse incision, but if a muscle-cutting incision (such as a Maylard incision*) is used, these arteries must be identified and ligated prior to transecting the rectus muscles.

2. **Intra-abdominal vessels**

- Uterine arteries. These arteries are on the lateral sides of the uterus in the broad ligament. They are most commonly injured when a low transverse uterine incision extends laterally.

C. Uterus

The uterus is a muscular organ that receives blood from the uterine arteries and the many collateral vessels (Figure 10.2).

D. Ureters/Bladder

The bladder is located anterior to the uterus, and a bladder flap is often made prior to the uterine incision in order to avoid injury. The ureters lie lateral to the cervix and may be

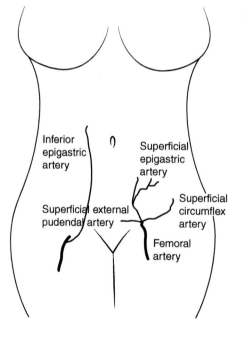

Figure 10.1 Abdominal wall blood vessels.

Inferior epigastric artery

Superficial epigastric artery

Superficial external pudendal artery

Superficial circumflex artery

Femoral artery

---

* This type of incision is rarely used in a cesarean, as a Pfannenstiel incision should generally not be converted to a Maylard.

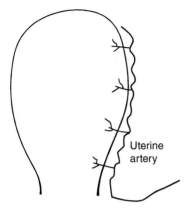

Figure 10.2 Location of uterine arteries with respect to the uterus.

Uterine
artery

damaged if there is lateral extension of the uterine incision and they are incorporated in clamps or sutures placed in this area to control bleeding. Making sure your initial uterine incision is not too lateral, as well as good technique with delivery of the fetus, will decrease the risk of the incision extending laterally.

Surgical Instruments

When in the OR, whether you are the surgeon or an assistant, you must be able to ask for the instrument you need in a way that the OR technician can provide it to you in a timely manner. To do this, you need to know the names of the basic instruments and what they are used for as well as what they look like, because sometimes you will be handed a different instrument than what you requested.

The basic surgical instruments used during a cesarean section are listed here. You will find photos of these instruments, with a description of their function and when they are used, in Appendix C, *Cesarean Talk-through*.

- Scalpel (usually a #10 blade for both abdominal and uterine incisions)
- Electrocautery (setting is commonly 40 cut / 40 coagulation)
- Suction (usually a Yankauer-type suction device)
- Pickups (Debakey or smooth pickups, Russian pickups, rat-tooth pickups)
- Clamps (Allis clamp, Kelly clamp, Hemostat, Pennington, ring forceps)
- Retractors (large, medium, small Rich retractors, bladder blade)
- Scissors (Metzenbaum, Mayo)
- Laparotomy sponges

Types of Uterine Incisions

The most common type of uterine incision is a low transverse uterine incision. Remember that the incision on the abdomen does not necessarily match the type of incision on the uterus. (This is a point that often confuses patients, medical students, and interns alike.) The type of uterine incision utilized may depend on the gestational age of the patient, the fetal lie, the location of the placenta, and the presence of uterine myomas or adhesions. Because the type of uterine incision made has implications for future pregnancies, it is important to clearly note in the operative report which type is made. Four common types of uterine incisions will be described here:

1. Low transverse
2. Low vertical
3. Classical
4. T-shaped

Low Transverse Incision (Figure 10.3a)

This is the most common uterine incision made during a cesarean section. It is used in term or near-term pregnancies with a developed lower uterine segment. The fetus may be in either a breech or a vertex presentation, and it may also be used with multiple gestations. In general, the uterine incision is repaired in two layers. The first is a running, locked suture, usually with 0-Vicryl. A second imbricating layer is then placed with a similar absorbable suture.

Subsequent pregnancies. These patients can labor with subsequent pregnancies. The risk of uterine rupture during trial of labor after cesarean (TOLAC) following one prior low transverse uterine incision is 0.2–0.9% (Cunningham *et al.* 2014).

Low Vertical Incision (Figure 10.3b)

This incision, while vertical like a classical incision, does not extend into the contractile portion of the uterus. It may be performed when one of the following situations is present:

1. Preterm fetus with an undeveloped lower uterine section
2. Anterior placenta previa
3. Scheduled cesarean hysterectomy
4. Back-down, transverse lie
5. Transverse lie with oligohydramnios
6. Myomas occupying the lower uterine segment

This type of incision is associated with increased blood loss and infection rates compared to a low transverse incision (Boyle and Gabbe 1996). While an incision may begin as a low vertical incision, it may extend spontaneously during delivery or be extended with bandage scissors if it is found not to be adequate for delivery. If this occurs, it must be clearly documented in the patient's record and the patient should not labor with her next pregnancy. Repair of this incision is done in two layers with an absorbable suture (usually 0-Vicryl).

(a)

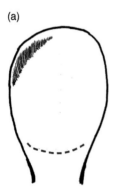

Figure 10.3a Low transverse uterine incision.

(b)

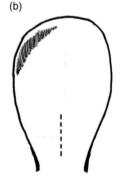

Figure 10.3b Low vertical uterine incision.

Subsequent pregnancies. These patients may be allowed to labor, although this is somewhat controversial. The risk of uterine rupture in future pregnancies is 1–7% (Cunningham *et al.* 2014).

Classical Incision (Figure 10.3c)

A classical incision extends vertically into the fundal region of the uterus. The incision is started as low as possible, but above the bladder, and then carried superiorly toward the fundus until it is large enough to allow for atraumatic delivery of the fetus. It is performed in the following situations:

1. Lower uterine segment cannot be entered because of adhesions or fibroids
2. Transverse lie with a large fetus
3. Very small fetus with a poorly developed (or very thick) lower uterine segment
4. Maternal morbid obesity where only the upper uterus can be accessed

This type of incision has to be repaired in layers because of the thickness of the tissue. The first two layers are usually closed with an absorbable suture such as 0-Vicryl. The surgical assistant helps by applying compression from the sides and trying to keep the edges closely approximated. Once the deep layers are closed, a smaller absorbable suture, often a 2-0 or 3-0 Vicryl, is used to close the uterine serosa.

Subsequent pregnancies. These patients should not be allowed to labor with subsequent pregnancies. The risk of uterine rupture in future pregnancies is 2–9% (Cunningham *et al.* 2014).

T-Shaped Incision (Figure 10.3d)

This incision is almost never made as the initial uterine incision, but rather occurs because a low transverse incision is found not to be adequate to deliver the fetus. At this point, bandage scissors are used to extend the incision upward toward the fundus from the middle of the original incision. (A variation of this is termed a J incision, in which the original incision is extended upward from one edge with bandage scissors.)

The most common reason for extending the incision in this manner is inadequate room because of fetal malpresentation or infant size. This is often chosen in place of further lateral extension, which risks involvement of the uterine vessels. Although the T-shaped incision

(c)

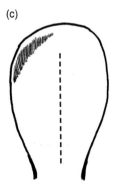

Figure 10.3c Classical uterine incision.

(d)

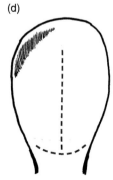

Figure 10.3d T-shaped uterine incision.

still does not pose as high a risk as a classical incision, it has been shown to be associated with higher risk of infection and blood loss, and lower 5-minute Apgar scores, when compared to the traditional low transverse incision (Patterson *et al.* 2002).

The upper portion of the incision is closed with the same technique as a classical incision, and the low transverse part as a low transverse incision.

Subsequent pregnancies. These patients should not be allowed to labor with subsequent pregnancies. The risk of uterine rupture in future pregnancies is 4–9% (Cunningham *et al.* 2014).

Potential Complications

Because a cesarean section is a laparotomy and major abdominal surgery, the patient must be counseled prior to the procedure, and you must be familiar with the incidence of potential complications that may occur. Some of the more common complications include the following:

Hemorrhage/Transfusion

Hemorrhage, which is defined as an estimated blood loss of > 1000 mL at time of cesarean section, a drop in hematocrit of 10%, or the need for a transfusion, occurs in approximately 6% of cesarean sections. This complication may occur secondary to uterine atony, abnormal placentation (e.g., placenta accreta) or laceration of blood vessels (most commonly the uterine arteries). Approximately 2–4% of women undergoing a primary cesarean section receive a blood transfusion (Hammad *et al.* 2014). This is more likely to occur when patients undergo a classical or T-shaped uterine incision.

Infection

Postoperative infections after a cesarean section usually include both wound infections and endometritis. The risk of infection depends on both the patient's individual risk factors and the circumstances surrounding the need for a cesarean section.

Maternal factors that increase the risk of a postoperative infection include the following:
1. Obesity
2. Diabetes
3. Malignancy
4. Malnutrition

Additional risk factors for postoperative infection include the following:
1. Prolonged rupture of membranes
2. Intra-amniotic infection
3. Manual removal of the placenta
4. Frequent vaginal examinations
5. Emergency cesarean section

A cesarean delivery is considered a clean-contaminated procedure and has an infection risk of up to 30% in the general population and up to 50% in morbidly obese women (Chauhan *et al.* 2001). It is important to note that the risk of postoperative infection is related to whether the patient was previously laboring or had intra-amniotic infection at the time of cesarean section. The overall incidence of wound infections after cesarean section has been reported to be approximately 4% (Chaim *et al.* 2000).

Damage to Bowel/Bladder

These complications are, fortunately, rare with cesarean section. The risk of injury is 1–3, 0.3, and 1 per 1000 for bladder, ureteral, and bowel injuries, respectively (Cunningham *et al.* 2014). Patients who have had previous abdominal surgery, severe adhesions or scarring from endometriosis or infection, or who require a cesarean hysterectomy are at increased risk of bowel or bladder injury during cesarean section. The risk of bladder injury is decreased by continuous drainage with a Foley catheter during the operation, which is why this step should always be taken, even with emergency deliveries.

Thromboembolic Disease

Deep venous thrombosis (DVT) with resultant pulmonary embolism (PE) is the leading cause of maternal mortality associated with cesarean section and is more than four times more likely to occur after cesarean section than after a vaginal delivery (Simpson *et al.* 2001). Attempts to prevent this complication include the use of pneumatic compression stockings, early ambulation after surgery, and even prophylactic anticoagulation in high-risk women.

Fascial Dehiscence

The risk of fascial dehiscence after cesarean section is approximately 0.3% (Hendrix *et al.* 2000). The most important risk factor for this complication, which occurs when the fascia comes apart after surgery and may allow protrusion of bowel through the incision, is wound infection. If a fascial dehiscence occurs, then the patient will require surgery to repair the defect.

Injury to the Baby

The uterus must be entered carefully, as it is possible to injure the fetus with the scalpel at this time. The overall incidence of this complication has been reported as between 1.1% and 1.5% (Wiener and Westwood 2002, Alexander *et al.* 2006). This risk appears to be the same regardless of the fetal presentation or whether the membranes are intact or ruptured. The type of incision may also make a difference, with fetal injury rates of 3.4% reported for a T or J incision, only 1.4% for a vertical uterine incision, and 1.1% for a low transverse incision (Alexander *et al.* 2006). If an injury does occur, it is important to inform the parents and have the pediatricians and a plastic surgeon evaluate the infant if needed.

Maternal Mortality

As with any abdominal surgery, there is a risk of maternal mortality. Even though this risk is low, especially with an elective cesarean section, it is still present and has been estimated to be approximately 2.2 per 100,000 operations for primary cesarean sections (Cunningham *et al.* 2014).

Retained Foreign Body

The risk of having a retained sponge or instrument is very low. One analysis of surgical cases over a 16-year period reported that the overall risk was between 1 in 8801 and 1 in 18,760 inpatient operations. This risk was increased if the procedure was an emergency or the patient had an elevated body mass index (Gawande *et al.* 2003). Care should be taken to ensure that counts of instruments and sponges are correct at the end of the procedure, and that if the procedure was an emergency and there was no count done, that abdominal films are done prior to completing the procedure.

Procedure

Preparing for Surgery

While the American College of Obstetricians and Gynecologists (ACOG) recommends that facilities should have the ability to perform a cesarean section within 30 minutes of the decision being made, the operation will proceed much more rapidly during an emergency, and can safely be delayed longer in non-acute situations (Berghella 2017).

Patient Counseling

After the decision has been made to perform a cesarean delivery, the patient and her partner should be counseled as to the risks and benefits of the operation, and the indications must be clearly explained. The depth of counseling will depend on the urgency of the clinical situation. For scheduled procedures, a longer explanation of the risks and benefits should occur and be documented. For emergency cases, a brief discussion of the most common potential complications (bleeding/transfusion/infection/damage to bowel or bladder) should occur. Ideally, the discussion regarding cesarean section should take place at the time of admission.

Things that should be brought up in counseling include the following:

1. Indication for the cesarean section
2. Potential complications:

   a. Hemorrhage
   b. Transfusion of blood products
   c. Damage to bowel, bladder, other abdominal organs
   d. Infection
   e. Hysterectomy
   f. Further surgery if complications occur
   g. Maternal death

A note should be made in the chart detailing the indication for the procedure as well as the fact that the patient was counseled, specifically mentioning the above elements (see Appendix B for an example).

Antibiotic Coverage

Antibiotics should be ordered and administered to the patient within 60 minutes of skin incision to decrease postoperative infection (ACOG 2011). If the cesarean section is performed as an emergency, then antibiotic coverage should be given as soon as possible following skin incision.

Options for antibiotic coverage include a first-generation cephalosporin (e.g., cephazolin), a second-generation cephalosporin, or ampicillin. Although studies have shown equal efficacy for both cephazolin and ampicillin, cephazolin's longer half-life makes it a better first-line choice. For patients with a well-documented and serious penicillin allergy, then clindamycin plus an aminoglycoside (e.g., gentamicin) is considered an appropriate option (ACOG 2011). Recent literature has recommended the addition of azithromycin 500 mg IV concurrently with standard cesarean section prophylaxis in women who undergo cesarean section during labor or after rupture of membranes (Tita *et al.* 2016).

Another consideration is patients who have been diagnosed with intra-amniotic infection (IAI). Typically, individuals who develop IAI prior to a cesarean section will have already been placed on antibiotics preoperatively, most commonly ampicillin and gentamicin. If they require a cesarean section, clindamycin should be added to the regimen (ACOG 2017a). Although the duration of treatment for IAI after delivery is debated, ACOG recommends at least one additional dose of antibiotic therapy postoperatively, with consideration of longer durations for patients with certain risk factors (ACOG 2017a).

In the Operating Room

After the patient is moved to the OR, it is important to document the fetal heart rate (FHR). In the case of fetal distress, this will help to gauge just how quickly the operation must proceed. After the FHR is documented, anesthesia is administered. In a non-emergency delivery, this usually means a spinal or epidural. This procedure will usually produce a surgical level of anesthesia in 10–20 minutes. In an emergency, general anesthesia may be given, or even IV sedation while the operation is started under local anesthesia (this technique is discussed below, under *Emergency Cesarean*).

When anesthesia has been administered, the FHR monitor is removed (if an FSE is on the fetal scalp, it is removed as well). A Foley catheter is inserted, a grounding pad is placed on the thigh, and the abdomen prepped. Additionally, new data suggest that a vaginal prep, most commonly with 10% povidone–iodine solution (Betadine), should also be performed. A systematic review and meta-analysis found that vaginal cleansing significantly decreased the risk of postpartum endometritis and fever in women undergoing cesarean section while laboring or after rupture of membranes (Caissutti *et al.* 2017). Although this study did not show a significant decrease in those women with planned cesarean section, given the low risk, vaginal cleansing should be considered in all women undergoing cesarean section.

While the aforementioned steps are being performed by the nursing staff, the surgeons scrub and gown. After the patient is prepped, the drape is placed by the surgeons and the appropriate suction and electrocautery attachments are handed off the field to be attached.

Description of the Operation

A final check is performed to ensure that anesthesia is adequate. This is usually done by grasping the skin with an Allis clamp at the level of the intended incision as well as near the umbilicus on both sides of the midline. If significant pain is experienced by the patient, then additional anesthesia is required.

Abdominal Incision

After adequate anesthesia is obtained, the skin is incised. The two main types of incisions used are the modified Pfannenstiel and the infra-umbilical vertical incision.

Modified Pfannenstiel. This is the most common incision for a cesarean section. It is a transverse, slightly curved incision made approximately two finger breadths above the superior edge of the pubic bone and extended slightly upward on either side to just past the lateral borders of the rectus muscles (Figure 10.4). It has the advantage of being stronger after repair than a vertical incision, and it usually gives a better cosmetic result as it is concealed near the hairline. The procedure for using a modified Pfannenstiel incision is as follows:

After the initial skin incision, the scalpel is used to carry the incision through the subcutaneous tissue down to the underlying fascia. The fascia is then incised in the midline and then, using Mayo scissors, the incision is extended in a transverse fashion on each side. At this point, Kocher clamps are used to grasp the superior edge of the fascia, and it is dissected off the underlying rectus muscles with sharp and blunt dissection. The inferior edges of the fascia are then grasped with Kocher clamps and dissection carried inferiorly to the symphysis. After this, the rectus muscles are separated in the midline and the underlying peritoneum is grasped with two clamps (usually either Kelly or mosquito clamps). Once the surgeon is sure there is no bowel, bladder, or other structures adherent to the peritoneum in that spot, it is incised with Metzenbaum scissors and the abdominal cavity entered.

Note: If additional room is needed for the operation, then a Pfannenstiel may be converted to a Cherney incision by sharply dissecting the tendinous insertion of the rectus abdominus muscles from their insertion into the pubic symphysis. The inferior epigastric arteries should be lateral to the insertion and do not need to be ligated. After the operation, the rectus abdominus muscles are then reattached using interrupted permanent sutures.

Vertical incision. Less often, this type of incision is used when rapid entry into the abdominal cavity is needed, such as in the case of fetal distress. It is also the preferred

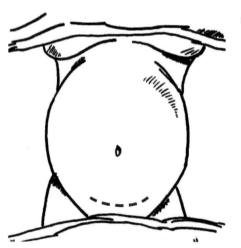

Figure 10.4 Pfannenstiel incision.

incision in patients with a coagulopathy, those who refuse transfusion, and those who are receiving systemic anticoagulation. It may also be used when the patient has had a previous vertical incision. It is usually started just below the umbilicus and extends inferiorly to approximately 2 cm above the pubic bone (Figure 10.5). The advantages of a vertical incision are that it facilitates more rapid access to the uterus, and it is associated with less blood loss and provides better exposure than a modified Pfannenstiel incision. The incision can be extended superiorly and directed around the umbilicus if additional exposure is needed. The procedure for a vertical incision is as follows:

A scalpel is used to make an incision in the midline from just below the umbilicus to approximately 2 cm above the pubic symphysis. The subcutaneous tissue is incised down to the sheath of the anterior rectus muscle. The fascia is then incised sharply with the scalpel and the incision is extended superiorly and inferiorly with either a scalpel or Mayo scissors. The rectus muscles are then split in the midline to expose the peritoneum, which is entered above the level of the bladder in the same way as previously described.

Creation of bladder flap. After the abdomen has been entered, a bladder blade is inserted to expose the lower uterine segment and the vesicouterine serosa is elevated and incised with Metzenbaum scissors in a curvilinear fashion just superior to the bladder. A clamp is then used to grasp the inferior part of the incision and a bladder flap is made bluntly, always applying pressure against the uterus and taking care not to injure the bladder anteriorly, or the blood vessels laterally. After this, the bladder blade is replaced between the newly formed bladder flap and the uterus.

Note: Creation of a bladder flap is often left up to surgeon preference. A randomized controlled trial evaluated outcomes following creation of bladder flap versus no bladder flap and found that creation of a bladder flap resulted in a longer incision-to-delivery interval without decreasing the risk of intraoperative or postoperative complications. This trial, however, did not look at long-term effects such as adhesions or bladder function, and therefore the decision to create a bladder flap should be determined on a case by case basis (Dahlke *et al.* 2013).

Figure 10.5 Vertical abdominal incision.

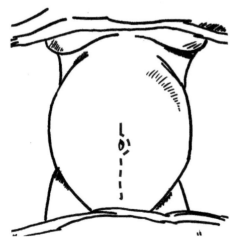

Uterine Incision

Prior to making the uterine incision, it is important to palpate the uterus to determine if it is significantly rotated. Assessing this will help prevent making an incision that is too lateral and should decrease the risk of extension into the uterine arteries. The uterus is then incised approximately 2–4 cm in a transverse direction in the center of the exposed lower uterine segment (other types of uterine incisions are discussed above). The incision site is then suctioned and palpated after each pass with the scalpel. This is done so that the fetus is not accidentally injured with entry into the uterine cavity. (If you get to the level of the membranes, then you can extend your incision with the membranes intact if desired.) After the uterine cavity is entered, with or without the membranes intact, the incision can be extended either sharply, with bandage scissors, or bluntly, with two fingers inserted into the uterus and traction exerted upward and slightly laterally. It is important that you pull in a mostly vertical/cephalad direction rather than laterally, as this has been shown to decrease the risk of extension of the incision into the lateral uterine vessels (Dahlke *et al.* 2013). While sharp extension is needed at times with an unlabored lower uterine segment, well-designed trials have shown that sharp extension is associated with increased blood loss; therefore, when possible, blunt extension of the uterine incision should be performed (Dahlke *et al.* 2013). The key in extending the uterine incision is to ensure you do not extend laterally into the uterine vessels.

It is also important to remember that with ruptured membranes or oligohydramnios, there may be very little fluid between the uterus and baby. In this case, you must take extra care not to injure the baby with the scalpel as you make your uterine incision.

Delivery of the Infant

The technique for this depends on the presentation of the fetus.

Vertex presentation. After the uterine incision has been extended, the surgeon's hand is inserted with fingers extended into the uterus inferior to the fetal head. (If the patient has been pushing prior to the operation, then an assistant may need to push the fetal head cephalad by inserting a hand into the vagina.) Once the fetal head is brought to the level of the hysterotomy, a moderate amount of fundal pressure is applied with either the surgeon's other hand or from an assistant, and the fetal head is gently brought through the uterine incision. The remainder of the infant body is then delivered using maneuvers similar to that of a vaginal delivery. Upon delivery of the infant, the umbilical cord is doubly clamped and cut and the infant handed off the field to the pediatricians.*

Breech presentation. The operator's hand is inserted in the same fashion as for a vertex presentation. The fetal buttocks are then elevated through the uterine incision, again with the assistance of a moderate amount of fundal pressure. The legs are delivered one at a time by splinting the fetal thigh with the fingers parallel to the femur and then sweeping the leg away from the midline. (If the fetus is in a footling breech position, then the feet are grasped and are then delivered through the incision to the level of the fetal back.) After this, the lower body of the fetus is rotated to a sacrum anterior position

---

* ACOG now recommends delayed cord clamping for 30–60 seconds upon delivery of the infant, for both vaginal and cesarean deliveries (ACOG 2017b). However, if the infant is in need of immediate resuscitation or the mother is hemorrhaging or hemodynamically unstable, then the umbilical cord should be immediately clamped and cut to provide the proper care to the mother and/or her infant.

if it is not already there and wrapped in a sterile blue towel. The infant is then delivered to the level of the scapula by gently rotating the trunk back and forth. The infant is then rotated so that one shoulder is superior, and that arm is then delivered by first splinting the arm with the fingers parallel to the humerus, and then sweeping it downward. The infant is then rotated to the other side, and the procedure repeated. After this, a Mauriceau–Smellie–Veit maneuver is performed, where the index and middle finger of one hand are placed on the fetal maxilla in order to flex the head and complete the delivery.*

Transverse presentation. When a fetus is in a transverse position, some thought must be given to what type of uterine incision will be made prior to beginning the operation. In general, a back-down transverse lie is an indication for a vertical uterine incision, as it can be very difficult or impossible to grasp the fetal feet through a low transverse incision with this presentation. If a transverse lie is present, then an intraoperative abdominal version may be attempted in order to allow a low transverse uterine incision to be made. This is performed in a similar manner to an external cephalic version (see Chapter 2). However, if this is not successful, or if the operator does not wish to attempt the maneuver, it is usually better to initially make a low vertical incision rather than be forced to convert a low transverse incision to a T- or J-shaped incision.

Delivery of the Placenta

After the infant has been delivered, the umbilical cord is doubly clamped and ligated and the infant is given to the waiting pediatrician. At this time the placenta is delivered, either by manual extraction or spontaneously with gentle traction on the cord. A prospective randomized study reported that the incidence of postoperative endometritis is significantly higher when the placenta is manually removed, so if it will deliver with simple traction on the cord, this is preferred (Berghella *et al.* 2005). In addition, blood loss is also significantly less when cord traction and oxytocin are used when compared to manual removal (Berghella *et al.* 2005).

Repair of the Uterus

After the placenta is removed, the uterus is exteriorized onto the abdomen and a laparotomy sponge can be used to clear all clots and debris from inside the uterus if desired. It is easier to hold the uterus in this position with a moist laparotomy tape draped over the fundus.

While you can repair a uterus without exteriorizing it, this step gives you better visualization and can allow you to notice uterine atony more quickly. If there is an extension of the uterine incision laterally, then you must exteriorize the uterus to determine how far the extension goes. Recent meta-analyses have shown that there is no statistically significant difference in febrile complications, surgical time, or intraoperative nausea, vomiting, or pain between the two types of closure; therefore, decision to exteriorize should be left up to the clinical judgment of the surgeon (Dahlke *et al.* 2013, Zaphiratos *et al.* 2015). There will be some cases where the uterus cannot be exteriorized because of adhesions or fibroids, which is why you must know your anatomy in order to prevent injury of the uterine vessels or ureters during your repair.

---

* The maneuvers to deliver a breech presentation during a cesarean section are the same as with a breech vaginal delivery, as described and illustrated in Chapter 14.

After the placenta is removed, clamps (which may be ring forceps, Pennington clamps, or Allis clamps) are placed at the lateral edges of the uterine incision, as well as at any point where there is significant bleeding along the incision. The incision is then closed with one or two layers of a locked, continuous #0 or #1 absorbable suture, most commonly either polyglactin (Vicryl) or chromic. Additional interrupted sutures (usually figure-of-eight) are thrown as necessary for hemostasis. After the uterus is repaired and good hemostasis is noted, the uterus, fallopian tubes, and ovaries are inspected and then replaced into the abdomen.

Data concerning single-layer versus double-layered uterine closure are somewhat inconsistent. While some studies have shown a significantly reduced risk of uterine rupture following double-layer closure, others have found no such difference. Given the somewhat inconsistent data and the minimal increase in operating time with a double-layer closure, most surgeons will perform a double-layer closure in women who desire future fertility and a single-layer closure for those women who are done with childbearing.

If a vertical incision is used on the uterus, then the repair is performed in several layers with the same types of sutures to reapproximate the incision. This will usually require two or three layers, and it is made easier if the assistant can compress the uterus with each throw to keep the two edges close together and prevent the suture from tearing through. After the muscular part of the uterus is together, the serosa is repaired in a running fashion with a smaller suture, such as a 3–0 Vicryl.

Closure of the Abdomen

With the uterus back in the abdomen, the incision is again visualized to ensure hemostasis. The gutters are irrigated and cleared of all clots and debris. Prior to closing the fascia, the scrub nurse should notify you that the sponge and instrument count is correct. If the count is incorrect, you must find the missing item. If the procedure was an emergency and therefore no count was performed, then radiology should be called in order to perform portable films of the abdomen. You should have these results before proceeding with closure of the abdomen.

Just as creation of a bladder flap may be controversial among providers, closure of a bladder flap is also a topic of debate. Although some feel that closure will decrease bladder adhesions for future surgeries, there is not convincing evidence for this, and a small study even showed it may result in more adhesion formation (Lyell *et al.* 2012). Ultimately, since data are lacking, the decision to create and close the bladder flap is ultimately left up to the surgeon. One important thing to note is that a bladder flap should be avoided if the patient has significant coagulopathy or disseminated intravascular coagulation (DIC), since there is a risk of creating a potential space for bladder hematoma formation. If one does wish to close the bladder flap, this is often done with 2–0 or 3–0 Vicryl or chromic in a running fashion.

In general, the peritoneum is not closed or reapproximated. While some physicians do prefer to close the peritoneum with a running suture of 2–0 or 3–0 Vicryl or chromic, data concerning outcomes of peritoneal closure versus non-closure are also inconsistent. A randomized controlled trial in 2012 found no difference in adhesion formation between closure and non-closure groups during subsequent repeat cesarean section (Kapustian *et al.* 2012). In contrast, a meta-analysis did show that peritoneal closure was associated with significantly less adhesion formation during subsequent surgery. Of note, this meta-analysis was not performed to evaluate peritoneal closure outcomes, but was merely a secondary analysis (Dahlke *et al.* 2013). It is important to note that non-closure is associated with shorter operating time, reduced hospital stay, and less postoperative fever (Dahlke *et al.* 2013). Therefore, it is up to the surgeon to weigh the risks of closure against the potential benefits.

If there is significant diastasis of the rectus abdominis muscles, some surgeons will place a few interrupted sutures of 2–0 chromic or Vicryl to reapproximate them in the midline. These throws are not tied tightly, as they are for reapproximation and not hemostasis. One secondary analysis did show that closure of the rectus muscles resulted in a decrease in dense adhesion formation (Lyell *et al.* 2012).

The fascia is then closed with a running suture of either a permanent or delayed-absorbable type.

Many surgeons prefer to use Vicryl for primary cesarean sections and either a delayed-absorbable monofilament suture such as PDS (polydiaxanone) or a permanent monofilament suture like polypropylene for repeat operations, vertical incisions, or other patients at increased risk for fascial dehiscence. After this, the subcutaneous tissue is irrigated with sterile water and any bleeding is stopped using electrocautery.

If the subcutaneous tissue is 2 cm or more in thickness, then closure is recommended (Dahlke *et al.* 2013). This may be performed in a running or interrupted fashion using 2–0 or 3–0 Vicryl. Of note, the placement of a subcutaneous drain has not been shown to reduce wound morbidity and is therefore not recommended regardless of tissue thickness.

The skin is then closed with either a subcuticular suture or staples, and as neither has been shown to be definitively superior the decision is left up to the surgeon (Dahlke *et al.* 2013). If subcuticular suture is chosen, 4–0 Monocryl is typically the suture of choice. A randomized controlled trial looking at subcuticular skin closure at the time of cesarean section found that Monocryl was associated with a decreased rate of wound complications when compared to Vicryl (Buresch *et al.* 2017).

Completing the Operation

After the skin is closed, the drapes are removed, the grounding pad taken off, and a vaginal exam performed to clear all clots from the uterus and vagina while the other hand massages the uterine fundus. This allows the operator to assess uterine tone. The patient is then transferred to a bed and taken to the recovery room.

A thorough "talk-through" of a cesarean section is included in Appendix C, which explains in detail every step performed and instrument used during a cesarean section. In conjunction with the above description of the operation, this will allow you to run through the procedure in your mind, focusing on what the next step is and what instruments you need to request.

Approach to Intraoperative Hemorrhage

This complication may occur secondary to uterine atony, abnormal placental implantation (e.g., placenta accreta), or laceration of blood vessels (most commonly the uterine arteries). Postpartum hemorrhage occurs in approximately 6% of cesarean deliveries. The risk of hemorrhage is higher with a classical or T-shaped uterine incision as compared to the more common low transverse incision.

The approach to stopping hemorrhage depends on the etiology of the hemorrhage. In general, bleeding will initially occur as a result of either uterine atony or extension of the uterine incision into other vessels, such as the uterine arteries.

Another consideration for hemorrhage is the onset of DIC, which may occur after a substantial blood loss has already occurred. If this is the case, then transfusion of blood products will be required to allow the patient to form clots in order to stop the bleeding.

Estimation of Blood Loss (EBL)

Deciding how much blood has been lost during a cesarean section is a very difficult thing to do, especially when there is a significant amount of amniotic fluid. In general, average blood loss at the time of a cesarean section is around 1000 mL. It is, however, possible to get a slightly better estimate when you consider the following rules of thumb:

- Make sure and tell the anesthesia provider when you are irrigating, so this fluid does not get counted in the EBL.
- Look at how much blood is in the suction, and then try to account for and subtract the amount of amniotic fluid (this will be an estimate).
- Count the laparotomy sponges and estimate the blood loss based on how much you see on each one (Table 10.1).

Lacerations

Bleeding from lacerations will generally be seen from the uterine incision or laterally if it extends into the uterine vessels.

Uterine Incision

If the bleeding is coming from the uterine incision, then you can place Pennington clamps on the edges where the vessels are bleeding the most while you prepare to close the incision. This will decrease your blood loss and allow you better visualization for the repair.

Uterine Arteries

If the bleeding appears arterial in nature and your incision extended laterally into the uterine artery, then you will need to perform an O'Leary stitch in order to stop the bleeding. To do this, first palpate the vessel inferior to where the bleeding is coming from, then use a 0-Vicryl suture and, going anterior to posterior, insert the needle into the broad ligament approximately 1 cm lateral to the vessel and then bring it through medially to where it exits in the uterine tissue (Figure 10.6). This is usually done with a single pass and not a figure-of-eight because the ureter runs about 2 cm lateral to the uterine artery and you must take care not to injure it.

Uterine Atony

This is the most common cause of bleeding at the time of a cesarean section. When this occurs, you should first administer medications in the same manner that you would if you had a postpartum hemorrhage after a vaginal delivery (see *Postpartum Hemorrhage* in

Table 10.1 Estimation of blood loss

	% Sponge covered	Amount of blood
Standard 18 × 18 surgical laparotomy sponge*	50%	25 mL
	75%	50 mL
	100%	75 mL
	100% + dripping	100 mL

* (Dildy *et al.* 2004)

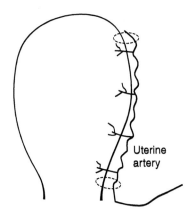

Figure 10.6 Uterine artery ligation and high uterine artery ligation.

Uterine artery

Chapter 14). If medications fail to improve the uterine tone and bleeding, then you may have to move on to the surgical methods listed below.

Surgical treatment of hemorrhage due to uterine atony is meant first to decrease the pulse pressure of the blood flow to the uterus and second to mechanically compress the uterus and stop the bleeding. A general order in which interventions are done is as follows:

1. **Bilateral O'Leary stitches.** These are performed as described above, but the sutures are thrown at the level of the internal cervical os. Remember this is a mass ligature and you do not need to dissect into the broad ligament to define the space you will be putting the stitch. This technique is effective in stopping hemorrhage in approximately 75% of cases. It must be done bilaterally, and care must be taken to avoid the ureters (Figure 10.6).
2. **Bilateral ovarian artery ligation.** A single suture of 0-Vicryl is thrown at the anastomosis of the ovarian and uterine vessels near the utero-ovarian ligament (Figure 10.6).
3. **Hypogastric artery ligation.** You will see many textbooks describe a technique where you can enter the retroperitoneum and divide the anterior division of the hypogastric artery. In practice, however, this has not been shown to be effective in most cases of postpartum hemorrhage.

4. **B-Lynch suture.** This intervention is an attempt to mechanically compress the uterus. While the original technique describes this being done with the uterine incision still open, it can be accomplished after the incision is closed. In practice, the uterine incision is almost always already closed when the suture is placed.

   A 0-chromic suture is used and inserted below the uterine incision at one of the lateral edges, then exits just above the incision. It is taken over the top of the uterus and then a horizontal suture is thrown on the posterior uterus. The suture is then brought back over the top of the uterus on the opposite side and inserted above the uterine incision on the opposite side the stitch was started, to exit below the incision. The assistant then compresses the uterus while the surgeon ties down the suture, which will keep the uterus in this position. See Figure 10.7 for an example of what this will look like.

   This technique is relatively easy to perform, with an overall success rate of approximately 75% (Cunningham *et al.* 2014).

5. **Hysterectomy.** If all other treatments (medications and sutures) have failed and the patient continues to bleed and becomes hemodynamically unstable, then you may have to proceed with a hysterectomy as a life-saving option. The technique for a cesarean hysterectomy is very similar to when the patient is not pregnant. Differences include the fact that the lateral vessels are engorged and often more difficult to adequately clamp. A supracervical hysterectomy is often performed, since, especially if the patient was in advanced labor, it may be difficult to identify the entire cervix and avoid the ureters.

Blood products may also be required during a postpartum hemorrhage to stabilize the patient. The specific blood products and recommendations for giving them can be found in Chapter 14.

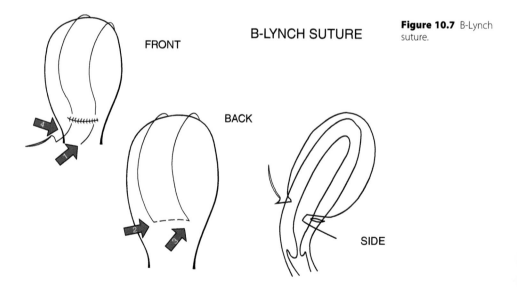

B-LYNCH SUTURE

FRONT

BACK

SIDE

Figure 10.7 B-Lynch suture.

Emergency Cesarean Section

A true emergency cesarean section is one that must be performed within minutes because of a potential life-threatening situation for the mother, the fetus, or both. When a true emergency exists, the baby can be delivered in under a minute from the time you make your incision. The delay that usually exists, therefore, is in making the decision and then transitioning the patient to the operating room and obtaining adequate anesthesia.

Potential Indications

An emergency cesarean section may be performed for either maternal or fetal indications, or for a combination. Some possible situations where an emergency cesarean section may be indicated include:

Fetal:

- Prolonged fetal bradycardia
- Umbilical cord prolapse

Maternal:

- Amniotic fluid embolism
- Myocardial infarction

Combined:

- Uterine rupture
- Hemorrhage (placental abruption/vasa previa/placenta previa)
- Trauma

Prevention

The best way to avoid an emergency cesarean section is to monitor any concerning FHR tracings closely so that you may intervene in such a manner as to prevent the situation from becoming a true emergency. While this will help you avoid an emergency cesarean in many cases, it will not help in those that do not have any specific warning signs, such as an amniotic fluid embolism or trauma.

Treatment

A well-rehearsed plan will help you to perform a rapid and safe emergency cesarean section.

Initial Actions

Take a quick moment and begin by considering your options.

1. **Determine the level of fetal/maternal distress.** If there is mild to moderate distress, then you may attempt conservative maneuvers (maternal position changes, administration of O_2 or terbutaline) as appropriate. If there is severe distress, or the mild/moderate distress worsens or does not respond to conservative maneuvers, then prompt intervention is required.

2. **Call for assistance.** When you have determined that an emergency cesarean delivery is indicated, alert the following personnel:
   - Staff provider
   - Anesthesia support
   - Nursing staff
   - OR technician
   - Pediatricians

3. **Counsel patient and family.** Briefly counsel the patient and her family on the need and indications for an emergency delivery while continuing to prepare to move the patient to the operating room.

4. **Unhook all monitors and the bed.** This step is often overlooked and results in a delay as the cables become entwined on something and are pulled out of the wall as you exit the room.

5. **Prep and scrub.** As the patient is coming out of the room, run ahead to the OR and make sure your gloves are out, and if they are not, then get them out. Tell the nurse to place a Foley and perform a very rapid prep (splashing the abdomen versus a quick scrub, as time permits). After making sure the patient is in the OR and on the operating table, quickly scrub for the procedure.

6. **Recheck the fetal heart rate before prepping the patient.** There are times when the FHR will have recovered, and then you can make the decision whether or not to proceed with the cesarean section or if you can wait. If it has recovered, then at least you can proceed in a more controlled manner and are more likely to be able to use conduction anesthesia rather than general anesthesia.

Anesthesia

The anesthesia provider should be one of the first people to arrive when an emergency cesarean section needs to be performed. Unless the patient has an extremely dense epidural, it is unlikely that time will permit you the 10–15 minutes needed to obtain an adequate level for the procedure. Although past data have indicated substantially higher maternal death rates associated with general versus neuraxial anesthesia, more recent literature has shown that the case-fatality rates have increased for neuraxial anesthesia and decreased for general anesthesia over time, with an overall non-significant difference between the two (Hawkins *et al.* 2011). Despite the recent data, it is important to keep in mind the other potential risks associated with general anesthesia, which include the potential for greater blood loss, early neonatal depression, and postoperative pain. Another key point to bear in mind is that the most common cause of general anesthesia-related death is secondary to failed intubation, which is 10-fold higher in pregnant women than in the non-pregnant population (Cunningham *et al.* 2014).

If, for whatever reason, there is a significant delay in obtaining an adequate level or administering a general anesthesia and there is severe fetal distress, the cesarean section can be started under local anesthesia. A dilute solution of lidocaine with epinephrine is prepared and injected. Typically, the solution is prepared by diluting 30 mL of 2% lidocaine with 1/200,000 epinephrine in 60 mL of normal saline. A total of 100–120 mL of the dilute solution is then injected along the intended skin incision, subcutaneous tissue, rectus sheath, and muscle. The surgeon should avoid injecting large volumes into the relatively nerve-free fatty tissue or otherwise risk increasing the total dose of anesthetic used (Cunningham *et al.* 2014). Obviously, it is often difficult to precisely measure solutions/dilutions during an emergency situation, and different sources may reference slightly different dilutions, but the key point is to remember not to exceed the maximum doses of each local anesthetic, which are listed in Table 10.2.

Operation

While the operation is the same as a routine cesarean section after the baby is delivered, the abdominal incision technique and entry into the abdomen are modified slightly.

Foley catheter placement. Make sure the OR nurse has placed a Foley catheter, even if this is being done while you make your incision. This will help to decrease the risk of bladder injury.

Choice of abdominal incision. After obtaining adequate anesthesia, make your abdominal incision. Your choices are either a Pfannenstiel or a vertical incision. The classic teaching is that a vertical incision is faster and associated with less blood loss. If the patient has had no previous abdominal surgery, however, it is usually just as quick, for most surgeons, to perform a transverse (Pfannenstiel) incision.

Initial incision. Make the initial incision deeper than normal, with the goal being to cut through all of the subcutaneous tissue and make your fascial incision with one, or at most two, passes with the scalpel.

Fascia. Once the fascia has been incised in the midline, you may perform a fascial "rip," where you simply place your fingers under the fascia on either side of the midline and then spread laterally. If this is too difficult, you may use pickups and Mayo scissors to incise the fascia as you normally do, just very quickly. In general, you will skip the step of placing Kocher clamps on the fascia and separating the underlying rectus muscles. (Note: when you dictate this part of the procedure, you should state that "the fascial incision was extended bluntly" rather than "a fascial rip technique was used.")

Entry into the abdomen. Bluntly separate the rectus abdominus muscles in the midline and then spread the peritoneum laterally with your fingers as superiorly as possible to minimize the risk of bladder injury, and enter the peritoneal cavity. If there are significant adhesions, you may or may not have time to dissect them away prior to entry into the peritoneum.

Bladder flap. As mentioned previously, surgeon preference determines whether a bladder flap will be created. This step may be skipped if the maternal or fetal situation is extremely emergent. However, if done very quickly, creation of a bladder flap will only take a few seconds.

Uterine incision. You will make the same type of uterine incision as during a routine cesarean section, i.e., a low transverse incision at term, and a classical incision for a significantly preterm fetus or back-down transverse presentation. (Take a deep breath when you get to the uterus and remember **not** to cut the baby!) After you have entered the

Table 10.2 Maximum doses of local anesthetics

Local anesthetic	Without epinephrine	With epinephrine
Lidocaine	5 mg/kg	7 mg/kg
Bupivacaine	3 mg/kg	3 mg/kg
Ropivacaine	2 mg/kg	2 mg/kg

(Adapted from ACOG 2017c)

uterine cavity, spread the incision with your fingers bluntly or with bandage scissors if necessary, and deliver the baby.

After delivery. After the baby is delivered, make sure to collect a segment of the cord for gases, then remove the placenta and inspect the following structures very carefully:

1. Uterus. Look for evidence of extension of the uterine incision as well as at the posterior side of the uterus to ensure the posterior wall is intact and was not injured or perforated during the delivery.

2. Bladder. Make sure you can clearly see where the bladder begins, so that you do not accidentally injure it during the uterine repair. Sometimes you will have to create a small bladder flap after the delivery to allow you to repair the uterine incision.

3. Intestines. Look to make sure there is no bowel in your field. If you see anything that resembles stool, it is a wise idea to run the bowel to look for evidence of injury.

After you have evaluated the above structures, you can proceed with your repair of the uterine incision. At this time, you should do the following:

1. Antibiotics. Make sure the anesthesia provider either has administered or is administering antibiotics, usually a cephalosporin, as the risk of infection is higher in patients undergoing an emergency procedure.

2. Call for x-ray. You will almost never get a count of instruments prior to starting an emergency cesarean section. Therefore, when you are closing the uterine incision, call to have x-ray come up. They will need to do a portable film of the abdomen and pelvis prior to closure of the fascia or at least before closing the skin. (Staples can potentially interfere with the interpretation of the film.) Make sure that you send someone with the film so that they can have the radiologist read it quickly. It is important to explain to them that you are attempting to rule out any retained instruments/sponges and that the patient is under anesthesia on the operating table so they cannot leave until the film is clear. A study by Gawande *et al.* (2003) reported that risk factors for retained instruments or sponges included an emergency procedure and an increased BMI.

Postoperatively

After the procedure, review the indications as well as how the operation went with the family. Make sure that your written and dictated operative notes are accurate, and note that the x-ray was negative for any retained instruments and sponges. Be very clear on the type of uterine incision that was made and any implications it has for future pregnancies. Also, try and dictate the operative report as soon as possible after the procedure. When writing postoperative orders, take into consideration the following:

1. **Antibiotics.** Continue antibiotics for 24–48 hours postoperatively, usually a cephalosporin, or, if the patient had intra-amniotic infection prior to the procedure, expand the coverage to triples (ampicillin/gentamicin/clindamycin).

2. **Feeding.** If you had to run the patient's bowel, then plan to advance the diet more slowly and monitor closely for evidence of a postoperative ileus.

3. **Pain control.** If the procedure was performed under general or local anesthesia, then postoperative pain control may become an issue. For these patients, patient-controlled analgesia (PCA) with hydromorphone or morphine may be a good option for postoperative pain control.

Postpartum

When seeing the patient postpartum, be vigilant for evidence of infection, both endometritis and wound infections, and have a low threshold to treat the patient or change antibiotics as needed.

Vaginal Birth After Cesarean (VBAC)

Brief History

Whereas women who had cesarean sections were told in the past that every subsequent delivery had to be by cesarean delivery, this began to change in the 1970s. As obstetric care for both the mother and infant improved, the VBAC rate in the United States, which was only 3% in 1981, increased significantly, with 27% of women with a previous cesarean delivery attempting VBAC in 1995 (Curtin 1997). However, because of the increasingly publicized cases of uterine rupture and more study into which patients are good candidates for VBAC, the rate of patients attempting VBAC subsequently decreased to only 8.5% (ACOG 2010).

Benefits of VBAC

Women who have a successful vaginal delivery after a cesarean section have less blood loss, fewer transfusions, fewer infections, a shorter recovery time and hospital stay, and usually no increased perinatal morbidity when compared to women who undergo cesarean delivery (ACOG 2009). Some women also feel that their previous cesarean section was a sign they "failed" in their task of having a normal delivery. The risk of postpartum infection and complications is also much lower in these patients, although their counterparts who undergo a repeat cesarean section are not at risk of the significant vaginal and anal sphincter lacerations that may occur during a vaginal delivery (see Chapter 11).

From a purely economic perspective, the prevention of a single major adverse neonatal outcome by performing a repeat cesarean section rather than attempting a VBAC requires 1591 cesarean deliveries at a cost of 2.4 million dollars by some estimates (Grobman *et al.* 2000).

Candidates

ACOG recommends that the following criteria be met before a patient is allowed to attempt a VBAC:

- History of only one or two previous low transverse cesarean deliveries
- No history of uterine rupture or other uterine scars or surgery (e.g., myomectomy with entry into the uterine cavity)
- Physician available during active labor to perform emergency cesarean if indicated
- Anesthesia support and facilities for emergency cesarean

Other patients for whom VBAC is controversial, but still considered acceptable in some institutions, include the following:

- Unknown uterine scar type
- Twin gestation
- Post-term pregnancy
- Suspected macrosomia
- History of a low vertical uterine incision

When you encounter patients such as these who desire VBAC, it is important to consult with their attending physician, as different staff will have different comfort levels with these patients.

Contraindications

Because of the serious complications, such as uterine rupture, that can occur while attempting a VBAC, patients with any of the following conditions should be delivered by repeat cesarean section:

- Prior classical uterine incision
- History of a T- or J-shaped uterine incision (see *Types of Uterine Incisions*, above)
- History of uterine surgery with entrance into the uterine cavity (e.g., during myomectomy)
- Medical or obstetric complications (maternal or fetal) that make vaginal delivery contraindicated
- Lack of facilities, physicians, and/or anesthesia support to perform an emergency cesarean section for fetal distress

Patient Counseling

Because there are risks associated with attempting a VBAC that can result in fetal distress, emergency surgery, and even hysterectomy, a specific counseling note should be placed on the patient's chart when she is admitted in labor. The counseling note should include the following items:

- The patient has been offered the option of a repeat cesarean section and she desires to attempt a VBAC.
- Risks of VBAC and uterine rupture have been discussed, as well as the potential complications of a cesarean section (as listed earlier in this chapter).
- It is also important to note in the chart that the risk of postpartum endometritis after a cesarean section during labor is slightly higher than with a primary cesarean section, and that this was explained to the patient.

A sample form for this counseling is located in Appendix B.

While the list of possible complications sounds horrible, remember that the incidence of any of these events is still very small. It is usually reassuring to the patient if you explain that they are rare occurrences and can comment on the general percentages mentioned previously.

Success Rates

Depending on the reference cited, overall VBAC success rates are reported to be between 60% and 80%. Patients who had their first cesarean for an indication such as fetal distress or malpresentation are more likely to be successful in their VBAC attempt than those who had a cesarean for arrest of descent (ACOG 2010). Factors that decrease the chances of a successful VBAC include labor augmentation or induction, maternal obesity, and fetal macrosomia. Several different VBAC success calculators may now be found online. They take into consideration factors such as maternal age, indication for prior cesarean section, ethnicity, and history of prior vaginal deliveries, among other things, that may ultimately affect the patient's success, and then calculate a relative VBAC success rate. These calculators may be helpful when determining whether a patient is a candidate for TOLAC as well as properly counseling a patient on her likely success rate. The Maternal–Fetal Medicine Units Network has an online VBAC calculator at https://mfmunetwork.bsc.gwu.edu/PublicBSC/MFMU/VGBirthCalc/vagbirth.html.

Labor Management

Because even those patients with a low transverse incision have up to a 1.5% chance of uterine rupture, their care in labor is slightly different than a patient who has never undergone a cesarean.

Initial evaluation. Once labor has started, the patient should be evaluated promptly, with most authorities recommending the use of continuous electronic fetal monitoring (ACOG 2010). Although some providers recommend early "internalization" with a fetal scalp electrode (FSE) and intrauterine pressure catheter (IUPC), there are no current data that suggest that these forms are superior to external monitoring (ACOG 2010). These patients require prompt attention and evaluation if any signs or symptoms of uterine rupture occur (see *Uterine Rupture* in Chapter 14).

Labor induction. Although labor induction is associated with decreased VBAC success rates when compared to spontaneous labor, induction is still an option. Induction of labor in VBAC patients can be done using several different methods. Most often, mechanical cervical dilators or oxytocin are chosen. It is important to note that misoprostol (prostaglandin E1) should **not** be used for induction or augmentation of labor in patients with a previous cesarean section or other scar on their uterus, as this significantly increases their risk of uterine rupture (ACOG 2009, 2010). Data on the risk of uterine rupture following induction with dinoprostone (prostaglandin E2) are limited. However, the prescription pamphlet of brand-name dinoprostone, Cervidil, explicitly states that the medication is contraindicated in patients in whom "prolonged contraction of the uterus may be detrimental to fetal safety or uterine integrity, such as previous cesarean section or uterine surgery (given the potential risk for uterine rupture and associated obstetrical complications, including the need for hysterectomy and the occurrence of fetal or neonatal death)."

Labor augmentation. In general, it appears that augmentation of labor using oxytocin is safe in patients attempting VBAC. Given the limited data with inconsistent outcomes and the overall low risk of uterine rupture with oxytocin augmentation, ACOG does support the use of oxytocin augmentation in TOLAC patients (ACOG 2010). It is important to note, however, that there appears to be a "dose response effect" where higher maximum doses of oxytocin are associated with increased risk of uterine rupture (ACOG 2010).

Anesthesia. Patients attempting VBAC should be allowed to have an epidural for pain control if desired. An epidural will not mask signs and symptoms of uterine rupture.

Providers should be aware that the first sign of uterine rupture is usually fetal distress and not maternal discomfort.

Potential Complications of VBAC

Uterine Rupture

The most serious complication that can occur during a TOLAC is uterine rupture. It is important to note for documentation purposes that a uterine rupture is different from a uterine dehiscence. Uterine rupture implies a complete opening in the uterus with at least part of the fetus being outside of the uterus, while dehiscence means there is at least a layer of serosa intact and the fetus remains in the uterine cavity. While many studies group these together, each should be documented accurately in the chart should they occur.

The risk of uterine rupture depends on the type of uterine incision that was made previously, as rupture of an unscarred uterus is extremely rare. Approximate risks of uterine rupture for different incisions are shown in Table 10.3.

If a patient has had a previous uterine rupture, then the risk of uterine rupture in subsequent pregnancies is reported to be between 6% and 32% depending on whether the initial rupture involved the lower uterine segment or the upper portion of the uterus, respectively (ACOG 2010).

It is also important to take into account when the patient's previous cesarean section was performed. A study of over 2400 women undergoing VBAC trials found that the risk of uterine rupture was three times higher in women whose VBAC trial was within 18 months of a prior cesarean section (Shipp *et al.* 2001). While the overall risk for these women was still low, at 2.25%, this is still higher than would be expected for a previous low transverse uterine incision and should be taken into consideration.

The clinical presentation of uterine rupture, as well as the management, can be found in Chapter 14, *Common Obstetric Complications and Emergencies*.

Repeat Cesarean Section

Even though the overall success rate for women attempting VBAC is excellent, there will still be some 20–40% of patients who will require a repeat cesarean section for

Table 10.3 Risk of uterine rupture associated with different uterine incisions

Incision	Incidence of uterine rupture
Low transverse incision	
• One prior	0.2–0.9%
• Multiple prior	0.9–1.8%
Low vertical incision	1–7%
Classical uterine incision	2–9%
T-shaped incision	4–9%
(Cunningham *et al.* 2014)	

a variety of indications. It is important to properly counsel your patients that although a successful VBAC conveys less risk than an elective repeat cesarean section, a failed TOLAC is associated with greater risk than an elective repeat cesarean section (ACOG 2010).

References

ACOG (2009). Induction of labor. *ACOG Practice Bulletin* **#107**, August 2009, reaffirmed 2016.

ACOG (2010). Vaginal birth after previous cesarean delivery. ACOG Practice Bulletin #115. *Obstet Gynecol* **116**: 450–63.

ACOG (2011). Use of prophylactic antibiotics in labor and delivery. ACOG Practice Bulletin #120. *Obstet Gynecol* **117**: 1472–83.

ACOG (2016a). Gynecologic care for women and adolescents with human immunodeficiency virus. ACOG Practice Bulletin #167. *Obstet Gynecol* **128**: e89–110.

ACOG (2016b). Fetal macrosomia. ACOG Practice Bulletin No. 173. *Obstet Gynecol* **128**: e195–209.

ACOG (2017a). Intrapartum management of intraamniotic infection. ACOG Committee Opinion #712. *Obstet Gynecol* **130**: e95–101.

ACOG (2017b). Delayed umbilical cord clamping after birth. ACOG Committee Opinion #684. *Obstet Gynecol* **129**: e5–10.

ACOG (2017c). Obstetric analgesia and anesthesia. ACOG Practice Bulletin #177. *Obstet Gynecol* **129**: e73–89.

Alexander JM, Levno KJ, Hauth J, *et al.* (2006). Fetal injury associated with cesarean delivery. *Obstet Gynecol* **108**: 885–90.

Berghella V (2017). Cesarean delivery: preoperative planning and patient preparation. *UpToDate.* www.uptodate.com/contents/cesarean-delivery-preoperative-planning-and-patient-preparation (accessed May 2018).

Berghella V, Baxter JK, Chauhan SP (2005). Evidence-based surgery for cesarean delivery. *Am J Obstet Gynecol* **193**: 1607–17.

Boyle JG, Gabbe SG (1996). T and J vertical extensions in low transverse cesarean births. *Obstet Gynecol* **87**: 238–43.

Buresch AM, Arsdale AV, Ferzli M, *et al.* (2017). Comparison of subcuticular suture type for skin closure after cesarean delivery. *Obstet Gynecol* **130**: 521–6.

Caissutti C, Saccone G, Zullo F, *et al.* (2017). Vaginal cleansing before cesearan delivery. *Obstet Gynecol* **130**: 527–38.

Chaim W, Bashiri A, Bar-David J, Shoham-Vardi I, Mazor M (2000). Prevalence and clinical significance of postpartum endometritis and wound infection. *Infect Dis Obstet Gynecol* **8**: 77–82.

Chauhan SP, Magann EF, Carroll CS, *et al.* (2001). Mode of delivery for morbidly obese with prior cesarean delivery: vaginal versus repeat cesarean section. *Am J Obstet Gynecol* **185**: 349–54.

Cunningham FG, Leveno KJ, Bloom SL, *et al.* (2014). *Williams Obstetrics*, 24th edn. New York: McGraw-Hill.

Curtin SC (1997). Rates of cesarean birth after vaginal birth after previous cesarean. *Monthly Vital Stat Rep* **45** (11 Suppl. 3).

Dahlke JD, Medez-Figueroa H, Rouse DJ, *et al.* (2013). Evidence-based surgery for cesarean delivery: an updated systematic review. *Am J Obstet Gynecol* **209**: 294–306.

Dildy GA, Paine AR, George NC, Velasco C (2004). Estimating blood loss: can teaching significantly improve visual estimation? *Obstet Gynecol* **104**: 601–6.

Gawande AA, Studdert DM, Orav EF, Brennan TA, Zinner MJ (2003). Risk factors for retained instruments and sponges after surgery. *N Engl J Med* **348**: 229–35.

Grobman WA, Peaceman AM, Socol ML (2000). Cost-effectiveness of elective cesarean delivery after one prior low transverse cesarean. *Obstet Gynecol* **95**: 745–51.

Hammad IA, Chauhan SP, Magann EF, Abuhamad AZ (2014). Peripartum complications with cesarean delivery: a review of Maternal–Fetal Medicine Units Network publications. *J Matern Fetal Neonatal Med* **27**: 463–74.

Hawkins JL, Chang J, Palmer SK, Gibbs CP, Callaghan WM (2011). Anesthesia-related maternal mortality in the United States: 1979–2002. *Obstet Gynecol* 117: 69–74.

Hendrix SL, Schimp V, Martin J, *et al.* (2000). The legendary superior strength of the Pfannensteil incision: a myth? *Am J Obstet Gynecol* 182: 1446–51.

Kapustian V, Anteby EY, Gdalevich M, *et al.* (2012). Effect of closure versus nonclosure of peritoneum at cesarean section on adhesions: a prospective randomized study. *Am J Obstet Gynecol* 206: 56.e1–4.

Lyell DJ, Caughey AB, Hu E, *et al.* (2012). Rectus muscle and visceral peritoneum closure at cesarean delivery and intraabdominal adhesions. *Am J Obstet Gynecol* 206: 515.e1–5.

Martin JA, Hamilton BE, Osterman MJ, Driscoll AK, Mathews TJ (2017). Births: final data for 2015. *Natl Vital Stat Rep* 66 (1).

Patterson LS, O'Connell CM, Baskett TF (2002). Maternal and perinatal morbidity associated with classic and inverted T cesarean incisions. *Obstet Gynecol* 100: 633–7.

Shipp TD, Zelop CM, Repke JT, Cohen A, Lieberman E (2001). Interdelivery interval and risk of symptomatic uterine rupture. *Obstet Gynecol* 97: 175–7.

Simpson EL, Lawrenson RA, Nightingale AL, Farmer RD (2001). Venous thromboembolism in pregnancy and the puerperium: incidence and additional risk factors from a London perinatal database. *BJOG* 108: 56–60.

Tita A, Szychowski JM, Boggess K, *et al.*; C/SOAP Trial Consortium (2016). Adjunctive azithromycin prophylaxis for cesarean delivery. *N Engl J Med* 375: 1231–41.

Wiener JJ, Westwood J (2002). Fetal lacerations at caesarean section. *J Obstet Gynaecol* 22: 23–4.

Zaphiratos V, George RB, Boyd JC, Habib AS (2015). Uterine exteriorization compared with in situ repair for Cesarean delivery: a systematic review and meta-analysis. *Can J Anaesth* 62: 1209–20.

Lacerations and Episiotomies

Allison Eubanks and Shad Deering

Introduction

Lacerations are a common occurrence during spontaneous vaginal deliveries and especially after operative vaginal deliveries. Several studies show lacerations occur in 53–85% of all deliveries depending on the patient and practice (Smith *et al.* 2013, Rogers *et al.* 2014). After delivery, it is important to fully inspect the cervix, vagina, and perineum and identify what lacerations, if any, are present and then repair them appropriately. Knowing how to perform an episiotomy is an important skill to have, but it must be used with care, as the procedure inevitably increases the risk of more extensive lacerations.

Types of Lacerations

Cervical

After delivery of the placenta, one hand should be placed into the posterior vagina and the cervix completely visualized. This is often made easier by grasping the anterior and/or posterior lip of the cervix with a ring forceps. (Make sure you have adequate lighting when examining for lacerations, and request additional lighting if needed.) If you notice profuse bleeding from the vagina, and you have good uterine tone, look closely for a cervical laceration, which could be as high as the upper third of the vagina. While one study noted cervical lacerations in as many as 50% of vaginal deliveries, most of these are less than 0.5 cm in length and do not require any treatment after delivery (Fahmy *et al.* 1991). One obstetric text even notes that "cervical lacerations of up to 2 cm must be regarded as inevitable in childbirth" (Cunningham *et al.* 2014).

If you identify a cervical laceration that is longer than 2 cm or one that is actively bleeding, then you should repair this immediately. In order to do this, first call for an assistant to provide retraction and right-angle retractors if needed, then grasp the cervix on either side of the laceration with ring forceps. Your assistant can retract so that you can identify the apex of the laceration and you then place your suture (usually either 2–0 chromic or 2–0 polyglactin [Vicryl]) just above the apex, which should control most of the bleeding and make visualization easier. You may either run this suture, which is often easier as you can use it for traction, or perform interrupted sutures. Be sure to only repair the laceration and not suture the cervix closed. Check to ensure the os is patent after your repair.

Vaginal/Perineal

Lacerations of the vagina and perineum are common during vaginal delivery. There are many factors that place a patient at risk for more significant lacerations, such as the following:

- Nulliparity
- Episiotomy
- Operative vaginal delivery
- Macrosomia, precipitous delivery
- Prolonged second stage
- Perineal body ≤ 2.5 cm

(Deering *et al.* 2004)

While some providers will attempt repair of lacerations before delivery of the placenta, these repairs can become dislodged after delivery of the placenta if you need to manually explore the uterus because of atony or retained membranes. If this happens, performing a repair a second time on tissue that has had sutures tear through it is not nearly as easy as the initial repair. For this reason it is generally recommended that repairs not be started until after the placenta has been delivered.*

Lacerations are classified as being first, second, third, or fourth degree (Table 11.1). It is important to know these, as you must accurately document what occurred in the medical record, as well as understand how to repair them. Missing a third- or fourth-degree laceration can result in anal incontinence and the formation of a rectovaginal fistula.

While first- and second-degree lacerations are usually repaired by junior providers with little trouble, when you have a third- or fourth-degree laceration, it is important to have a senior resident or staff present for help in identifying anatomy and providing adequate exposure. Repair techniques are discussed later in this chapter.

---

* An exception to this is if you have a specific vessel or area that is bleeding profusely. In this case, an interrupted suture to prevent continued hemorrhage is advised rather than waiting for the placenta to deliver.

Table 11.1 Classification of vaginal/perineal lacerations

First degree	Involves the vaginal fourchette, perineal skin, or vaginal mucous membranes
Second degree	Involves skin plus the fascia and muscles of the perineal body*
Third degree	Involves the skin, fascia/muscles of perineal body, plus at least some portion of the anal sphincter 3a: Less than 50% of external anal sphincter thickness torn 3b: More than 50% of external anal sphincter thickness torn 3c: Both external and internal anal sphincter torn
Fourth degree	Laceration extends into the rectal mucosa and involves the entire sphincter complex and anal epithelium

* By definition, any episiotomy is at least a second-degree laceration as it incises the fascia/muscles of the perineal body.

Periurethral

Sometimes, after delivery, there will be bleeding from the anterior portion of the vagina near the urethral opening. Most of the time this will stop with direct pressure, but if it does require sutures for hemostasis, then it is prudent to place a straight catheter or Foley catheter into the urethra. This will allow you to avoid the urethra while you throw either interrupted or figure-of-eight sutures for hemostasis. Afterwards, you can leave a Foley catheter in place if there was an extensive repair, or, if you remove the catheter, warn the patient that it will be painful to urinate for the next few days, and monitor her for urinary retention in the postpartum period.

Episiotomy

An episiotomy is an incision in the perineum made in an attempt to enlarge the vaginal opening during delivery. While there was a time in obstetric practice when episiotomies were cut with nearly all deliveries, this is no longer the case. Arguments that a clean cut is easier to repair than a jagged tear, that it protects the woman against pelvic relaxation, or that it prevents fetal injury at delivery have not been borne out in studies. It is also well established that performing a midline episiotomy significantly increases the risk of a third- or fourth-degree laceration. Because of this, the incidence of episiotomy during delivery has decreased significantly in recent years. In 2012, episiotomies were estimated to have been performed in only 12% of deliveries in the United States (Friedman *et al.* 2015).

Indications

Indications for an episiotomy all involve the need for a larger vaginal opening for delivery. Some commonly cited reasons for making an episiotomy include:

- Shoulder dystocia
- Macrosomic fetus
- Breech vaginal delivery
- Operative vaginal delivery (forceps or vacuum)
- Occiput posterior presentation

It is important to note that these are not absolute indications, and the increased risk of an extension of the incision must be taken into account when making the decision to perform an episiotomy. For example, whereas in the past it was recommended that an episiotomy be cut with every operative vaginal delivery, studies have demonstrated that this increases the risk of third- and fourth-degree lacerations and may not be necessary in all cases (Coombs *et al.* 1991, Helwig *et al.* 1993). In these situations, clinical judgment must be used with regards to when to perform an episiotomy.

Another thing to consider is the medical-legal matter of informed consent with this procedure, because of the potential for long-term morbidity that can result from a significant extension of an episiotomy. Prior to performing an episiotomy, preferably at the time of admission to the labor and delivery unit, you should talk with the patient about the possibility of her requiring one, as well as the potential complications. These complications are discussed in detail later in this chapter.

While there is adequate clinical evidence to argue against performing routine episiotomies, the bottom line when it comes to making an episiotomy is that the benefit of widening the vaginal opening must be weighed against the potential complications and the clinical situation.

Anatomy

With a midline episiotomy, the incision will involve the vaginal mucosa, perineal body, and the inferior portion of the bulbocavernosus muscle in the perineum (Figure 11.1). If the episiotomy extends during delivery, it can disrupt the anal sphincter and rectal mucosa. A mediolateral episiotomy will transect the junction of the bulbocavernosus and transverse perineal muscles. It is important to understand the anatomy well, as these structures must be identified during the repair (Figure 11.2).

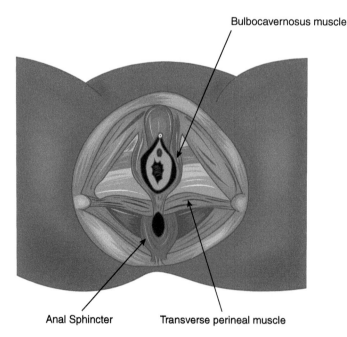

Bulbocavernosus muscle

Figure 11.1 The anatomy of the perineum and muscles.

Anal Sphincter   Transverse perineal muscle

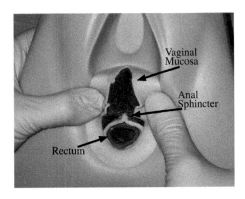

Figure 11.2 Anatomy of perineum and episiotomy.

Types of Episiotomies

An episiotomy should always be noted in the delivery record, as well as any extensions that occur. You must also be specific about the type of episiotomy. The most common types of episiotomies are a midline episiotomy and a mediolateral episiotomy although a modified mediolateral episiotomy is also sometimes used.

Midline Episiotomy (Figure 11.3a)

In the United States, a midline episiotomy (MLE) is almost always used, whereas a mediolateral episiotomy is commonly employed in other parts of the world. When an MLE is cut, the fingers of the non-dominant hand are placed between the baby and the perineum and scissors are then used to make a midline incision in the perineum into the perineal body. Care is taken not to incise the anal sphincter or cut the fetus at the time the incision is made.

Mediolateral Episiotomy (Figure 11.3b)

A mediolateral episiotomy is made the same way as a MLE in terms of how the hands are positioned, but the scissors are angled at approximately 60 degrees towards the ischial tuberosity in an attempt to direct any extension that may occur with delivery around the anal sphincter (Kalis *et al.* 2012).

Modified Mediolateral Episiotomy (Figure 11.3c)

A modification of the MLE that is sometimes used is called a modified mediolateral episiotomy. In doing this, the incision is initially directly inferior, just like an MLE, for approximately 2 cm, and then directed laterally at a 45-degree angle. This is meant to prevent the incision from severing the junction of the bulbocavernosus and transverse perineal muscles while still directing the incision, and hopefully any extension, lateral to the anal sphincter.

(a)

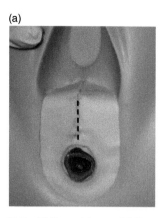

Figure 11.3a Midline episiotomy (MLE).

(b)

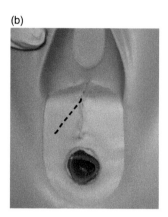

Figure 11.3b Mediolateral episiotomy.

(c)

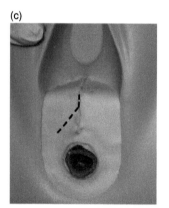

Figure 11.3c Modified mediolateral episiotomy.

Repair of Lacerations and Episiotomies

Repairing lacerations caused by delivery can be a time-consuming procedure. It may take longer to do a proper repair of a fourth-degree laceration than to complete an uncomplicated cesarean section. It is extremely important to correctly identify all lacerations that are present in order to prevent complications, such as postpartum hemorrhage, immediately after delivery, and the potential long-term complications of a rectovaginal fistula or anal incontinence from unidentified injuries or improper repairs. Before doing these types of repairs on your own you should review all pertinent anatomy and perform several with an experienced senior physician.

It is imperative that you actively seek someone out to help you with this and not assume a resident or staff will sit down and teach you these skills. A recent study reported that nearly 60% of residents in the United States did not receive any didactic teaching on either episiotomy repair techniques or pelvic floor anatomy during their residency (McLennan *et al.* 2002). It is a good knowledge of anatomy as well as the ability to recognize and adequately repair lacerations that will prevent future debilitating complications.

Anesthesia

The amount of anesthesia required will depend on the extent of suturing that must be done. In general, a working epidural is almost always adequate for repair. It may need to be re-bolused by the anesthesia provider after delivery if an extensive repair is required. If the patient does not have an epidural, then injecting local anesthetic into the tissue where you will place sutures usually works well. If this is not adequate, then intravenous medications can help. The maximum doses for some common local anesthetics are as follows:

- Bupivacaine: 3 mg/kg
- Lidocaine: 4.5 mg/kg
- Lidocaine with epinephrine: 7 mg/kg

See Chapter 8, *Obstetric Analgesia and Anesthesia*, for additional information on options for anesthesia for laceration repairs.

Suture Choice

The type of suture used depends on physician preference and the tissues that are to be repaired (Table 11.2).

A recent analysis of the medical literature comparing synthetic sutures, such as polyglactin, versus catgut or chromic sutures for perineal repairs found that the synthetic sutures were associated with less pain in the immediate postpartum period as well as a decreased risk of repair dehiscence (Kettle and Johanson 2000). In addition, there were no long-term differences in residual perineal pain or dyspareunia.

Repair Techniques

First-Degree Laceration

First-degree lacerations may or may not need to be repaired. Examine them closely and apply pressure for several minutes if there is only a small amount of bleeding present. If hemostasis cannot be achieved this way, then interrupted sutures of 3–0 Vicryl or chromic can be used. Also, if there is a wide space created by the superficial laceration, it may be reapproximated using interrupted sutures. Always remember the principle, "The enemy of good is better" (which simply means that additional sutures when there is no bleeding can result in additional bleeding or a hematoma).

Table 11.2 Recommended suture choices for episiotomy repair

	Negative GBS and no diagnosis of intra-amniotic infection	Positive GBS or diagnosis of intra-amniotic infection
Vaginal mucosa	3–0 Vicryl or 3–0 Monocryl	3–0 Monocryl
Perirectal fascia	3–0 Vicryl or 3–0 Monocryl	3–0 Monocryl
Anal sphincter	2–0 Vicryl or 2–0 Monocryl	2–0 Monocryl
Anal mucosa	3–0 Vicryl or 4–0 Monocryl	4–0 Monocryl

Vicryl = polyglactin; Monocryl = polyglecaprone; GBS, group B streptococcus.

Second-Degree Laceration

Second-degree lacerations should always be repaired. If the vaginal portion of the laceration is deep, then it is prudent to place one finger into the rectum and ensure there are no small "buttonhole" defects in the rectum that communicate with the floor of the laceration. If these are present, you actually have a fourth-degree laceration and, if you do not repair it properly, you may have a fistula form between the rectum and vagina and the repair will break down. Also, after placing a finger in the rectum it is wise to change gloves to prevent bringing fecal matter into the repair.

In order to repair a second-degree laceration, start by placing a suture at the vaginal apex. This is done using either 2–0 or 3–0 Vicryl, Monocryl, or chromic suture as previously discussed. Continue your repair toward the hymen in a running and locked manner for hemostasis (Figure 11.4a).

Once you reach the hymenal ring you can continue the repair in one of two ways:

Technique 1

1. Turn the needle so that it is parallel with the vagina and go from the hymen area out towards yourself on the perineum (Figure 11.4b).
2. Close the incised muscles/fascia of the perineum with the same suture in a running fashion (Figure 11.4c).
3. Ensure the suture comes through the posterior apex of the incision in the subcutaneous tissue.
4. Run the suture to close the subcutaneous tissue back to the hymenal ring (Figure 11.4d).
5. Turn the needle to be parallel with the vagina and place the suture from outside the hymenal ring to inside the vagina.
6. Take a small amount of vaginal tissue lateral to your suture and tie (Figure 11.4e).

Technique 2

1. Tie the vaginal suture at the hymenal ring.
2. Close the incised muscles/fascia of the perineum with interrupted sutures (using the same type of suture as in the vagina).

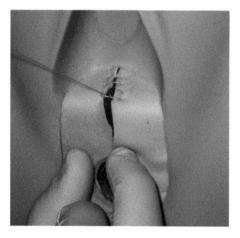

Figure 11.4a Initial repair of vaginal portion of episiotomy.

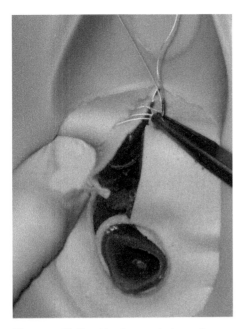

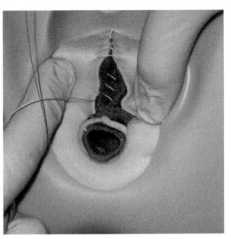

Figure 11.4c Closure of deep portion of muscular tissue.

Figure 11.4b Transition from vaginal to perineum with episiotomy repair.

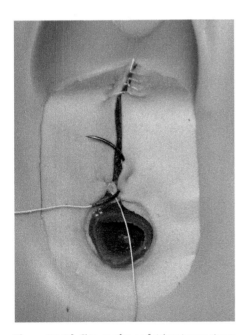

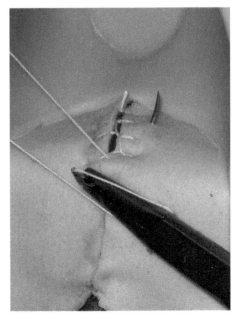

Figure 11.4d Closure of superficial perineum tissue.

Figure 11.4e Transition back to vaginal tissue to tie final suture.

3. Close the subcutaneous tissue by starting at the inferior apex and then tie near the hymenal ring.

At the end of either of these repairs, place a finger into the rectum to ensure there are no sutures penetrating the rectum or any hematomas present. If there is a suture that has gone into the rectum, it should be removed in order to prevent a potential fistula from forming.

Third-Degree Laceration

When you confirm you have a third-degree laceration, place a finger into the rectum to check for a fourth-degree extension. Change gloves, then identify both ends of the anal sphincter. These can often retract laterally, and you may need to use Allis clamps to grasp them (Figure 11.5a). After you have identified the sphincter, the ends are reapproximated using three or four either interrupted or figure-of-eight sutures, usually 2–0 Vicryl, Monocryl, or polydiaxanone (PDS). After the anal sphincter is reapproximated, the repair is the same as for a second degree. Figure 11.5b shows the initial suture placed in the anal sphincter.

Another technique that has been taught is to actually overlap the torn distal ends of the anal sphincter during the repair. However, a meta-analysis has shown no significant difference in perineal pain, dyspareunia, or incontinence at 12 months postpartum between overlap and end-to-end repairs (Fernando *et al.* 2013).

Fourth-Degree Laceration

When you discover a fourth-degree laceration, you should ensure you have the following:

Adequate anesthesia. Usually an epidural is required for this type of repair. Otherwise, IV sedation in addition to local anesthetic is usually needed, but this will often require the assistance of an anesthesiologist. (See Chapter 8 for information on potential medications that can be used.) It is also advisable to inject bupivacaine 0.25% with epinephrine into the perineum around the repair for postoperative pain relief.

Adequate visualization. If you cannot adequately visualize the apex of the laceration in the rectum, then you may need to transfer the patient to the operating room for better lighting and positioning. (The OR table is equipped for stirrups, which will improve

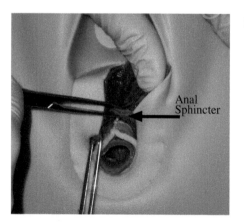

Figure 11.5a Grasping the anal sphincter.

Anal
Sphincter

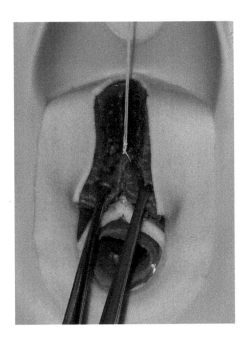

Figure 11.5b Repair of the anal sphincter.

visualization considerably.) Additional retractors and an assistant will also make the repair easier. Some retractors that may be helpful include the Breisky–Navratil vaginal retractor, right-angle retractors, and long Deaver retractors.

Adequate support staff present. While repairs should be completed as soon as possible, if necessary it is acceptable to wait for adequate anesthesia support and appropriately trained staff to help with repair. Studies show that, as long as bleeding is under control, packing the area and waiting up to 12 hours results in no long-term differences in anal incontinence 1 year postpartum (Nordenstam *et al.* 2008).

During the repair, make sure that you keep track of the patient's vital signs, urine output, and blood loss. It is easy to concentrate on the repair and not notice continued bleeding until the patient has sustained a significant hemorrhage.

When starting the repair, identify the apex of the rectal injury. (If you need to put a sponge into the vagina to keep your view of the field, try and use a laparotomy tape and leave the blue tag on the outside so you do not forget it at the end of the repair.)

Reapproximate the edges of the rectal mucosa and muscularis with a continuous suture of either 3–0 polyglactin (Vicryl) or 4–0 polyglecaprone (Monocryl) on an SH needle. After this, perform your repair of the anal sphincter as previously described and shown in Figure 11.5. When closing the remaining vaginal portion of the laceration, be sure to close the deep tissue overlying the rectum and do not leave any dead space where a hematoma could form. The rest of the repair is the same as for a second-degree laceration. After the repair is complete, make sure all sponges are removed from the vagina and perform a gentle rectal exam to ensure you have not significantly constricted the lumen, left any significant gaps in the repair, or put sutures into the rectum. Make sure that you write appropriate postpartum orders, to include stool softeners, the application of an ice pack to the perineum for the next 24–48 hours, and sitz baths twice daily. There is also some literature to support the use of prophylactic antibiotics in these patients at the time of repair (usually a single dose of a second-generation cephalosporin) and for the first few days after delivery to prevent infection or breakdown of the repair (Buppasiri *et al.* 2014). (See Appendix B, *Sample Notes and Orders.*)

Complications of Lacerations and Episiotomies

Both lacerations that occur spontaneously and those that result from an episiotomy can cause a number of complications. It is important not only to recognize the acute problems, such as postpartum hemorrhage, but also to be aware of and monitor for those that are delayed for several days or weeks, such as infection, hematomas, and fistulas. Some of the more common complications are discussed below.

Third/Fourth-Degree Lacerations

The incidence of third- and fourth-degree lacerations is increased when an episiotomy is performed. This risk is higher with a midline episiotomy than with a mediolateral episiotomy, although the risk is increased with both. One study showed the risk of deep perineal tears almost doubles with a midline episiotomy (14.8%) versus a mediolateral episiotomy (7.0%) (Sooklim *et al.* 2007).

There have been studies that demonstrate that mediolateral episiotomies can be protective against third- and fourth-degree lacerations in primiparous women. However, one study of over 43,000 patients demonstrated that it would require 48 episiotomies to prevent one severe tear (Anthony *et al.* 1994). When the other complications of an episiotomy, such as hemorrhage and infection, are taken into account, it cannot be recommended that a mediolateral episiotomy be made routinely for this indication.

Hemorrhage

All types of lacerations, including episiotomies, are associated with an increased risk of postpartum hemorrhage. Compared with delivering over an intact perineum, the increased blood loss has been estimated to be between 300 mL and 600 mL (Thacker and Banta 1983, Rockner *et al.* 1989). Another study that used the change in hematocrit to define a postpartum hemorrhage demonstrated that both midline and mediolateral episiotomies are associated with an increased risk of postpartum hemorrhage (Coombs *et al.* 1991). When evaluating a patient for a postpartum hemorrhage and the uterus is firm, you must consider and inspect for cervical and vaginal lacerations.

Infection

When you consider the amount of trauma that can occur with a vaginal delivery, the normal bacteria in the vagina, and the lochia that flows through the vagina after delivery, it is remarkable that infections of episiotomies are relatively uncommon. When these do occur, it may be a superficial wound infection or a deeper abscess which can form from a hematoma. Risk factors associated with infection include infected lochia, fecal contamination, and poor hygiene of the incision site. Third- and fourth-degree tears have a higher rate of infection than first- and second-degree tears. In fact, a recent review shows that 20% of women with a third- or fourth-degree tear will develop an infection (Lewicky-Gaupp *et al.* 2015).

When an infection or episiotomy breakdown occurs, it will usually happen in the first 7 days after delivery (Sanz 2001). The incidence of episiotomy infection has been reported to be between 0.35% and 10% (Myers-Helfgott and Helfgott 1999).

In general, whenever a patient who had lacerations repaired after delivery complains of increasing pain and/or fevers, the repair should be inspected and examined. This most commonly occurs on postpartum day three or four. Erythema, a tender, fluctuant mass, or purulent drainage may be present. If a superficial infection is present, then it should be treated with antibiotics. If an abscess or infected hematoma is present, it must be incised, drained, and the area surgically debrided and then antibiotics administered.

Antibiotic Prophylaxis

While there has been considerable discussion regarding the need for antibiotics when a patient experiences a third- or fourth-degree laceration, this has previously been left up to the discretion and preference of the patient's physician. A randomized study, however, suggests that patients who have a third- or fourth-degree laceration should receive a single dose of a second-generation cephalosporin after delivery as this will decrease the incidence of perineal wound complications from 24% to 8% (Duggal *et al.* 2008).

Hematoma

If an episiotomy is not properly repaired, or if the soft-tissue dead space of a deep laceration is not properly closed, then bleeding may continue into this potential space. A hematoma can form, which has the potential to cause significant discomfort as well as to become a nidus for infection. When present, a hematoma can often be felt on gentle digital examination of both rectum and vagina. The incidence of hematomas after delivery has been reported to be between 1 in 300 and 1 in 1000 deliveries (Gilstrap *et al.* 2001). If the hematoma continues to expand, it can even dissect into the retroperitoneum, which should be considered when a patient has a falling hematocrit and an expanding hematoma.

When the hematoma is small to moderate in size and not expanding, if the patient is hemodynamically stable, it may be conservatively managed. The patient is given oral pain medication and may use a heating pad for comfort. If it is expanding or the patient is unstable, then it should be evacuated and, after identifying and correcting any bleeding with hemostatic sutures, a vaginal packing can be placed for up to 24 hours. The patient is then reexamined to ensure it has not reaccumulated. It is important to note that nearly half of women with hematomas that require surgical treatment will require a transfusion (Zahn and Yeomans 1990).

Rectovaginal Fistula

This is a rare complication, but can occur when an infected hematoma erodes through the rectovaginal septum, or when an unrecognized injury into the rectum occurs and is not repaired. This latter injury allows for fecal contamination of the incision, which then progresses to become a fistula. This unrecognized "buttonhole" lesion of the rectum has been reported to occur in approximately 0.1% of deliveries in older literature (Graber and O'Rourke 1957). It can be avoided by performing a rectal exam on all patients with a tear after a delivery to examine for its presence.

Repair Breakdown

Fortunately, breakdown of a repair is an uncommon occurrence with first- and second-degree lacerations, seen in only around 4% of cases (Sanz 2001). When it does occur, it is usually associated with a concurrent infection over 75% of the time (Ramin *et al.* 1992). Patients with third- and fourth-degree tears can experience a wound breakdown up to 25% of the time (Lewicky-Gaupp *et al.* 2015). While in the past, repair of the breakdown was performed after waiting at least 3–4 months, it has been demonstrated that, with appropriate preoperative care including IV antibiotics, bowel preparation, and aggressive cleansing of the wound, early repair of an episiotomy breakdown (usually within 1 week) is associated with good outcomes (Hankins *et al.* 1990, Ramin *et al.* 1992).

Anal Incontinence

In general, anal incontinence only occurs when there has been damage to the anal sphincter, i.e., with third- and fourth-degree lacerations. When a third-degree laceration occurs, the incidence of long-term anal incontinence has been reported as high as 40%, with recent data confirming this number (Poen *et al.* 1998, Fornell *et al.* 2005). The risk of sustaining a third- or fourth-degree laceration is increased in patients who are nulliparous, or who have an instrumental vaginal delivery, a macrosomic infant, or an episiotomy.

References

Anthony S, Buitendijk S, Zondervan K, *et al.* (1994). Episiotomies and the occurrence of severe perineal lacerations. *Br J Obstet Gynaecol* 101: 1064–7.

Buppasiri P, Lumbiganon P, Thinkhamrop J, Thinkhamrop B (2014). Antibiotic prophylaxis for third- and fourth-degree perineal tear during vaginal birth. *Cochrane Database Syst Rev* (10): CD005125.

Coombs CA, Murphy E, Laros R (1991). Factors associated with postpartum hemorrhage with vaginal birth. *Obstet Gynecol* 77: 69–76.

Cunningham FG, Leveno KJ, Bloom SL, *et al.* (2014). Obstetrical complications. In *Williams Obstetrics*, 24th edn. New York: McGraw-Hill.

Deering SH, Carlson N, Stitely M, Allaire AD, Satin AJ (2004). Perineal body length and perineal lacerations at delivery. *J Reprod Med* 49: 306–10.

Duggal N, Mercado C, Daniels K, *et al.* (2008). Antibiotic prophylaxis for prevention of postpartum perineal wound complications. *Obstet Gynecol* 111: 1268–73.

Fahmy K, el-Gazar A, Sammour M, Nosair M, Salem A (1991). Postpartum colposcopy of the cervix: Injury and healing. *In J Gynaecol Obstet* 34: 133–7.

Fernando RJ, Sultan AH, Kettle C, Thakar R (2013). Methods of repair for obstetric anal sphincter injury. *Cochrane Database Syst Rev* (12): CD002866.

Fornell EU, Matthiesen L, Sjödahl R, Berg G (2005). Obstetric anal sphincter injury ten years after: subjective and objective long term effects. *BJOG* 112: 312–16.

Friedman AM, Ananth CV, Prendergast E, D'Alton ME, Wright JD (2015). Variation in and factors associated with use of episiotomy. *JAMA* 313: 197–9.

Gilstrap LC, Van Dorsten PV, Cunningham FG (2001). Puerperal hematomas and genital tract lacerations. In *Operative Obstetrics*, 2nd edn. New York, McGraw-Hill.

Graber E, O'Rourke J (1957). Rectal injuries during vaginal delivery. *Am J Obstet Gynecol* 73: 301–4.

Hankins G, Hauth J, Gilstrap L, *et al.* (1990). Early repair of episiotomy dehiscence. *Obstet Gynecol* 75: 48–51.

Helwig J, Thorp J, Bowes W (1993). Does midline episiotomy increase the risk of third and fourth degree lacerations in operative vaginal deliveries? *Obstet Gynecol* 82: 276–9.

Kalis V, Laine K, de Leeuw J, Ismail K, Tincello D (2012). Classification of episiotomy:

towards a standardisation of terminology. *BJOG* **119**: 522–6.

Kettle C, Johanson RB (2000). Absorbable synthetic versus catgut suture material for perineal repair. *Cochrane Database Syst Rev* (2): CD000006.

Lewicky-Gaupp C, Leader-Cramer A, Johnson LL, Kenton K, Gossett DR (2015). Wound complications after obstetric anal sphincter injuries. *Obstet Gynecol* **125**: 1088–93.

McLennan MT, Melick CF, Clancy SL, Artal R (2002). Episiotomy and perineal repair: an evaluation of resident education and experience. *J Reprod Med* **47**: 1025–30.

Myers-Helfgott MG, Helfgott AW (1999). Routine use of episiotomies in modern obstetrics. *Obstet Gynecol Clin North Am* **26**: 305–25.

Nordenstam J, Mellgren A, Altman D, *et al.* (2008). Immediate or delayed repair of obstetric anal sphincter tears: a randomised controlled trial. *BJOG* **115**: 857–65.

Poen AC, Felt-Bersma RJ, Strijers RL, *et al.* (1998). Third-degree obstetric perineal tear: Long-term clinical and functional results after primary repair. *Br J Surg* **85**: 1433–8.

Ramin S, Ramus R, Little B, *et al.* (1992). Early repair of episiotomy dehiscence associated with infection. *Am J Obstet Gynecol* **167**: 1104–7.

Rockner G, Walhbberg V, Olund A (1989). Episiotomy and perineal trauma during childbirth. *J Adv Nurs* **14**: 264–8.

Rogers RG, Leeman LM, Borders N, *et al.* (2014). Contribution of the second stage of labour to pelvic floor dysfunction: a prospective cohort comparison of nulliparous women. *BJOG* **121**: 1145–54.

Sanz LE (2001). Managing episiotomies and their complications. *Contemporary OB/GYN* **46** (5).

Smith LA, Price N, Simonite V, Burns EE (2013). Incidence of and risk factors for perineal trauma: a prospective observational study. *BMC Pregnancy Childbirth* **13**: 59.

Sooklim R, Thinkhamrop J, Lumbiganon P, *et al.* (2007). The outcomes of midline versus medio-lateral episiotomy. *Reprod Health* **4**: 10.

Thacker SB, Banta HD (1983). Benefits and risks of episiotomy: an interpretative review of the English language literature, 1860–1980. *Obstet Gynecol Surv* **38**: 322–38.

Zahn CM, Yeomans ER (1990). Postpartum hemorrhage: placenta accreta, uterine inversion and puerperal hematomas. *Clin Obstet Gynecol* **33**: 422–31.

12

Neonatal Resuscitation

Mary Kathryn Collins and Shad Deering

Introduction

In most deliveries, the baby will cry and breathe spontaneously soon after birth. In some deliveries, however, the baby will come out blue, apneic, and significantly depressed. Although you are not expected to be an expert in pediatrics, it is incumbent upon you to know when and how to resuscitate a newborn baby, as it may take several minutes for the pediatricians to arrive. While fewer than 1% of term and late preterm infants require extensive resuscitative measures, there should be at least one individual, capable of initiating resuscitation, present at every delivery whose sole responsibility is the neonate. In the case of higher-risk neonates, additional personnel with qualifications and capabilities appropriate for the anticipated situation should be present.

Apgar Scores

Apgar scores are routinely assigned at 1 and 5 minutes of life. Should the score continue to be below 7, they should continue to be assigned at 10, 15, and 20 minutes. Apgar scores take into account five variables, which are listed in Table 12.1 (ACOG 2015). While many parents may focus on Apgar scores, they are a subjective evaluation of the infant and are meant to guide you in your resuscitation of the baby, not to predict long-term outcomes. Also, remember that you never wait for a 1-minute Apgar to begin resuscitation.

Resuscitation

Apnea

When a baby is born and not breathing, this is called apnea. There are two different types of apnea, primary and secondary. Primary apnea is the initial response of a baby to asphyxia,

Table 12.1 Apgar scores

Score	0	1	2
Activity (tone)	Limp	Some flexion	Active flexion
Pulse (bpm)	Absent	< 100 bpm	> 100 bpm
Grimace (reflex irritability)	None	Grimace	Cry or withdrawal to stimulus
Appearance (skin color)	Blue or pale	Body pink, extremities blue	Completely pink
Respirations	Absent	Weak cry	Strong cry

The Apgar score is named for Virginia Apgar (1909–1974), but it also functions effectively as a mnemonic for the five elements that make up the score: Activity, Pulse, Grimace, Appearance, Respirations.

or oxygen deprivation. It will often resolve without intervention and will always respond to stimulation alone. Secondary apnea occurs after several minutes of asphyxia and will not resolve spontaneously or with stimulation alone. Secondary apnea requires respiratory intervention, such as positive-pressure ventilation (PPV). The most important thing to remember when an apneic infant is born is that *you cannot differentiate between primary and secondary apnea based on the fetal heart rate (FHR) tracing preceding birth or the physical exam*, so you must begin resuscitation efforts immediately. Always assume that apnea is secondary apnea.

Preparing for a Delivery

As with nearly everything in obstetrics, it is important to try and anticipate when a baby may require resuscitation. If there is a concerning FHR tracing prior to delivery, an operative delivery of any kind is being performed, narcotics have been given to the mother within two hours of delivery, or the fetus is preterm, then pediatricians should be called prior to the delivery. A list of other potential situations where you should be concerned about a depressed infant being delivered can be found in Table 12.2.

In addition to the staff, the environment should be considered. Premature newborns should have the room temperature at around 26 °C (78.8 °F), with a goal of 36.5 °C (97.7 °F) axial temperature. Exothermic mattresses or heat-resistant plastic wrapping may be used to prevent hypothermia. It is essential to ensure that the proper equipment is available for resuscitating a newborn, and to know where this is kept. The standard equipment required is listed in Table 12.3.

It is also necessary to check the equipment prior to delivery. Besides ensuring you have the proper equipment, check the following:

1. Turn on the oxygen and make sure you have good flow.
2. Check that you can get a good seal with the mask by placing it on your hand, and ensure the pressure-release valve works when you squeeze the bag.
3. Open the laryngoscope and check the light to ensure it functions and is properly secured. (You will use a size 0 blade for preterm infants and size 1 blade for term infants.)

Table 12.2 Antepartum factors that can be associated with delivery of a depressed neonate

- All cesarean sections, especially urgent and emergency ones
- Operative vaginal delivery (forceps or vacuum)
- Premature labor
- Precipitous labor
- General anesthesia
- Maternal narcotic administration within 2 hours of delivery
- Placental abruption
- Placenta previa
- Intra-amniotic infection
- Meconium-stained amniotic fluid
- Fetal anomalies

Table 12.3 Infant resuscitation equipment

Suction equipment	Bulb suction DeLee suction 8 F feeding tube and 20 mL syringe Meconium aspirator
Bag and mask	Infant resuscitation bag with a pressure-release valve Face masks (newborn and premature sizes with cushioned rims) Oral airways Oxygen supply with tubing and flow meter
Intubation equipment	Laryngoscope with blades (size 0 and 1) Functioning batteries in laryngoscope Secured and functioning light Endotracheal tubes, sizes 2.5, 3.0, 3.5, 4.0 mm Stylet

4. Make sure you have the proper size endotracheal tube (ETT) for the size of baby you expect. ETT sizes for different weights and gestational ages as recommended by the American Academy of Pediatrics are listed in Table 12.4.

Algorithm for Evaluation and Resuscitation

The algorithm for neonatal evaluation and resuscitation is described in detail in the following paragraphs and is also illustrated in the flow diagram shown in Figure 12.1.

When an infant is born, note the tone of the infant and whether or not the infant is attempting to breathe. A term infant that has good muscle tone and is breathing or crying may remain with the mother while continuing to be evaluated. However, if the infant is apneic or has poor tone, you may consider quickly clamping and cutting the cord and taking the infant over to the warmer. At present, there is insufficient evidence for recommending a definite approach to cord clamping for newborns who need resuscitative efforts. In the setting of a vigorous or term or preterm newborn, evidence suggests that delayed cord clamping for 30–60 seconds may be beneficial (ACOG 2017a).

Table 12.4 Endotracheal tube sizes

Gestational age	Fetal weight	Endotracheal tube size (mm)
< 28 weeks	< 1000 g	2.5 mm/5 F
28–33^{+6} weeks	1000–2000 g	3.0 mm/6 F
34–37^{+6} weeks	2000–3000 g	3.5 mm/8 F
> 38 weeks	> 3000 g	4.0 mm/10 F

If the infant is apneic or has poor tone, ensure the pediatricians are in the room, and if not instruct one of the nurses or assistants to contact the pediatricians and have them come immediately. Most institutions have a "code" button in the delivery room that will alert the pediatric resuscitation team. Make sure you know where this is if your hospital has one.

After clamping and cutting the cord, place the infant on the radiant warmer with the head towards you. Quickly dry and clean the infant with a warm towel, which will provide gentle stimulation. Evaluate for respirations and position the infant on its back, with the neck slightly extended to open the airway. (Please note that this is not the exaggerated "sniffing position" that adult resuscitation may require, as that position can close off the infant's airway.) In vigorous newborns routine suctioning of the oral or nasopharynx is not necessary and therefore should not be performed unless there is an obvious airway obstruction or PPV is required. This includes infants who are delivered through meconium-stained amniotic fluid, as this has not been shown to change prevalence or outcomes in meconium aspiration syndrome (ACOG 2017b). Should the airway need to be cleared, the mouth should be suctioned first so when suctioning the nose if the child gasps there is less chance of aspiration. Care should be taken, as damage can be done to the mucosa as well as a reflex bradycardia from deep or vigorous suctioning. After the airway has been evaluated, proceed with the evaluation and resuscitation in the following order: *respiratory effort, heart rate, color.*

Respiratory effort. Normal spontaneous respirations for newborns range from 30 to 60 breaths per minute. If apnea is present, always presume secondary apnea and start PPV with O_2. When PPV is required, the initial breaths should be 20–25 cmH$_2$O, and then subsequent breaths should be 5 cmH$_2$O for normal lungs. The ventilation rate should be 40–60 per minute (when performed without compressions, which are addressed under *Heart rate*, below).

With regards to the concentration of oxygen to use for PPV, it is important to consider gestational age. Newborns born at 35+ weeks EGA should be started on 21% oxygen (room air). Infants less than 35 weeks EGA should begin with 21–30% oxygen. In circumstances where infant oxygen saturation levels are not in the target range despite adequate ventilation (Table 12.5), free-flow oxygen may begin at 30% and be adjusted as needed to achieve the oxygen saturation target. If the newborn has labored breathing, or if oxygen saturation cannot be achieved despite 100% free-flow oxygen, consider a trial of continuous positive airway pressure (CPAP).

If your ventilation efforts and oxygen therapy are not improving the oxygen saturation level, you should perform a list of checks using the mnemonic Mr. SOPA (Table 12.6).

Table 12.5 Target oxygen saturation levels after delivery

1 min	60–65%
2 min	65–70%
3 min	70–75%
4 min	75–80%
5 min	80–85%
10 min	90–95%

Table 12.6 Mr. SOPA (actions to ensure proper ventilation)

M	Adjust MASK to ensure good seal
R	REPOSITION by adjusting head to slightly extend neck and open airway
S	SUCTION if secretions are present in nose and mouth
O	OPEN mouth slightly and move jaw forward
P	Increase PRESSURE until you see chest rise
A	Consider AIRWAY ALTERNATIVE

Adapted from AAP/AHA 2015 Neonatal Resuscitation Guidelines (Wyckoff *et al.* 2015).

Heart rate. If the infant is breathing spontaneously, then check the heart rate with a stethoscope over the left side of the chest. This has been found to be more accurate than palpating the umbilical stump (which has a tendency to underestimate the heart rate). A normal heart rate is between 100 and 180 beats per minute (bpm). Despite normal respiration, if the heart rate is less than 100 bpm, then PPV should be initiated. If there is no reliable pulse identified after 10 seconds, or the heart rate remains below 60 bpm after 30 seconds of effective ventilation, chest compressions should be initiated while ventilation efforts continue, using 100% oxygen. This should be performed at a 3:1 rate, pausing compressions for ventilations, i.e., 90 compressions then 30 ventilations. When chest compressions are required, ECG monitoring is recommended, as pulse oximetry may not accurately measure the newborn's pulse.

Chest compressions should be performed over the lower half of the sternum, with avoidance of the xiphoid process as it can cause trauma to the infant's internal organs. Maximum effectiveness can be achieved by depressing the chest one-third to one-half of the anterior–posterior diameter. In the two-thumb technique, hands are placed around the thorax and both thumbs compress the sternum while the fingers support the infant's back. The goal rate for compressions is 120/minute, which should continue for 60 seconds prior to checking the heart rate. If at that time the heart rate has not increased, endotracheal intubation should be performed and epinephrine should be administered. However, if the heart rate is > 100 bpm, you can discontinue the PPV and go to the next step of evaluating the infant's color (see Figure 12.1).

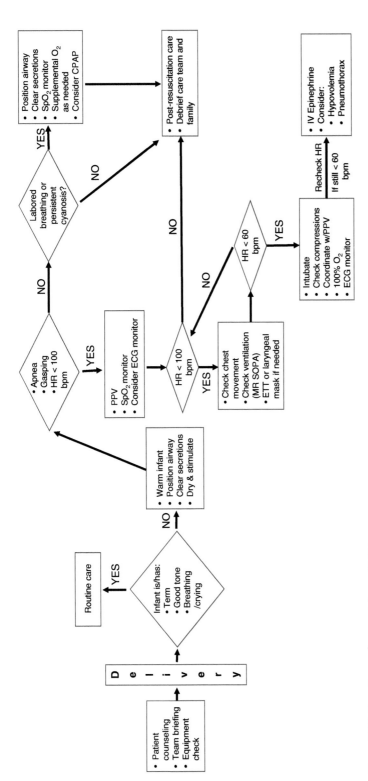

Figure 12.1 Flow diagram for neonatal resuscitation (adapted from Weiner and Zaichkin 2016).

Note: an increased heart rate is the most sensitive indicator of successful response to resuscitative steps.

Color. Evaluate the infant's color. Check for central cyanosis, which means the infant will appear blue over the abdomen and truncal area, as opposed to acrocyanosis, which means that cyanosis is only present in the extremities. If central cyanosis is present, and there are spontaneous respirations and a heart rate of over 100 bpm, then administer free-flow oxygen by face mask. As the infant's color improves, you can gradually remove the oxygen.

Medications for Resuscitation

Usually, by the time medications are required, the pediatric team will have arrived. But, just in case, it is good to know the indications and initial medications needed during a resuscitation. In rare circumstances, if the heart rate remains < 60 bpm after 60 seconds of chest compressions with PPV using 100% oxygen, assuming effective ventilation, then medications should be administered. This is shown in the flow diagram in Figure 12.1.

Common medications and fluids given during resuscitation are listed in Table 12.7. The first medication given in this situation is always epinephrine, and the first dose can be administered intravenously or through the endotracheal tube if vascular access has not yet been established. Intravenous administration is the preferred route, as efficacy and safety are currently unproven for endotracheal epinephrine. Hence, if there is no appropriate response to an initial endotracheal dose, an additional dose may be given once vascular access is established without waiting the typical 3–5 minutes.

Volume expanders should be reserved for newborns who have known or suspected blood loss. Normal saline (or, if anemia is known/suspected, O negative packed red blood cells [PRBCs]) should be given, with an initial dose of 10 mL/kg over 5–10 minutes through umbilical catheter or interosseous needle.

Of note, these recommended medications represent changes from previous guidelines. For instance, lactated Ringers is no longer recommended as a form of volume expander. For newborns with respiratory depression born to mothers with opiate use, there is also insufficient evidence for the efficacy and safety of naloxone and there are potential adverse reactions including pulmonary edema, cardiac arrest, and seizures.

Umbilical Artery Blood Acid–Base Analysis

Whenever an infant is born it is prudent to obtain a sample of cord in case arterial blood sampling is needed for analysis. This information provides a much more objective measure of the infant's acid–base status at the time of delivery as compared to Apgar scores. The goal is to determine the degree of acidosis, if any, that is present, and what type of acidosis it is, i.e., respiratory, metabolic, or mixed. This is important because if the acidosis is respiratory it is probably secondary to an acute event, whereas a metabolic acidosis reflects a more chronic process.

Table 12.7 Medications used in neonatal resuscitation

Medication	Concentration and preparation	Dosage	Route of administration	Weight	IV volume	Rate of administration
Epinephrine	1:10,000	0.01–0.03 mg/kg 0.1–0.3 mL/kg	IV (preferred)	1 kg	0.1–0.3 mL	Give rapidly Repeat every 3–5 minutes
		0.05–0.1 mg/kg 0.5–1.0 mL/kg	ETT	2 kg	0.2–0.6 mL	
				3 kg	0.3–0.9 mL	
				4 kg	0.4–1.2 mL	
Volume expanders	Type O negative PRBC or normal saline	10 mL/kg	IV	1 kg	10 mL	Give over 5–10 minutes Indicated for shock
				2 kg	20 mL	
				3 kg	30 mL	
				4 kg	40 mL	
Dextrose	0.1 g/mL	0.2 g/kg 2 mL/kg	IV	1 kg	2 mL	Check bedside glucose May require dilution with sterile water
				2 kg	4 mL	
				3 kg	6 mL	
				4 kg	8 mL	

ETT, endotracheal tube; IM, intramuscular; IV, intravenous; PRBC, packed red blood cells.

Basic Physiology

The pH of fetal blood is directly correlated with the concentration of base, or bicarbonate (HCO_3-), and inversely related to the concentration of carbonic acid (H_2CO_3) that is present. This is shown in the Henderson–Hasselbalch equation:

$$pH = pK + \log\frac{HCO_3\,(\text{base})}{H_2CO_3\,(\text{acid})}$$

The carbonic acid dissociates to a hydrogen ion (H^+) and bicarbonate (HCO_3-).

As long as there is adequate placental perfusion, oxygen is supplied to the fetus and carbon dioxide (CO_2) and acid metabolites are removed by the placenta and the fetus is able to maintain its normal acid–base balance. When, for whatever reason, this process is interrupted, fetal acidosis may occur. This is first seen with the accumulation of CO_2.

An acidosis is classified as respiratory, metabolic, or mixed depending on the levels of PCO_2 and bicarbonate (HCO_3-) present. Table 12.8 demonstrates these different combinations.

Respiratory acidosis, which is associated with an accumulation of CO_2 with a normal level of HCO_3-, is most commonly caused by an abrupt decrease in either uteroplacental or umbilical perfusion. The presence of respiratory acidosis is not predictive of long-term injury. Some potential causes for this are:

- Maternal hypoxia from narcotic administration
- Hypotension from the administration of regional anesthesia
- Uterine hyperstimulation
- Magnesium sulfate toxicity
- Umbilical cord compression
- Placental abruption

A metabolic acidosis may occur in the presence of either a chronic or prolonged metabolic imbalance. In this situation, the PCO_2 is relatively normal and the HCO_3- level is decreased. Some potential causes of a metabolic acidosis include chronic uteroplacental insufficiency, fetal growth restriction, and maternal acidemia from diabetes, preeclampsia, or chronic hypertension (Thorp and Rushing 1999).

The presence of a metabolic acidosis results in both a decreased amount of buffer base and an excess of acid. This results in a base deficit, which is also measured on a standard blood gas analysis.

When respiratory acidosis occurs for a prolonged period of time, it may result in a mixed acidosis, which is characterized by both elevated PCO_2 and decreased HCO_3- levels. When either a severe metabolic or mixed acidosis is present, there is a much higher risk of fetal problems.

Table 12.8 Fetal acidosis

Type of acidosis	PCO_2(mmHg)	HCO_3- (mEq/L)
Respiratory	Elevated	Normal
Metabolic	Normal	Low
Mixed	Elevated	Low

Technique

The umbilical cord is clamped immediately after the infant is delivered, and a 10–20 cm length of cord is obtained and set aside on the delivery table. There are conflicting data in regards to the effects of delayed cord clamping and cord gases, and thus more studies are required (ACOG 2017a). If it is necessary to obtain an arterial blood sample, then a 1–2 mL heparin-flushed syringe is used to aspirate one of the umbilical cord arteries. If you cannot obtain an adequate sample, then you can aspirate from an artery on the chorionic surface of the placenta (the arteries should be visible as they cross over the veins). After this, obtain a similar sample from the umbilical vein. The samples then undergo laboratory evaluation for acid–base assessment. It is worthwhile trying to obtain both arterial and venous samples, as it is not uncommon for a specimen to clot. The sample is stable at room temperature for 30–60 minutes (Strickland *et al.* 1984).

While some people have recommended sending blood gases with every delivery, this is probably not a cost-effective or necessary procedure. Since you cannot always predict which infants will have low Apgar scores based on antepartum monitoring, following the procedure in Figure 12.2 will ensure you can send a sample if needed by clamping the cord at every delivery until the 5-minute Apgar is assigned.

Normal Values

The normal values from over 3500 infants after vaginal delivery, as well as the accepted normal ranges, are listed in Table 12.9. Note that the normal pH for the umbilical vein is higher than for the umbilical artery. This is because the umbilical artery samples blood directly from the fetus and is a better measure of fetal acid–base status, whereas the umbilical vein is more representative of maternal status.

Umbilical cord gases may be affected by multiparity, living at high altitude, and smoking, with all of these patients having slightly elevated pH values. These differences are, however, rarely significant (Riley and Johnson 1993, Thorp and Rushing 1999). However, blood gas values may change with delayed cord clamping, which is important to recognize given the new recommendation to do this with infants that you do not anticipate requiring resuscitation. In these cases, you should realize that the arterial pH may be slightly lower when sampled (by approximately 0.03) and the base excess lower (by 1.3 mmol/L) (Wiberg *et al.* 2008).

Table 12.9 Normal mean blood gas values

	Arterial blood value (± SD)	Arterial range	Venous blood value (± SD)	Venous range
pH	7.27 (± 0.069)	7.15–7.38	7.34 (± 0.063)	7.20–7.41
PCO₂ (mmHg)	50.3 (± 11.1)	35–70	40.7 (± 7.9)	33–50
HCO₃– (mEq/L)	22.0 (± 3.6)	17–28	21.4 (± 2.5)	15–26
Base excess (mEq/L)	–2.7 (± 2.8)	–2.0 to –9.0	–2.4 (± 2)	–1.0 to –8.0

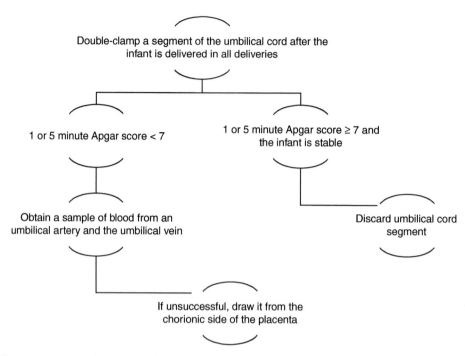

Figure 12.2 Protocol for umbilical cord gas collection during delivery.

Interpretation of Results

After obtaining the values from the samples (assuming you were able to obtain both arterial and venous samples), compare the pH values to ensure they are labeled correctly (the pH should be higher in the venous sample). After doing this, determine whether the pH is in the normal range and what categories the PCO_2 and HCO_3- fall into (normal, elevated, or low). If the pH is low, then look at Table 12.8 to determine what type of acidosis, if any, is present.*

If a metabolic or mixed acidosis is present, the base deficit should also be noted. The risk of significant newborn complications increases with the amount of the base deficit, with infants with values greater than 16 mmol/L having a fourfold higher incidence than those with a level between 12 and 16 mmol/L (Low 1997).

The umbilical PO_2 is not predictive of fetal outcome, as normal newborns may be hypoxic according to this value until extrauterine respirations are well established.

As a final note, there is much confusion over certain terms used to describe the depressed neonate, and the word "asphyxia" is often misused. It is extremely important for medicolegal reasons to be precise in your notes. The American College of Obstetricians and Gynecologists (ACOG 1995) gives the following definitions:

---

* While there is much disagreement about what pH cutoff should constitute fetal acidosis, many experts suggest a cutoff of < 7.10 for defining acidosis at birth. It should be noted that the risk of perinatal morbidity or mortality does not increase unless the pH is < 7.00 (Freeman and Nelson 1988, Fee *et al.* 1990).

- Hypoxemia: decreased oxygen content in the blood
- Hypoxia: decreased level of oxygen in the tissue
- Acidemia: increased concentration of hydrogen ions in the blood
- Acidosis: increased concentration of hydrogen ions in the tissue
- Asphyxia: hypoxia with evidence of a metabolic acidosis

References

ACOG (1995). Umbilical artery blood acid–base analysis. *ACOG Technical Bulletin #216*, November 1995.

ACOG (2015). The Apgar score. *ACOG Committee Opinion #644*, October 2015.

ACOG (2017a). Delayed umbilical cord clamping after birth. *ACOG Committee Opinion #684*, January 2017.

ACOG (2017b). Delivery of a newborn with meconium-stained amniotic fluid. *ACOG Committee Opinion #689*, March 2017.

Fee SC, Malee K, Deddish R, Minogue JP, Socol ML (1990). Severe acidosis and subsequent neurologic status. *Am J Obstet Gynecol* **162**: 802–6.

Freeman JM, Nelson KB (1988). Intrapartum asphyxia and cerebral palsy. *Pediatrics* **82**: 240–9.

Low JA (1997). Intrapartum fetal asphyxia: definition, diagnosis, and classification. *Am J Obstet Gynecol* **176**: 957–9.

Riley RJ, Johnson JWC (1993). Collecting and analyzing cord blood gases. *Clin Obstet Gynecol* **36**: 13–23.

Strickland DM, Gilstrap LC, Hauth JC, Widmer K (1984). Umbilical cord pH and PCO_2: effect of interval from delivery to determination. *Am J Obstet Gynecol* **148**: 191–3.

Thorp JA, Rushing SR (1999). Umbilical cord blood gas analysis. *Obstet Gynecol Clin North Am* **26**: 695–709.

Weiner GM, Zaichkin J (2016). *Textbook of neonatal resuscitation*. Elk Grove Village, IL: American Academy of Pediatrics.

Wiberg N, Kallen K, Olofsson P (2008). Delayed umbilical cord clamping at birth has effects on arterial and venous blood gases and lactate concentrations. *BJOG* **115**: 697–703.

Wyckoff MH, Aziz K, Escobedo MB, *et al.* (2015). 2015 American Heart Association Guidelines Update for Cardiopulmonary Resuscitation and Emergency Cardiovascular Care. *Circulation* **132** (18 Suppl. 2): S543–60.

Postpartum Care

Sierra Seaman and Shad Deering

Routine Care after Spontaneous Vaginal Delivery

Rounds

After a vaginal delivery the infant and mother are monitored for several hours to ensure both are stable before being transferred to the postpartum service for the remainder of their stay. For mothers who are doing well, you will see them at least once a day on rounds to check on their recovery and issues. Important questions to ask include:

1. **How is the mother feeling?**

   - Most new mothers will be expectedly tired after having been through labor. Be sure to ask if they were able to get any sleep.

2. **How much bleeding (lochia) is there?**

   - In general, she should not be passing large clots, and should not be soaking more than one pad per hour. If she is, then it is important to investigate this further by checking vital signs, fundal height, uterine tone, and for vaginal lacerations that are bleeding. If the patient is dizzy or lightheaded (i.e., orthostatic symptoms) then you must find the etiology quickly and should order a stat CBC. See Chapter 14 for more details on postpartum hemorrhage.

3. **Any fevers or chills?**
   - If the patient has fevers or chills, then a further investigation is required to determine the etiology. Postpartum fever evaluation is discussed later in the chapter.

4. **Is the mother able to void spontaneously?**
   - It is not uncommon for a patient to have difficulty urinating after delivery, especially after an operative vaginal delivery or an epidural. However, it is important to monitor for urinary retention, as an overdistended bladder that is neglected or unnoticed for a long period of time may result in damage to bladder innervation. This complication is discussed later.

5. **How is the mother's pain?**
   - Uterine cramping. This is a normal but sometimes painful postpartum phenomenon that occurs as the uterus begins to contract back to its pre-pregnancy size. Cramping is often worse while breastfeeding, as oxytocin is released with nipple stimulation and causes the uterus to contract. It is usually worst in the first 2–3 days postpartum, and improves over time. It is best treated with analgesics such as ibuprofen. In cases where this is not adequate, a mild narcotic, such as Percocet (which is a combination of acetaminophen and oxycodone) can be given. During the physical exam, you must make sure the patient's complaint of uterine cramping is not actually a manifestation of endometritis, which will demonstrate significant uterine tenderness with palpation.
   - Perineal pain. Patients who had significant lacerations may have dysuria and pain in the perineal region. This is again best treated with ibuprofen and/or acetaminophen, but mild narcotics may be required. Ice during the first few days and warm sitz baths are also helpful in relieving pain and swelling and promoting healing. Any complaint of a significant increase in pain should be investigated with a gentle physical exam to look for evidence of infection or a hematoma.
   - Headache. This is a common complaint after delivery. It may simply be due to a lack of sleep, but it is important to look for other causes such as a post-epidural/spinal headache or preeclampsia.

6. **Is the baby breastfeeding? How is the baby feeding?**
   - Difficulty with breastfeeding is one of the more frustrating things a new mother may encounter. Taking the time to discuss this and address any concerns is important for the mother to continue and bond with the baby. Many units have a lactation consultant that you can consult. This is discussed in more detail later in this chapter.
   - While the pediatricians will almost always round at a different time, if you discover any issues with the baby, you may need to contact them after you have seen the patient.

A sample postpartum note is contained in Appendix B, *Sample Notes and Orders*.

Physical Exam

The physical exam should generally include a brief exam of the heart, the lungs, and the head and neck if there are specific complaints such as headache or sinus congestion. The breasts should be examined if there have been any fevers or if the patient complains of tenderness or engorgement.

The abdominal exam after a vaginal delivery focuses on palpation of the uterus and ensuring that it is firm and appropriately contracted. The fundal height is usually described in relation to the umbilicus in centimeters. Postpartum, the fundus is expected to be within 2 cm (usually measured with your fingers, with each finger breadth being counted as 1 cm) above the umbilicus or lower. Often, the fundal height is increased by a full bladder. In the absence of significant bleeding, simply checking the fundal height again after the patient has urinated usually results in an exam that falls within the normal range. If it does not, this should raise some concern for retained clots in the uterus and should prompt further evaluation of lochia.

It is also important to evaluate the uterus for tenderness. In general, the uterus may be mildly tender, especially with contractions during breastfeeding, but it should not be significantly tender to palpation. If it is, then you must consider the possibility of endometritis.

The perineum should be inspected if there was a significant laceration or repair, or if the patient complains of significant or increasing pain in that area. Care and evaluation of the perineum is discussed below.

The extremities should be evaluated for edema, which can be a normal finding when bilateral, especially in the lower extremities. Concerning findings are unilateral edema accompanied by significant pain, erythema, or a palpable cord on examination. Because pregnancy and the postpartum period are marked by a hypercoagulable state, deep venous thrombosis should be in your differential diagnosis. If the patient has hypertension and worsening edema, then also consider the possibility of postpartum preeclampsia.

Episiotomy/Laceration Care

If either an episiotomy was made or a laceration requiring sutures occurred, then the patient should be asked about increasing pain or discomfort in that area each day. An ice pack should be applied just after delivery and continued for several hours to help reduce swelling. The area should also be visually inspected to monitor for early signs of infection. If the patient has fevers, chills, or increasing discomfort in the area, then a gentle digital exam is needed to evaluate for hematomas. A rare but potentially fatal infection, necrotizing fasciitis, can occur, and requires immediate surgical debridement for best outcomes.

Pain Medication

Most women will not require any pain medication other than ibuprofen or acetaminophen after an uncomplicated vaginal delivery. Women who have significant lacerations and repairs may require mild narcotics, such as oxycodone. Of note, codeine is no longer recommended in breastfeeding mothers as the conversion into morphine is rapid and can lead to high levels of morphine in breast milk (ACOG 2017).

Routine Care after Operative Vaginal Delivery

Care after an operative vaginal delivery is the same as after a spontaneous vaginal delivery with the following small differences:

1. Always inspect the perineum, especially since operative vaginal deliveries are more likely to have had an episiotomy or more extensive lacerations and there is the potential for vaginal hematomas.
2. Examine the infant. With a vacuum delivery, inspect the fetal scalp (and take off the hat if the child has one on during rounds) and look for evidence of a hematoma. For forceps deliveries, make sure and note any facial marks and if they have diminished, as they will usually begin to fade in the days after delivery.
3. Be aware of the potential for urinary retention and ask the mother if she is having any difficulty with urination.

Routine Care after Cesarean Section

Rounds

After a cesarean section, the mother and infant are taken to a recovery room where they are monitored for several hours. As long as she remains stable, the mother is transferred to the postpartum service. The questions you will ask a postoperative patient are the same as after a vaginal delivery, with the following additions:

1. Are you having any nausea or vomiting?
2. Are you dizzy or lightheaded?
3. Have you been able to ambulate?
4. Have you had any drainage from your incision?
5. Is the pain from your incision controlled with pain medications?
6. Are you passing flatus?

A cesarean section is a major abdominal surgery. Patients should be evaluated daily for postoperative bleeding and return of bowel function. Note any symptoms that could be related to hypovolemia from bleeding, such as dizziness or lightheadedness, especially with ambulation. Vital signs are, as always, vital information. Watch for tachycardia and hypotension as these could be signs of previously unrecognized blood loss. Urine output, which should be at least 0.5 mL/kg/hour, is another way to monitor the patient's hemodynamic status and should be reviewed every shift and included in progress notes. If urine output is adequate, the Foley catheter can generally be removed 12–24 hours postoperatively.

Physical Exam

The physical exam after a cesarean delivery is essentially the same as after a vaginal delivery, with the addition of an incision to monitor.

Incision Care

At the end of a cesarean section, the incision is covered with a sterile dressing. This dressing should be left in place for 24–48 hours before removal. On postoperative day one, evaluate the dressing for any staining or active drainage beyond the bandage. On postoperative day two, after removing the bandage, inspect to be sure the incision is clean, dry, and intact.

Look for areas of erythema, and note any drainage coming from the incision. If erythema is present, you can mark the extent of it with a pen to compare at the next exam. A small amount of serosanguinous drainage is common, and a piece of 4 × 4 gauze can be placed over this and checked later. Frank bleeding, a significant increase in drainage, or purulent discharge will need to be evaluated immediately. If any of these are present, make sure the team is aware – and if you are a student or resident, have the staff see the incision. Wound infections and treatment are discussed in detail in Chapter 10.

Pain Medication

After a cesarean section, many patients receive a long-acting narcotic in their epidural, which will usually provide adequate analgesia for the next 12–24 hours. If they do not, then patient-controlled analgesia (PCA), which is a pump that administers a small dose of a narcotic when the patient pushes a button, can be used for the initial postoperative period. Another option is using IV narcotics on an as-needed, or PRN, basis. A non-steroidal medication such as ketorolac can be given as well if there was not excessive bleeding during the cesarean section.

When the patient is able to tolerate oral intake, a non-steroidal medication, such as ibuprofen, is given on a schedule, e.g., 800 mg PO every 8 hours. A mild narcotic such as Percocet (see Appendix A, *Medication Database*) can be given every 4–6 hours as needed to control breakthrough pain.

Foley Catheter Management

The Foley catheter is usually removed on postoperative day one. It is an important tool for monitoring hemodynamic status. If the patient is not making adequate urine or is hemo-dynamically unstable then the Foley should remain in place until she is stable.

After the catheter is removed, it is important the patient have a "due to of void," which means you will check to make sure she has been able to urinate within 4–6 hours in order to prevent her bladder from becoming overdistended. If the patient is not able to void by that time, then further evaluation with a bladder scan or straight catheterization should be performed, or the Foley catheter can be replaced and removed again the next day. If the patient has continued urinary retention, she will need further evaluation.

Return of Bowel Function

In the past, patients were not given anything by mouth after a cesarean section until they had flatus, owing to the belief that this would prevent a postoperative ileus. This notion has been challenged in recent years by several studies showing that early feeding for both gynecologic abdominal surgery and cesarean sections is associated with decreased time in the hospital and no significant increase in the incidence of postoperative ileus (Soriano *et al.* 1996, Fanning and Andrews 2001, Patolia *et al.* 2001, Ljungqvist *et al.* 2017). Also, patients do not need to have a bowel movement before leaving the hospital. If patients are tolerating PO without issues of emesis or distension, this is reassuring of proper bowel function.

Breastfeeding

Breast milk is the ideal food for new infants and decreases the risk of infection, including diarrhea, otitis media, urinary tract infections, and many other common infant infections.

There are also studies that show it may be protective against sudden infant death syndrome and the development of type 1 diabetes (AAP 1997). In 2011, as many as 79% of new mothers were breastfeeding in the initial postpartum period (CDC 2016). Although breastfeeding has so many proven benefits, it can be frustrating at first, and it is important to encourage continued trials of breastfeeding and provide support in the form of teaching with providers or lactation consultants to maximize chances for success. Unfortunately, it is not recommended for all women to breastfeed. Contraindications to breastfeeding are listed below.

Contraindications

- HIV infection is a contraindication to breastfeeding in developed countries, as the infection may be transmitted to the infant
- Active HSV infection of the nipple
- Active, untreated tuberculosis
- Patients with an infant with galactosemia
- Patients undergoing treatment for breast cancer
- Patients taking illicit drugs or who abuse alcohol

Maternal medications. Most antibiotics and medications do not pose a problem for breastfeeding. The *Medication Database* in Appendix A includes notes on the safety of each with breastfeeding. If you are using another medication, then a helpful reference is the book *Drugs in Pregnancy and Lactation*, which is currently in its 11th edition (Briggs *et al.* 2017). For online resources, LactMed (https://toxnet.nlm.nih.gov/newtoxnet/lactmed.htm) is another excellent resource.

Common Challenges

It is important to know how to manage common complications in order to allow the mother to continue to breastfeed. With appropriate and prompt care, most problems can be overcome.

Sore nipples/fissures. These complications usually result from incorrect positioning of the infant and poor latching-on rather than prolonged nursing (Berens 2001). If the nipple appears infected, then treatment with an antibiotic to cover *Staphylococcus aureus* should be started (see Appendix A, *Medication Database*). In addition, the use of over-the-counter topical creams, such as those containing lanolin, may be helpful.

Mastitis. This infection occurs in 1–2% of lactating women and is most common in the first and fifth weeks postpartum (ACOG 2007). Some risk factors include missed feedings, nipple fissures, and untreated breast engorgement. Clinically, the patient will usually complain of the rapid onset of fever, unilateral breast pain, and myalgia. The most common responsible organism is *Staphylococcus aureus*, which accounts for almost half of cases. A narrow-spectrum antibiotic, such as dicloxacillin or a cephalosporin, is the first-line therapy and should be given for 10–14 days. (If the patient is allergic to penicillins and cephalosporins, then erythromycin can be given.) See Appendix A, *Medication Database*, for more information on these antibiotics. The patient should continue to breastfeed, as the milk is not harmful and both penicillins and cephalosporins are safe in breastfeeding. If this is too uncomfortable for the patient, then the infected breast should be expressed by hand if possible.

Mastitis should be treated early and aggressively, because delaying treatment increases the risk of developing a breast abscess.

Breast abscess. Between 5% and 11% of women with mastitis will go on to develop a breast abscess (Berens 2001). The symptoms are essentially the same as mastitis, but a fluctuant mass is present. It is diagnosed by either a palpable mass or failure to respond to antibiotic treatment for a presumed mastitis within 48–72 hours.
The most common treatment of a breast abscess is surgical incision and drainage, with continued antibiotic treatment. If multiple abscesses are present, all must be drained and meticulous hemostasis obtained to prevent hematomas from forming. After surgery, breast milk from the affected breast is generally disposed of for the first 24 hours. Breastfeeding after surgery from the infected breast can be restarted after this time as long as there is not drainage from the incision onto the nipple. Another therapy that has been utilized for breast abscesses involves the drainage of the abscess by needle aspiration guided by ultrasound (Irusen *et al.* 2015).

Galactocele. This is caused by plugged milk ducts that create a tender, palpable lump in the breast. It is not accompanied by evidence of infection such as fevers, chills, or erythema. Some risk factors include missing a feeding, overabundant milk supply, and poor latch-on (Berens 2001). Treatment is symptomatic and includes increasing the frequency of feeding, massaging the area during feeding, and applying a moist, warm compress to the area. The galactocele should generally resolve within 72 hours. If signs of infection become evident, then patients should be evaluated for mastitis or an abscess.

Bloody nipple discharge. This can be a normal finding during the third trimester because of increased vascularity of the breast, or during the postpartum period from nipple trauma. It is not harmful to the infant, and should resolve spontaneously within approximately 7 days. If the bloody discharge lasts longer than this, or appears to be coming from a single duct, then further evaluation, including a breast exam, cytologic evaluation of the discharge, and possibly mammography or ultrasound, should be pursued, as this can be a presenting symptom of a malignant tumor.

Breast mass. When a breast mass is found postpartum, and it is not felt to be due to a galactocele or breast abscess, then further workup is required. Fortunately, the incidence of breast cancer in breastfeeding mothers is only 1 in 3000 to 1 in 10,000 patients, and there is no difference in survival rates when compared to non-pregnant women (Berens 2001). The same diagnostic workup, including breast exam, fine-needle aspiration, mammography, and ultrasound as required, is acceptable and safe in breastfeeding patients.

Contraception issues. The immediate postpartum period is an ideal time to initiate contraception, as patients are known to not be pregnant. Contraception is particularly important in the immediate postpartum period, as 45% of women are sexually active within 6 weeks after delivery when most patients have their routine postpartum visit. Early contraception can help avoid unintended and close-interval pregnancy (ACOG 2016). When breastfeeding is used exclusively, lactational amenorrhea can be an effective form of contraception. This method is also beneficial in that it does not affect the milk supply. Barrier methods such as condoms also do not affect the milk supply, but they are less effective. Progesterone-only contraceptives may be started as soon as the patient is discharged from the hospital and do not affect the milk supply. Depot medroxyprogesterone acetate can be given prior to hospital discharge, especially in patients who may not follow up for a postpartum visit, but is normally given at 4–6 weeks postpartum. Combination birth control pills (OCPs), which contain estrogen, are not generally started until 6 weeks after delivery because of the concern about the risk of venous thromboembolism (VTE) in the immediate postpartum period. When available, use of long-acting reversible contraception (LARC) is preferred. With success rates of more than 99%, this is the most effective form of contraception. Both implants and intrauterine devices (IUDs) are safe to use in the immediate postpartum period (ACOG 2016). IUD placement should ideally take place in the delivery room within 10 minutes of the delivery of the placenta, and the device may be placed either manually or with a ring forceps, with or without the guidance of ultrasound. In the case of a cesarean section, IUD placement occurs after the uterus has good tone and before the completion of the hysterotomy. IUD insertion is contraindicated in patients with signs of infection (intra-amniotic infection, endometritis). Patients should be counseled that expulsion rates are higher postpartum, up to 24%, and if expulsion is suspected, a backup contraceptive method should be used and they should come to see their provider for an exam. Implants have no increased risk associated with postpartum use.

Common Postpartum Infections and Complications

Postpartum Fever

If a patient develops a fever in the postpartum period, she should be examined closely for a source. One useful memory aid that can help you remember what to look for is:

Wind: atelectasis or sinus/upper respiratory infections (atelectasis is more common after a cesarean delivery, especially if the patient has not been ambulatory)

Water: urinary tract infection

Walking: thrombophlebitis

Wound: infection of the incision or episiotomy

Wonder drug: medication-induced fevers

Womb: endometritis

Woman: mastitis

A thorough review of systems and a physical exam should be performed. If a source is not obvious, such as endometritis, then a urinalysis and culture, and a complete blood count with differential should be sent and acetaminophen administered. If the fever continues to increase or the patient's condition worsens, then two sets of blood cultures and a chest x-ray should be done as well.

When a source is found, the infection should be treated with the appropriate antibiotics, and the patient should not be discharged until she has been afebrile for at least 24 hours.

Endometritis

This is much more common in patients who undergo a cesarean delivery. It generally presents with fevers and chills in combination with significant uterine tenderness on abdominal exam. Please refer to Chapter 14 for a complete discussion of the diagnosis and treatment of this infection.

Mastitis

See under *Breastfeeding* above.

Preeclampsia

While the cure for preeclampsia is delivery of the placenta, it is possible for patients to develop preeclampsia in the postpartum period. Early postpartum preeclampsia develops within 48 hours of delivery, and late-onset postpartum preeclampsia is generally defined as having an onset between 48 hours and 4 weeks after delivery. This complication is also discussed in detail in Chapter 14.

Postpartum Blues

Mild depressive symptoms, referred to as the postpartum blues, are common in the first week after delivery. Symptoms include anxiety, difficulty concentrating, labile mood swings, insomnia, and weepiness. The hallmark characteristic of postpartum blues is that symptoms only last for a few days or weeks and do not meet criteria for a diagnosis of major depression. Treatment is initially supportive, and you should reassure the patient that this is most likely a transient phase. Ensure the patient does not have any suicidal ideations and that she is able to care for the infant prior to discharge, and arrange early follow-up and provide phone numbers so that she can contact her provider if she continues to experience problems.

If the symptoms persist beyond a week, the diagnosis of postpartum depression should be considered. Between 10% and 15% of new mothers may experience postpartum depression up to 1 year after birth (ACOG 2013). In addition to tearfulness and emotional lability, patients may feel hopeless or worthless or have difficulty caring for themselves or their child. As with major depression outside of pregnancy, a patient must have five depressive symptoms for at least 2 weeks for the diagnosis to be made. In more severe cases, patients have suicidal ideation or homicidal ideation (usually toward the child). Postpartum psychosis occurs in 1–2 per 1000 births. Patients may present with delirium, hallucinations, or delusions and have a higher risk for suicide and infanticide. These rare but severe cases require emergency evaluation and hospitalization (Wesseloo *et al.* 2016).

Urinary Retention

It is not uncommon for women to have difficulty voiding after either vaginal delivery or a cesarean section. It is important to diagnose this, as prolonged urinary retention and overdistention of the bladder can result in permanent damage and voiding problems. Urinary retention is usually diagnosed when a patient has been unable to void for 4–6 hours after a Foley catheter has been removed and when an enlarged bladder, which feels like a cystic mass in the lower abdomen on exam, is palpated.

A differential of the causes of urinary retention after delivery that must be considered includes the following:

- Effects of medication/anesthesia
- Vaginal hematoma causing obstruction
- Urethral obstruction by sutures from laceration repair

A physical exam can usually rule out a hematoma or suture as the etiology of urinary retention.

Treatment of urinary retention initially consists of a physical exam and then placing a Foley catheter to provide drainage of the bladder. If the catheter is placed in the afternoon, it is often left in place overnight and removed the next morning. After the catheter is removed, immediately after the first time the patient urinates, a post-void residual is checked by an in-and-out catheterization. If the residual is less than 200 mL, then the Foley does not need to be replaced. If it is more than this, the Foley is either replaced or post-void residuals continue to be checked, ensuring the patient does not go more than 4 hours between voids. If the residuals do not decrease and are consistently greater than 200 mL, then a Foley catheter may be replaced to rest the bladder and voiding trials conducted again the next day.

If the patient is still unable to void appropriately when she meets all other discharge criteria, then she may either be taught how to self-catheterize or have a Foley catheter inserted with a leg bag attached to go home with. Close follow-up and bladder trials are important to monitor for return of normal function.

Fortunately, it is uncommon for urinary retention to persist more than a couple of days after delivery. One study of over 8000 deliveries found the incidence of persistent urinary retention, which was defined as present if the patient was still unable to void spontaneously on the third postpartum day, to be only 0.05% (Groutz *et al.* 2001). Risk factors for this included VBAC, a prolonged second stage of labor, epidural analgesia, and delayed diagnosis and intervention.

Wound/Episiotomy Infections

When the normal bacterial content of the vagina and the continued normal lochia that occurs after delivery are considered, the incidence of episiotomy infections is surprisingly low.

While an episiotomy infection often presents with increased pain, erythema, fevers, and chills, an abdominal wound infection can present with an increased amount of drainage in addition to erythema, fever, and chills.

Please see the following chapters for a complete discussion of these problems:

- Chapter 10: Wound infections after cesarean section
- Chapter 11: Episiotomy infections

Postpartum Hemorrhage

While this usually occurs at the time of delivery, it may occur while the patient is on the postpartum ward. This complication is addressed in detail in Chapter 14.

Discharge Issues

Discharge criteria. Prior to discharge, the following conditions must be met:

- The patient is able to ambulate
- She can spontaneously void (or if not, then she must have a catheter, or learn how to self-catheterize as described above)
- She can tolerate a regular diet
- She is hemodynamically stable
- There is no evidence of serious infection that requires inpatient treatment

- Adequate follow-up for both mother and child has been arranged
- All immunizations/Rhogam have been given as indicated
- Contraception has been discussed

Timing of discharge. The time from delivery to discharge differs between vaginal deliveries and cesarean deliveries, but the same criteria as listed above must be met for the patient to leave the hospital.

- Vaginal delivery. If there are no complications, then patients are usually not kept any longer than 48 hours. In some cases, patients may leave as early as 24 hours after delivery, if they desire, as long as the infant is cleared for discharge.
- Cesarean delivery. Patients may be discharged when they meet the discharge criteria above. This will occur in most patients by 72 hours, but there are times when they will have slow return of bowel function and need to stay another day.

Immunizations. Patients who are rubella non-immune should be vaccinated prior to discharge. You can reassure the parents that breastfeeding is not a contraindication to the immunization and does not place the infant at risk of contracting the disease (APGO 1999).

Rhogam. If the mother is Rh-negative and the infant is Rh-positive, then prior to discharge, the patient should receive the standard dose of 300 mcg of anti-D immune globulin (Rhogam) in order to prevent isoimmunization and complications with subsequent pregnancies.

Contraception. While this may be the last thing on a new mother's mind, it is important to discuss contraception prior to discharge. If the patient is breastfeeding on demand, then ovulation is usually suppressed, but in the non-lactating mother, ovulation usually occurs between 3 and 10 weeks after delivery. In general, the following options are available for women who are not using lactational amenorrhea for contraception:

- Barrier methods.
- Progestin-only oral contraceptive pills may be given to patients at the time of discharge, or at any time postpartum. Ovulation generally does not return before 3 weeks postpartum even in non-lactating women.
- Combination oral contraceptive pills (OCPs) may be started at 6 weeks postpartum.
- Depot medroxyprogesterone acetate is generally given prior to discharge from the hospital or at approximately 6 weeks postpartum.*
- Intrauterine device (immediate placement postpartum or interval placement).**
- Hormonal implant (immediate placement postpartum or interval placement).**

---

* An additional benefit of the depot medroxyprogesterone over OCPs is that adolescents are much less likely to discontinue this form of birth control as compared to OCPs. In one study, 72% of women under the age of 18 discontinued OCPs within a year, compared to 44% using depot medroxyprogesterone (Templeman et al. 2000).

** Remember, if your patient chooses an interval placement of a LARC device, an immediate form of birth control (any of the choices listed above) should be provided until the postpartum visit when the device can be placed.

Resuming coitus. For patients who had a cesarean section, abstinence is recommended for 4–6 weeks to permit adequate healing of the incision. For patients who had a vaginal delivery, data do not support a specific time period that must lapse before coitus is resumed. For women with significant vaginal lacerations, 4 weeks of abstinence are generally recommended for wound healing. For those without lacerations, coitus can generally be resumed 2–3 weeks postpartum, depending on the patient's desire and level of comfort. Breastfeeding patients should be informed that they may experience vaginal dryness postpartum because of decreased estrogen production, and vaginal lubricant can be recommended.

References

AAP (1997). Breastfeeding and the use of human milk. American Academy of Pediatrics. Work Group on Breastfeeding. *Pediatrics* **100**: 1035–9.

ACOG (2007). Breastfeeding: maternal and infant aspects. *ACOG Educational Bulletin* **#361**, February 2007.

ACOG (2013). Postpartum depression. *ACOG Educational Bulletin* **AP091**, December 2013.

ACOG (2016). Immediate postpartum long-acting reversible contraception. *ACOG Committee Opinion* **#670**, August 2016.

ACOG (2017). Practice advisory on codeine and tramadol for breastfeeding women. https://www.acog.org/Clinical-Guidance-and-Publications/Practice-Advisories/Practice-Advisory-on-Codeine-and-Tramadol-for-Breastfeeding-Women (accessed May 2018).

APGO (1999). *Immunization for Women's Health.* APGO Educational Series on Women's Health Issues. Washington, DC: Association of Professors of Gynecology and Obstetrics.

Berens PD (2001). Prenatal, intrapartum, and postpartum support of the lactating mother. *Pediatr Clin North Am* **48**: 356–75.

Briggs GG, Freeman RK, Towers CV, Forinash AB (eds.) (2017). *Drugs in Pregnancy and Lactation*, 11th edn. Philadelphia, PA: Wolters Kluwer.

CDC (2016). Breastfeeding report card: United States 2014. Atlanta, GA: Centers for Disease Control and Prevention. www.cdc.gov/breastfeeding/pdf/2014breastfeedingreportcard.pdf (accessed May 2018).

Fanning J, Andrews S (2001). Early postoperative feeding after major gynecologic surgery: Evidence-based scientific medicine. *Am J Obstet Gynecol* **185**: 1–4.

Groutz A, Gordon D, Wolman I, *et al.* (2001). Persistent postpartum urinary retention in contemporary obstetric practice: definition, prevalence and clinical implications. *J Reprod Med* **46**: 44–8.

Irusen H, Rohwer AC, Steyn DW, Young T (2015). Treatments for breast abscesses in breastfeeding women. *Cochrane Database Syst Rev* (8): CD010490.

Ljungqvist O, Scott M, Fearon KC (2017). Enhanced recovery after surgery: a review. *JAMA Surg* **152**: 292–8.

Patolia DS, Hilliard RLM, Toy EC, Baker B (2001). Early feeding after cesarean: Randomized trial. *Obstet Gynecol* **98**: 113–16.

Soriano D, Dulitzki M, Keidar N, *et al.* (1996). Early oral feeding after cesarean delivery. *Obstet Gynecol* **87**: 1006–8.

Templeman CL, Cook V, Goldsmith LJ, Powell J, Hertweck P (2000). Postpartum contraceptive use among adolescent mothers. *Obstet Gynecol* **95**: 770–6.

Wesseloo R, Kamperman AM, Munk-Olsen T, *et al.* (2016). Risk of postpartum relapse in bipolar disorder and postpartum psychosis: a systematic review and meta-analysis. *Am J Psychiatry* **173**: 117–27.

Common Obstetric Complications and Emergencies

Devon M. Rupley, Kristen Elmezzi and Shad Deering

Introduction

While the vast majority of deliveries are uncomplicated, when complications do occur, they happen quickly and often without warning. Rapid and effective interventions can be life-saving for both mother and baby. Always remember that every delivery is an emergency waiting to happen.

This chapter covers some of the most common obstetric complications and emergencies as well as their treatments, to prepare you for when these occur.

Intra-amniotic Infection

Intra-amniotic infection (IAI), also sometimes referred to as chorioamnionitis, is an infection involving the amnion, chorion, placenta, or fetus. In an effort to reduce the ambiguity around the diagnosis and treatment of clinical chorioamnionitis, in 2015 the National Institute of Child Health and Human Development recommended replacing the term chorioamnionitis with "triple I" (intrauterine inflammation or infection or both). It is defined as the following:

- Maternal fever (two documented temperatures of > 38.0 °C at least 30 minutes apart) with one or more of the following:

  - Fetal tachycardia (> 160 bpm for over 10 minutes)

- Maternal WBC > 15,000 in the absence of recent corticosteroids
- Purulent fluid from the cervical os
- Biochemical or microbiologic amniotic fluid results indicating microbial invasion of amniotic fluid

(Higgins *et al.* 2016, Tita 2017)

Incidence
IAI is reported to occur in 1–4% of all births in the US and complicates 7% of term PROM deliveries (Tita and Andrews 2010, Tita 2017). The incidence is significantly higher (5–10%) in preterm deliveries (Chapman *et al.* 2014, Kim *et al.* 2015).

Clinical Picture
Traditionally, patients with IAI present with a constellation of non-specific findings including maternal fever and abdominal pain or uterine tenderness. It is also common to find fetal tachycardia.

Risk Factors
- Prolonged duration of membrane rupture
- Prolonged labor with either a second stage > 2 hours or active labor > 12 hours
- Multiple digital examinations with ruptured membranes
- Nulliparity
- GBS colonization or bacterial vaginosis
- Alcohol and tobacco use
- Internal monitors (FSE or IUPC)
- Meconium-stained amniotic fluid
- Epidural anesthesia

(Tita and Andrews 2010)

Causes
IAI is typically a polymicrobial infection secondary to ascending genital microbes. The most common bacteria identified are *Ureaplasma urealyticum* and *Mycoplasma hominis*, followed by *Gardnerella vaginalis, Bacteroides*, Group B streptococcus, and *Escherichia coli* (Tita and Andrews 2010).

Complications
IAI is associated with increased risk of cesarean delivery, endometritis, wound infection, and pelvic abscess. It also nearly doubles the risk of postpartum hemorrhage and increases the risk for significant maternal bacteremia. Intrauterine infection is associated with higher rates of neonatal sepsis, pneumonia, respiratory distress, perinatal death, and long-term neurodevelopmental disability (Tita and Andrews 2010).

Treatment

The treatment of IAI depends on the clinical status of the mother and fetus. Isolated maternal fever may be monitored, especially immediately following epidural anesthesia initiation. If the patient meets criteria for IAI, ampicillin (2 g IV q6h) and gentamycin (5 mg/kg once daily) should be initiated. If the patient requires a cesarean section for delivery, then you should consider adding either clindamycin (900 mg) or metronidazole (500 mg) to the patient's regimen and continue this for at least one additional dose of antibiotics and often for 24 hours after delivery. Antibiotics can typically be discontinued after vaginal delivery if the patient clinically improves. Discontinuation of antibiotics after one additional dose following delivery can also be considered in patients who underwent cesarean delivery, depending on the clinical status of the patient (i.e., if she remains afebrile and does not have additional risk factors) (Higgins *et al.* 2016).

Additional Potential Antibiotic Regimens

Mild penicillin allergy:

Cefazolin 2 g IV q8h + gentamycin (5 mg/kg IV q24h or 2 mg/kg IV then 1.5 mg/kg q8h)

Severe penicillin allergy:

Clindamycin 900 mg IV q8h or vancomycin 1 g IV q12h + Gentamycin (5 mg/kg IV q24h or 2 mg/kg IV then 1.5 mg/kg q8h)

Alternative regimens:

Ampicillin–sulbactam 3 g IV q6h
Piperacillin–tazobactam 3.375 g IV q6h or 4.5 g IV q8h
Cefotetan 2 g IV q12h
Cefoxitin 2 g IV q8h
Ertapenem 1 g IV q24h

(ACOG 2017a)

Endometritis

Endometritis is a postpartum infection of the decidua and surrounding tissues.

Incidence

Endometritis is rare following vaginal delivery, occurring in only 1–3% of patients, but the incidence increases to up to 27% with cesarean delivery (Mackeen *et al.* 2015).

Clinical Picture

Patients usually present in the first several days postpartum. Endometritis is typically a clinical diagnosis made after other sources of infection (mastitis, cellulitis, surgical site infection, or urinary tract infection) are ruled out. Findings may include:

- Fever (> 100.4 °F or 38.0 °C)
- Uterine tenderness
- Foul-smelling lochia
- Leukocytosis

Risk Factors

The most common risk factor is cesarean delivery, especially if the procedure is done following onset of labor. Additional risk factors include:

- Cesarean delivery
- Bacterial vaginosis
- Intra-amniotic infection
- Prolonged rupture of membranes
- Prolonged labor
- Multiple vaginal examinations with ruptured membranes
- Meconium staining of amniotic fluid
- Manual placental removal
- Low socioeconomic status
- Maternal diabetes
- Severe maternal anemia

Causes

Endometritis is typically a polymicrobial infection from common bacteria from the genital tract (Chen 2018). Direct seeding of the uterine cavity, through cesarean section, manual removal of placenta, or internal monitoring increases the likelihood of endometritis. Prolonged duration of labor, especially with ruptured membranes, also increases the incidence.

Treatment

While prevention through administration of preoperative antibiotics within 60 minutes prior to skin incision for cesarean delivery is the best way to avoid endometritis, antibiotics must be quickly started if it is diagnosed. Initial treatment includes the administration of broad-spectrum antibiotics, usually gentamycin (2 mg/kg IV then 1.5 mg/kg IV q8h or 5 mg/kg q24h)* plus clindamycin (900 mg IV q8h) until the patient has been afebrile for 24–48 hours and has clinically improved (decreased fundal tenderness). If the patient does not improve after 48 hours of antibiotics, the addition of ampicillin (2 g q6h) or penicillin, or vancomycin in the penicillin-allergic patient, should be considered (Faro 2005).

Other regimens that have been reported for the treatment of postpartum endometritis include cefoxitin (2 gm IV q6h) or ampicillin–sulbactam (3 gm IV q6h).

---

* In the postpartum period, gentamycin is generally given as 5 mg/kg IV q24h, and multiple studies have demonstrated that this regimen is less expensive, requires less nursing time, and is as safe and effective as the q8h dosing (Del Priore *et al.* 1996, Mitra *et al.* 1997).

Hemorrhage

Significant bleeding may occur during the antepartum, peripartum, and postpartum periods. Obstetric hemorrhage is the most common cause of maternal death worldwide, and postpartum hemorrhage (PPH) is one of the top five causes of maternal mortality globally (Belfort 2017).

Antepartum Hemorrhage

Vaginal bleeding is most common in the first trimester, complicating 20–40% of pregnancies (Norwitz 2016). Antepartum bleeding, occurring after 20 weeks' gestation, complicates 4–5% of pregnancies. Common causes include:
- Placental abruption (30%)
- Placenta previa (20%)
- Cervical dilation from labor
- Vasa previa
- Uterine rupture

(Norwitz 2016)

In general, bleeding due to cervical change is rarely significant enough to result in fetal or maternal distress, but may alert the physician to the presence of labor. It is essential that digital exams are not performed during the evaluation of bleeding during the second or third trimester of pregnancy until placenta previa has been ruled out, as digital exam may precipitate a catastrophic hemorrhage.

The evaluation and workup of patients presenting with antepartum hemorrhage should proceed as follows:
- Obtain a thorough maternal history (onset and amount of bleeding, any evidence of rupture of membranes, trauma or motor vehicle accident, history of bleeding problems, medication use such as aspirin or heparin).
- Assess maternal hemodynamic status (vital signs, CBC, fibrinogen, PT/PTT).
- Assess fetal status (fetal heart rate): continuous monitoring if > 24 weeks, monitor for contractions.
- Perform abdominal ultrasound and determine placental location; if there is any possibility of a placenta previa, perform vaginal ultrasound.
- If no evidence of a placenta previa, then perform a speculum examination and digital examination to look for cervical source of bleeding (e.g., polyps, cervicitis, or dilation).

Placenta Previa

A placenta previa is defined as placental tissue either covering the cervical os or being in close proximity to the internal os (< 2 cm). Some common nomenclature relating to different degrees of placenta previa are listed in Table 14.1.

Incidence

Two percent of pregnancies will demonstrate evidence of placenta previa on ultrasound at around 20 weeks' gestation, but 90% of these resolve prior to delivery (Lockwood and Russo-Stieglitz 2017). At term, the incidence of placenta previa is 5 per 1000 pregnancies (Creswell *et al.* 2013). Typical management when a placenta previa is diagnosed early in pregnancy is to give the patient bleeding precautions and recommend pelvic rest (i.e., no intercourse or anything in the vagina) and ordering repeat transvaginal ultrasound around 28 weeks' gestation to reassess placental location.

Table 14.1 Placenta previa

Complete previa	Placental tissue covers the entire internal cervical os
Partial previa	Placental tissue partially covers the internal cervical os
Marginal previa	Placental tissue is up to the edge of the internal cervical os
Low-lying placenta	Placental edge is < 2 cm from the internal cervical os

(Oyelese and Smulian 2006)

Clinical Picture

Classically, patients with placenta previa present with painless vaginal bleeding; however, many patients may also have uterine contractions at the time of diagnosis. Bleeding can range from minimal to life-threatening and quickly progress to maternal shock, fetal distress, and even fetal demise. Patients typically present with bleeding in the third trimester, with around 30% of patients presenting prior to 30 weeks and 44.6% having their first bleed after 30 weeks (Dola *et al.* 2003). Placenta previa is associated with a risk of placenta accreta (where the placenta is abnormally attached to the uterus and does not completely detach after delivery, often resulting in significant bleeding and potentially requiring hysterectomy to correct) of 1–5%, in the setting of no prior uterine surgery. This risk goes up significantly when the patient has had a cesarean section. As more women are delivering by cesarean section, the incidence of placenta accreta is increasing.

Risk Factors

- Maternal age > 40
- Multiparity
- Previous uterine curettage
- Previous cesarean delivery
- Smoking
- Male fetus
- Multiple gestation
- Malpresentation

Cause

Placenta previa occurs when the placenta implants in very close proximity to or overlying the cervical os. This may be idiopathic or occur as a result of previous uterine scarring from procedures like uterine curettage or cesarean section.

Diagnosis

The diagnosis is generally made by ultrasound. While an abdominal ultrasound is quite accurate for making the diagnosis, transvaginal ultrasound examination is not only safe and effective, but more accurate and should be performed when this condition is suspected on abdominal ultrasound. Digital exams should be avoided until placenta previa is ruled out to avoid catastrophic hemorrhage from disruption of placental vessels.

Treatment

The initial treatment is stabilization of the mother and assessment of fetal status. If there is profuse hemorrhage in conjunction with fetal distress in a viable (i.e., > 23-week) fetus, then rapid delivery by cesarean section may be warranted. If the patient is beyond 34 weeks' gestation, then delivery is generally indicated regardless of the quantity of bleeding. If the patient is less than 34 weeks and hemodynamically stable with no evidence of fetal distress, then corticosteroids may be administered for fetal lung maturity and careful monitoring undertaken in an attempt to prolong pregnancy.

Regarding mode of delivery, when placenta previa is present a cesarean section is the route of delivery to prevent the catastrophic hemorrhage that would occur with continued dilation and labor. In general, cesarean section is recommended if the placental edge is within 2 cm of the internal cervical os, or if there is already active bleeding. In a patient in labor or at term, if the distance is at least 1 cm, the risk of significant bleeding before delivery is only approximately 3%, and it has been shown that more than two-thirds of women will be able to have a vaginal delivery with minimal problems (Oyelese 2010).

Placental Abruption

A placental abruption occurs when the placenta prematurely separates from the uterine wall. As separation happens, bleeding occurs and is clinically evident in approximately 80% of cases. Thus, 20% of abruptions are concealed, meaning that though there is bleeding happening, no visible vaginal bleeding occurs. This is important to remember when evaluating a patient with risk factors and a clinical picture concerning for abruption. Placental abruption accounts for approximately one-third of all cases of antepartum hemorrhage, and the amount of vaginal bleeding correlates poorly with degree of abruption.

Incidence

Placental abruption occurs in approximately 1% of all deliveries in the United States, with the majority, 40–60%, occurring in patients beyond 37 weeks (Tikkanen 2011).

Clinical Picture

Placental abruption usually presents with painful vaginal bleeding, strong uterine contractions, uterine tenderness, and fetal distress as evidenced by a non-reassuring fetal heart rate (FHR) tracing. Because a large of amount of blood can be stored behind the placenta, the amount of hemorrhage seen is not an accurate gauge of actual blood loss. As mentioned previously, in 20% of patients, the bleeding will be concealed – so strong suspicion of abruption must be maintained for any patient presenting with abdominal pain and fetal distress.

Risk Factors

- Previous abruption (10–15-fold increased risk)
- Cocaine/methamphetamine abuse
- Trauma: blunt abdominal trauma from motor vehicle accidents, falls, or domestic abuse
- Chronic hypertension (5-fold increased risk)
- Preeclampsia/eclampsia
- Preterm premature rupture of membranes (PPROM)

- Increased maternal age and parity
- Cigarette smoking
- Multiple gestations
- Intra-amniotic infection
- Polyhydramnios

(Ananth *et al.* 1996)

Diagnosis

This is generally a clinical diagnosis, although laboratory evaluation and ultrasound are helpful in confirming the presence of abruption.

Physical Examination

The maternal examination consists of assessing the patient for other causes of vaginal bleeding (which should ideally begin with an ultrasound) to exclude the possibility of a placenta previa, cervical polyps, or labor as the source of bleeding. It is also important to look for evidence of uterine contractions and tenderness to palpation in the absence of a fever. The patient should be evaluated for evidence of hypovolemic shock, with vital signs and urine output monitored closely. A large-bore IV should be started if fluid resuscitation is needed or anticipated. Evaluation of the FHR tracing should also be done.

Laboratory Evaluation

Maternal labs should include a CBC, fibrinogen level, and PT/PTT, both to evaluate the patient's hemodynamic stability and to look for evidence of disseminated intravascular coagulopathy (DIC). A fibrinogen of < 200 mg/dL and/or a platelet count of < 100,000 are both highly suspicious for an abruption. Fortunately, DIC occurs in a small number of abruptions.

Note: The Kleihauer–Betke test, D-dimer, and CA-125 have been used in an attempt to make the diagnosis of abruption. They are, however, of questionable benefit and do not need to be performed routinely (Atkinson *et al.* 2015).

Ultrasound

It is imperative to rule out a placenta previa by ultrasound evaluation in settings of vaginal bleeding in patients without prior ultrasounds, as digital examination could precipitate a catastrophic bleed. While it is often possible to see a retroplacental hemorrhage on sonogram, clot appearance depends on when the ultrasound is done, as the blood at first may appear similar to placental tissue and may not become hypoechoic for nearly a week. If you visualize what appears to be a significant hemorrhage, this increases your suspicion for abruption, but if you do not see it you cannot rule it out completely.

Treatment

Treatment depends both on the gestational age as well as the extent of the abruption. In a preterm fetus (i.e., < 34 weeks' gestation) in the setting of mild abruption with no evidence of fetal distress or maternal instability, conservative management, which includes close monitoring and the administration of corticosteroids, is a reasonable approach. Tocolysis may be considered in stable cases to decrease the contractions that often accompany abruption; however, this is best done in consultation with a maternal–fetal medicine specialist.

In a patient at or near term who presents with abruption, delivery should be undertaken. A vaginal delivery is preferable in the patient who is stable, but a cesarean is required should there be significant fetal distress, life-threatening hemorrhage, or evidence of DIC. The care team should be ready to implement appropriate fluid resuscitation and administer blood products, which usually include packed red blood cells (PRBCs), fresh frozen plasma (FFP), and platelets to prevent further compromise.

Postpartum Hemorrhage (PPH)

Postpartum hemorrhage (PPH) is a common obstetric emergency, and is one of the top causes of maternal mortality across the world. The incidence of PPH increased 26% between 1994 and 2006 (Callaghan *et al.* 2010). PPH complicates 1–5% of all deliveries, so obstetric care teams must be ready to recognize and treat this common and potentially devastating pregnancy complication (Belfort 2017).

Primary PPH occurs within the first 24 hours following delivery, while secondary, or delayed, PPH occurs from 24 hours to 12 weeks after delivery. PPH is defined as an estimated blood loss (EBL) of 1000 mL or blood loss associated with signs or symptoms of hypovolemia within 24 hours of delivery, regardless of the route of delivery (ACOG 2017c). While the average blood loss at vaginal and cesarean deliveries has been reported as 500 mL and 1000 mL respectively, it is important to recognize that blood loss at delivery is often significantly underestimated, by as much as 50%.

Incidence

The incidence of PPH differs based on the type of delivery, occurring after approximately 3% of vaginal and 6% of cesarean deliveries (Rossen *et al.* 2010). For women with a history of a previous PPH, the risk of recurrence is as high as 15% (Oberg *et al.* 2014).

Clinical Picture

Healthcare providers are inaccurate when it comes to estimating blood loss at time of delivery. Clinical signs including tachycardia and hypotension, as well as patient-reported symptoms of shortness of breath, chest pain, or altered mental status, should alert providers to be concerned for increasing blood loss.

Risk Factors

There are multiple risk factors for PPH, including:

- Previous PPH
- Higher-order pregnancy
- Grand multiparity
- Preeclampsia
- Prolonged second or third stage of labor
- Prolonged use of oxytocin
- Episiotomy and operative vaginal delivery
- Maternal obesity

- Placental abruption or placenta previa
- Intra-amniotic infection
- Birth weight > 4000 g
- Coagulopathy

Causes

The most common causes of PPH are uterine atony (80% of cases), retained placental tissue, and cervical or vaginal lacerations. Initial evaluation should be to rule out these common causes.

Prevention

Active management of the third stage of labor, which includes early cord clamping, maternal oxytocin administration after delivery of the infant, and controlled cord traction to facilitate placental delivery, can significantly decrease the risk of PPH (ACOG 2017c).

Treatment

The treatment of PPH should include efforts to both stabilize the mother and correct the underlying cause of hemorrhage. As hematocrit does not drop immediately following a hemorrhage and will not equilibrate until nearly 12 hours later, treatment of hypovolemia with either intravenous fluids or blood products should be based on the patient's clinical status and not on EBL or lab values. In settings concerning for PPH, initial steps that should be taken are:

- Call for additional assistance (nursing staff/anesthesia)
- Assess vital signs with appropriate monitors
- Ensure IV access and administer fluid bolus
- Determine cause through:
    - Assessment of uterine tone to rule out atony
    - Manual exploration of uterus for retained products
    - Examination of vagina and cervix for lacerations

See Figure 14.1 for a complete treatment algorithm for postpartum hemorrhage.

Treatment by Etiology

Lacerations

Lacerations are often not evident on first assessment, given impaired visibility due to location and redundant tissue present in the vagina. If there is continued bleeding and good uterine tone, it is important to rule out cervical lacerations as the cause of PPH. If lacerations are noted to be present and bleeding, then you can apply pressure and repair them to stop the hemorrhage. Techniques for repair of lacerations are discussed in detail in Chapter 11.

Of note, if lacerations are suspected, it may be appropriate to move to the OR to allow for better visualization and facilitate repair.

Retained Placenta

To evaluate for retained products of conception, perform a manual sweep of the uterus during a bimanual exam. Transabdominal ultrasound can be a helpful tool for confirming all products are removed, as products of conception will appear as an echogenic mass or as a significantly thickened endometrial stripe.

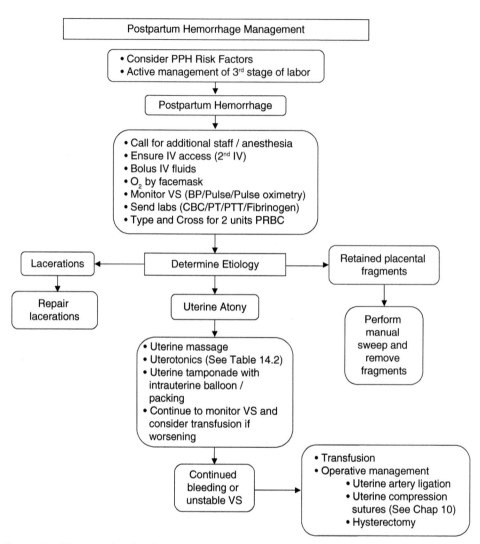

Figure 14.1 Treatment algorithm for postpartum hemorrhage (PPH).

Uterine Atony

If uterine palpation reveals poor tone consistent with atony, then you should proceed in the following manner:

1. Perform bimanual uterine massage with one hand on the maternal abdomen and the other in the vagina, to facilitate compression of the uterus.
2. Administer uterotonic medications (Methergine, Hemabate, misoprostol) to correct uterine atony (see Table 14.2 for doses and contraindications).
3. Reassess the patient's vital signs and blood loss. If there is continued bleeding and evidence of hypotension and your initial medical interventions are not working, consider

Table 14.2 Medications and dosages of uterotonics for postpartum hemorrhage

Medication	Dose	Contraindications
Methylergonovine (Methergine)	0.2 mg IM or into myometrium every 2–4 hours	Hypertension, preeclampsia, asthma, Raynaud's syndrome
Prostaglandin F2-alpha (carboprost/Hemabate)	250 mcg IM or into myometrium every 15 minutes (up to 8 doses)	Asthma, renal disorders, pulmonary hypertension
Misoprostol (Cytotec, PGE1)	800–1000 mcg per rectum × 1 dose	Known hypersensitivity to NSAIDs, active gastrointestinal bleeding
Tranexamic acid (TXA)	1 g IV over 10 minutes 2nd dose can be given if continued bleeding within 24 hours	Subarachnoid hemorrhage, acute intravascular clotting, hypersensitivity to TXA

either an intrauterine balloon for tamponade or uterine packing. This is most often done with a Bakri balloon, which is made and marketed specifically for PPH. After it is inserted, you can fill it with up to 500 mL of saline to compress the inside of the uterus. If the patient had a vaginal delivery, then you should place vaginal packing into the vagina to help make sure the Bakri stays in the uterus, because the cervix will still be dilated. If this intervention stops the bleeding, then the device is left in place for approximately 24 hours while the patient is monitored. When removing the Bakri, some providers take down the balloon slowly (100 mL per hour until empty) while others may just deflate and remove it.

4. If the patient continues to bleed despite your interventions and is unstable, surgical intervention in the OR is appropriate. Counsel the patient and family of likely interventions, and discuss the need for hysterectomy as a last resort prior to moving to the OR. When the decision is made to move to the OR, notify the following teams:

- Anesthesia
- Nursing personnel
- OR technician

A comprehensive discussion of the surgical treatment of PPH, or hemorrhage during a cesarean section, can be found in Chapter 10.

When managing a patient with PPH, it is often helpful to place a Foley catheter to monitor urine output, as this will give you a gauge of her intravascular volume. You should also obtain a follow-up CBC 12 hours later.

Use of Blood Products

The use of blood products in patients who experience a significant PPH can be life-saving. Most institutions now have a massive transfusion protocol (MTP) that can be activated to make blood products rapidly available. It is important to review this at your hospital because delays during a significant hemorrhage can result in increased morbidity.

Patients who refuse blood transfusions, such as Jehovah's Witnesses, are at increased risk for maternal mortality from PPH, with one study reporting a 44-fold increase in the risk of death from hemorrhage in this population (Singla *et al.* 2001). However, because a transfusion involves some risk to the patient in terms of viral infection and transfusion reactions, treatment should be carefully considered and the appropriate products ordered. The most commonly used blood products on labor and delivery include packed red blood cells (PRBCs), platelets, fresh frozen plasma (FFP), and cryoprecipitate. In the setting of massive blood loss, PRBC, platelets, and FFP are usually given in a 1:1:1 ratio.

Packed red blood cells (PRBCs). Most patients who suffer a significant hemorrhage will first receive a transfusion of PRBCs. They are indicated when a patient is hemodynamically unstable (hypotensive) due to hemorrhage, especially if the hemoglobin level falls to less than 7 g/dL (although remember you should not wait for lab results to treat an unstable patient). While red blood cells are critical to transport oxygen to tissues in the body, care must be taken to monitor the patient for pulmonary edema when multiple transfusions are required. In general, the patient's hemoglobin and hematocrit typically increase by 1 g/dL and 3%, respectively, per unit transfused.

Platelets. Platelets should be transfused when there is evidence of hemorrhage as a result of either thrombocytopenia or platelet dysfunction. Platelets may also be given in the face of massive transfusion of PRBCs and abnormal bleeding, as a dilutional thrombocytopenia can occur in this situation. While a patient is considered thrombocytopenic if the platelet count falls below 100×10^9/L, concern for bleeding during cesarean section is minimal as long as the level does not fall to below 50×10^9/L. When platelets are less than 20×10^9/L, prophylactic transfusion to prevent spontaneous bleeding should be administered. A single unit of platelets will increase the patient's platelet count by approximately 7.5×10^9/L.

Fresh frozen plasma (FFP). FFP is extracted from whole blood and contains significant amounts of fibrinogen as well as multiple clotting factors. This is given when disseminated intravascular coagulation (DIC), vitamin K deficiency, or clotting factor deficiencies related to liver disease (and therefore vitamin-K-dependent clotting factors) are present. It typically increases the fibrinogen level by 10–15 mg/dL per unit transfused. The goal of treatment with FFP in the presence of DIC or hypofibrinogenemia is a fibrinogen level of at least 100 mg/dL. (Of note, this is the only blood product with clotting factors V, XI, and XII.)

If you need FFP, understand that it takes at least 30 minutes to be thawed and made available in most blood banks, so advance warning must be provided if hemorrhage is anticipated. (Of note, this is the only blood product with clotting factors V, XI, and XII.)

Cryoprecipitate (cryo). Cryo is a concentrated fraction of FFP that is rich in factors VII, XIII, fibrinogen, and von Willebrand's factor. Because it is a small amount of volume as compared to FFP (40 mL vs. 250 mL) it is a more efficient way to raise the fibrinogen level, which may be especially important in a patient with DIC who is at risk for pulmonary edema secondary to fluid overload from multiple transfusions of PRBCs. One unit of cryoprecipitate will increase the fibrinogen level by 10–15 mg/dL. In most cases, cryoprecipitate is given specifically for the treatment of von Willebrand's disease, factor VII deficiency, or hypofibrinogenemia.

See Table 14.3 for a comparison of the different blood products.

Table 14.3 Blood products

Blood product	Contains	Indications	Volume (mL)	Effect
Packed red blood cells	Red cells, some plasma	Increase red cell volume	300	Increase Hct 3%/unit Increase Hgb 1 g/unit
Platelets	Platelets, some plasma, few RBC/WBC	Hemorrhage from thrombocytopenia	50	Increase platelet count by 7.5×10^9/L/ unit
Fresh frozen plasma	Plasma, clotting factors	Treatment of coagulation disorders	250	Increase total fibrinogen 10–15 mg/ dL/unit
Cryoprecipitate	Fibrinogen, factors V, VIII, XIII, von Willebrand's factor	Hemophilia A, von Willebrand's disease, hypofibrinogenemia	40	Increase total fibrinogen 10–15 mg/ dL/unit

Complications of Blood Transfusions

While the transfusion of blood products is often life-saving in obstetrics, there are risks involved, and it is important to discuss these with the patient when blood products are required. Adverse reactions that may occur generally involve acute transfusion reactions or, rarely, transmission of infectious agents to the recipient.

Acute hemolytic transfusion reaction. This most commonly results from a clerical error that allows for the transfusion of incompatible blood products. It usually presents with a fever, which may be accompanied by nausea, emesis, dyspnea, back pain, and discomfort at the infusion site. It may progress to shock, DIC, or acute renal failure. Acute hemolytic transfusion reaction is rare, with an incidence of 1 in 25,000 transfusions, and the risk of a fatal acute hemolytic reaction is 1 in 600,000. If there is any suspicion of a hemolytic reaction, then the transfusion should be stopped, the blood product returned to the blood bank with a description of the possible reaction, and supportive care of the patient should be undertaken.

Febrile non-hemolytic transfusion reaction. This complication occurs in approximately 1 in 10,000 transfusions. Patients generally experience a headache, shaking chills, or a fever within an hour of transfusion initiation. If any of these symptoms occur, then the transfusion should be stopped and the blood product sent back to the blood bank for testing. A hemolytic reaction should be ruled out by demonstrating no evidence of hemolysis (i.e., absence of hemoglobinemia or hemoglobinuria, and a negative direct antiglobulin test). Patients should receive acetaminophen for the fever and be given supportive care. Febrile transfusion reactions can often be prevented through pre-transfusion administration of antihistamines (Benadryl) and acetaminophen.

Anaphylactic reaction. Anaphylactic reactions, which are characterized by urticaria, angioedema, dypsnea, nausea or abdominal cramping, and even shock, occur with

Table 14.4 Incidence of viral infection after transfusion (per unit infused)

INFECTION	RISK
Hepatitis B	1:205,000
Hepatitis C	1:1,000,000 to 1:2,000,000
HIV 1–2	1:1,000,000 to 1:2,000,000

(NHLBI 2012)

approximately 1 in 150,000 units of blood transfused. When this happens, transfusion should be stopped and products sent to the laboratory. Treatment of the patient involves stabilizing the airway and administering antihistamines and epinephrine as needed.

Infections. Although all blood products are screened prior to administration to patients, the possibility of acquiring an infection, usually viral, still exists. Current estimates of these risks can be found in Table 14.4.

Magnesium Toxicity

Magnesium sulfate is used routinely on labor and delivery, both for seizure prophylaxis in patients with preeclampsia and for fetal neuroprotection in patients where delivery is imminent prior to 32 weeks. In addition, some providers utilize magnesium for its tocolytic effects, though this is now uncommon. Magnesium usage is contraindicated in patients with neuromuscular disease (e.g., myasthenia gravis), and since magnesium is cleared through the kidney, dosing should be adjusted in patients with renal impairment to prevent magnesium intoxication. Therapeutic serum levels of magnesium are between 4 and 8 mg/dL. (Note that some labs will report magnesium levels in mEq/L.)

Clinical Picture

Some common side effects of magnesium administration include:

- Nausea/emesis
- Headache
- Dry mouth
- Intense flushing
- Drowsiness
- Blurred vision
- Decreased FHR variability

Clinical signs and symptoms that are indicative of potential magnesium toxicity include the following:

- Absent deep tendon reflexes (DTRs)
- New-onset hypotension
- Pulmonary edema

- Respiratory depression

Serum magnesium levels at which different complications may occur include:

- ECG changes: 6–12 mg/dL
- Decreased DTRs: 12 mg/dL
- Respiratory depression: 18 mg/dL
- Cardiovascular collapse: > 30 mg/dL

Risk Factors

The most significant risk factor for magnesium toxicity is renal insufficiency, as magnesium is cleared through the kidneys. In patients with elevated creatinine, normal loading doses of magnesium should be given to achieve therapeutic levels, but the maintenance dose can be decreased or held. If you are concerned about magnesium toxicity, then you can check magnesium serum levels.

Treatment

1 gram (10 mL of 10% solution) of calcium gluconate IV given over 3 minutes will reverse the effects of magnesium sulfate. Additional actions should include:

- Stop magnesium infusion.
- Administer supplemental oxygen and continuously monitor mother with pulse oximetry (intubation if necessary for respiratory failure).
- Administer diuretics (furosemide 20–40 mg IV) as needed for pulmonary edema.

Malpresentation

Breech Presentation

A breech presentation occurs when either the fetal buttocks or lower extremities are the presenting part rather than the fetal head. Regardless of the type of breech presentation, the recommended mode of delivery is generally a cesarean section.

Incidence

The incidence of breech presentation decreases with increasing gestational age. Twenty-five percent of fetuses are in breech presentation under 28 weeks, but at term only approximately 3–4% of all fetuses will be in some form of breech presentation (Hickok *et al.* 1992).

Clinical Picture

Breech presentation can be suspected via Leopold's maneuvers or during cervical examination. Upon initial presentation to the labor unit patients should have an ultrasound to confirm presentation.

Risk Factors

- Preterm gestation
- Uterine abnormalities (bicornuate uterus or uterine septum)
- Placenta previa
- Multiparity

- Polyhydramnios
- Fetal anomalies (hydrocephaly)
- Multiple gestation
- CNS structural anomalies (anencephaly)
- Large fibroids
- Short umbilical cord

Treatment

In general, breech presenting fetuses are delivered via cesarean section, especially if patients present with ruptured membranes or in labor. Depending on the clinical scenario, an external cephalic version (ECV), which is usually performed around 36 weeks and attempts to turn the fetus to the vertex position through external manipulation, may be offered (see Chapter 2 for a description of an ECV). If the patient declines this intervention, or the ECV is unsuccessful, then a cesarean section is most often performed. ACOG now recommends that the route of delivery should depend on the experience level of the provider, and acknowledges that a planned vaginal breech delivery may be acceptable under hospital protocols if the patient is counseled that short-term perinatal outcomes may be worse when compared to cesarean section (ACOG 2006).

Regardless of whether a vaginal delivery of a breech fetus is imminent when a patient presents or is planned, technique is important to ensure the best outcome possible. Equipment and preparation should include the following:

1. Call for additional staff (obstetrics/pediatrics/anesthesia).
2. Ensure adequate anesthesia.
3. Move to the operating room if possible.
4. Have Piper forceps in the room.

Below is a description of the general techniques needed for vaginal breech delivery.

- As the mother pushes, the infant's buttocks will present at the introitus. No assistance should be given to the infant at this point. Allow the mother to push and deliver the buttocks and, if the legs are flexed, the lower limbs as well. If the legs are extended, then flex each leg at the knee and move it laterally to deliver each foot (Figure 14.2a).
- At this point, wrap the infant's body in a sterile towel and continue to have the mother push while applying gentle downward traction with your thumbs on the fetal sacrum and fingers in the groin (Figure 14.2b). When the infant has delivered to the level of the scapula, the shoulders should be rotated to the anterior–posterior plane and the arms/shoulders delivered individually. If they do not come spontaneously, then placing a finger over the shoulder into the antecubital fossa and sweeping it across the body will help facilitate delivery (Figure 14.2c).
- After the shoulders are delivered, the fetal head is delivered either by the placement of Piper forceps or with a Mauriceau–Smellie–Veit (MSV) maneuver, with care to make sure to avoid hyperextension of the infant's cervical spine (Figures 14.2d, 14.2e). The MSV maneuver includes hooking fingers over the fetal neck with one hand and placing the fingers of the other hand on the fetal maxilla while an assistant provides suprapubic pressure, with all of this done to ensure the fetal head remains flexed during the delivery. An episiotomy may be helpful in this situation to provide more room posteriorly.
- If you cannot deliver the infant with the MSV, then Piper forceps may be placed to ensure the fetal head remains flexed during delivery. If there is fetal head entrapment, which is

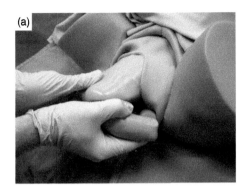

Figure 14.2a Delivery of fetal legs.

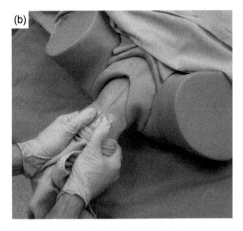

Figure 14.2b Hands on bones and groins.

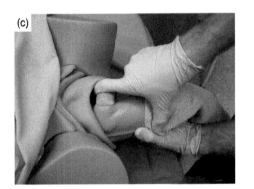

Figure 14.2c Delivery of fetal arms.

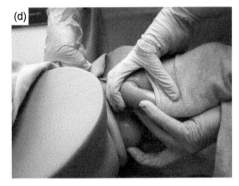

Figure 14.2d Mauriceau–Smellie–Veit maneuver.

Figure 14.2e Mauriceau–Smellie–Veit demonstration.

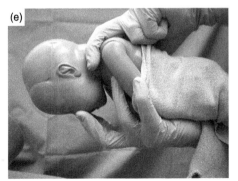

more common in preterm deliveries when the cervix does not completely dilate but allows the rest of the breech fetus to deliver, then it may be necessary to cut the cervix with surgical scissors at roughly 2, 6, and 10 o'clock to allow the head to deliver (these are called Dührssen incisions).

Transverse Lie

A transverse lie occurs when the fetal spine is perpendicular to the mother's spine, and it may be referred to as either a "back-up" or "back-down" transverse lie depending on the orientation. It is often suspected by visual inspection of the maternal abdomen when the uterus appears unusually wide.

Incidence

A transverse lie is an uncommon finding in singleton pregnancies, but it is encountered often in twin gestations with the second twin.

Clinical Picture

This abnormal presentation is usually first suspected at the time of Leopold's maneuvers or cervical examination, although the appearance of the maternal abdomen or an abnormally small fundal height can also alert you to this possibility.

Risk Factors

- Uterine abnormalities
- Large myomas
- Polyhydramnios
- Placenta previa
- Preterm fetus
- Multiple gestation

Treatment

Similar to a breech presentation, an ECV may be offered to those patients who have intact membranes and are not in active labor. ECV may also be attempted during early labor if membranes are intact. If the patient declines the ECV or it is not successful, then a cesarean section is performed, as the fetus cannot deliver vaginally in this position (refer to the section on uterine incisions and transverse presentation in Chapter 10). These fetuses are at increased risk of complications if they go into labor or rupture membranes, as the risk of umbilical cord prolapse is significantly increased with a back-up transverse lie.

Oligohydramnios

Oligohydramnios is a term used to describe a decreased amount of amniotic fluid surrounding the fetus. As amniotic fluid is an indirect measure of fetal perfusion and renal function, a significantly decreased amount should lead to further testing and/or other interventions.

The most common definition of oligohydramnios is an amniotic fluid index (AFI – see Chapter 2) of less than 5 cm or a single maximum vertical pocket (MVP) less than 2 cm. More recently, the use of MVP rather than AFI for diagnosis of oligohydramnios has become more common, as this is associated with a reduction in unwarranted interventions without an increase in adverse perinatal outcomes (ACOG 2014).

Incidence

Oligohydramnios occurs in between 1% and 3% of pregnancies, depending on the definition used (Gilbert 2017).

Clinical Picture

Laboring patients who have oligohydramnios are more likely to have FHR abnormalities (typically variable decelerations from cord compression) leading to cesarean section than patients with a normal amount of amniotic fluid.

In the preterm fetus, long-standing oligohydramnios may result in muscle contractures, lung hypoplasia, and even skeletal deformations. These severe problems, however, are usually seen only when the process begins early in the second trimester.

Causes

Maternal
• Uteroplacental insufficiency (placental abnormalities or hypertensive disorders)
• Antiphospholipid syndrome
• Dehydration

Fetal
• Rupture of membranes (term or preterm)
• Prolonged pregnancy
• Fetal growth restriction
• Renal agenesis

(Gilbert 2017)

Treatment

The treatment of a patient with oligohydramnios depends on the etiology and gestational age of the patient.

Preterm (< 37 weeks). After ensuring that PPROM has not occurred, these patients should undergo antepartum testing including an NST, AFI, growth assessment, and BPP once or twice weekly to ensure that there is no evidence of fetal compromise. If there is evidence of fetal distress, then further testing or delivery is indicated. The patient is usually delivered once she reaches 36–37 weeks gestational age (ACOG 2014).

Term. When a term patient is diagnosed with oligohydramnios, she is usually induced unless she is already in labor. During labor, variable decelerations (indicative of umbilical cord compression) may be present, which may require starting an amnioinfusion. Although amnioinfusion may reduce the number of variable decelerations, there is little evidence that its use reduces perinatal morbidity of mortality rates, or cesarean delivery rates (Gilbert 2017).

Gestational Hypertension

Gestational hypertension (GHTN) is defined as new-onset elevation in blood pressure after 20 weeks gestational age without evidence of proteinuria or severe symptoms of preeclampsia.

ACOG recommends blood pressures be taken with the patient comfortably seated in the upright position with legs uncrossed and arm and back supported. The blood pressure cuff should be at the level of the right atrium (level of the sternum) and the patient should be resting for at least 5 minutes prior to taking the blood pressure (ACOG 2013).

Incidence

GHTN occurs in 6–29% of nulliparous women and 2–4% of multiparous women (Sibai 2017).

Clinical Picture

These patients develop elevations in blood pressure, with systolic BP > 140 mmHg and/or diastolic BP > 90 mmHg. To meet criteria for GHTN, a patient must have two elevated blood pressures at least 4 hours apart.

When GHTN is suspected, the patient should be evaluated for evidence of preeclampsia with laboratory testing (CBC, AST/ALT, uric acid, serum creatinine, urine protein/creatinine ratio). If this is negative and the patient has GHTN, then patients generally are managed expectantly and delivered between 37 and 38 weeks gestational age. This involves weekly laboratory evaluation for preeclampsia, twice-weekly antepartum testing, and serial sonograms for fetal growth. It is important to watch these patients closely, as they are at increased risk of progressing to preeclampsia (Spong *et al.* 2011, Cunningham *et al.* 2014).

Preeclampsia

Preeclampsia is a common occurrence in obstetrics and is characterized by the development of hypertension and proteinuria after 20 weeks' gestation. Although proteinuria is a common finding, preeclampsia may be diagnosed in the presence of elevated blood pressures with any of the following:

- Thrombocytopenia (platelet count < 100×10^9/L)
- Renal insufficiency (serum creatinine > 1.1 mg/dL or doubling of baseline creatinine in the absence of other renal abnormalities)
- Impaired liver function (transaminases elevated to twice normal baseline concentrations)
- Pulmonary edema
- Cerebral or visual symptoms (e.g., headaches)

It is described as either with or without severe features and may be complicated by generalized seizures (eclampsia).

Incidence

Occurs in 3–10% of nulliparous pregnancies, varies in multiparous pregnancies (Cunningham *et al.* 2014).

Clinical Picture

Patients present after 20 weeks' gestation with persistently elevated blood pressures (systolic BP > 140 and/or diastolic BP > 90 on two occasions at least 4 hours apart) and proteinuria (defined as at least 300 mg in a 24-hour specimen), protein/creatinine ratio ≥ 0.3 (Table 14.5), or urine dipstick > +1 (used only if other methods are not available) (Markham and Funai 2014). Preeclampsia is further classified as either with or without severe features. This is important in terms of management, especially in the preterm fetus. Severe features are listed below.

Severe Features

- Systolic BP ≥ 160 mmHg or diastolic BP ≥ 110 mmHg*
- Thrombocytopenia (platelet count < 100×10^9/L)
- Impaired liver function:
  - Elevated liver enzymes (to twice normal concentration)
  - Severe persistent right upper quadrant pain not accounted for by alternative diagnoses

- Renal insufficiency:
  - Serum creatinine concentration > 1.1 mg/dL

    or
  - Doubling of the serum creatinine concentration in the absence of other renal disease

- Pulmonary edema
- New-onset cerebral or visual symptoms (e.g., headaches, scotomata)

Table 14.5 Urine protein/creatinine ratio

Send a single urine sample (at least 200 mL if possible) for a spot urine protein and spot urine creatinine measurement

Timing of specimen collection (morning, afternoon, evening, etc.) does not matter

Calculate the ratio (make sure and check the units that your lab reports the results in as you may have to convert them to match)

$$\text{Urine protein/creatinine ratio} = \frac{\text{Urine spot protein (mg/dL)}}{\text{Urine spot creatinine (mg/dL)}}$$

Interpret the results

• If the result is > 0.19, then a 24-hour urine collection is usually obtained

• A result of ≥ 0.30 is considered consistent with proteinuria for the diagnosis of preeclampsia

(Stout *et al.* 2013)

---

* **Either** the systolic **or** diastolic values can be elevated in the severe range to meet this definition. It **does not have to be both.**

Risk Factors

- Nulliparity
- Age > 40 years
- Pregnancy with assisted reproductive techniques (including in vitro fertilization)
- Interpregnancy interval > 7 years
- Family history of preeclampsia
- Obesity
- Gestational diabetes mellitus
- Multifetal gestation
- Preeclampsia in previous pregnancy
- Fetal growth restriction, placental abruption, intrauterine fetal demise
- Chronic hypertension
- Renal disease
- Type 1 diabetes mellitus

(Sibai 2017)

Causes

The cause of this disease is still unknown.

Treatment

The only treatment for preeclampsia, with or without severe features, is delivery. The decision to deliver a patient, however, is dependent both on the severity of the disease and on the gestational age.

Preeclampsia Without Severe Features

If preeclampsia is diagnosed after 37 weeks then delivery is indicated. The treatment of preeclampsia between 34 and 37 weeks' gestation may be to deliver the patient, but conservative management and close monitoring are usually undertaken in cases of preeclampsia without severe features until 37 weeks. If there is any evidence of progression to preeclampsia with severe features, however, then delivery is indicated. Induction of labor should be started at 37 weeks gestational age for all women with preeclampsia without severe features.

With regards to route of delivery, it is important to note that preeclampsia is not by itself an indication for cesarean section, and that a cesarean should only be performed for obstetric indications (see Chapter 10).* In patients with preeclampsia without severe features, magnesium sulfate for seizure prophylaxis is not necessarily given during labor. Magnesium sulfate therapy should, however, be initiated for seizure prophylaxis if severe features develop while the patient is in labor or immediately postpartum.

---

* When patients have preeclampsia with severe features and delivery is indicated, vaginal delivery may be accomplished, although cesarean section may need to be performed. Mode of delivery should be determined based on gestational age, fetal presentation, cervical exam, and maternal/fetal indications (ACOG 2013).

Preeclampsia With Severe Features

When a patient has preeclampsia with severe features and is at least 34 weeks along, then delivery is indicated and a course of corticosteroids should be started if they have not already been given. Maternal stabilization may be performed for 48 hours in some cases to allow maximum benefit of steroid therapy. If preeclampsia with severe features develops prior to 34 weeks, then a decision must be made about whether or not conservative management may be attempted, which includes antihypertensive medications, inpatient monitoring, and the administration of corticosteroids for fetal lung maturity. Consultation with a maternal–fetal medicine specialist is recommended in these cases.

Regardless of gestational age, when the decision is made to deliver, the patient with severe features is given magnesium sulfate for seizure prophylaxis. A loading dose of 4–6 grams is administered followed by a continuous infusion of 1–2 grams per hour. After delivery, the patient is continued on magnesium sulfate for 24 hours postpartum (ACOG 2013).

Chronic Hypertension with Superimposed Preeclampsia

Diagnosing superimposed preeclampsia in women who have hypertension at their baseline can be challenging. Because of this, baseline preeclampsia labs, including assessment for proteinuria, should be done in the first trimester so they can be compared to labs later in pregnancy if there is worsening hypertension. When a woman with hypertension diagnosed prior to 20 weeks' gestation develops proteinuria after 20 weeks, she meets the criteria for chronic hypertension with superimposed preeclampsia. Alternatively, this diagnosis can be made in women with proteinuria before 20 weeks of gestation and any of the following:

- Sudden worsening of hypertension or a need for increasing doses of antihypertensive therapy
- Increase in liver enzymes to twice normal baseline levels
- Platelet levels below 100×10^9/L
- Severe persistent right upper quadrant pain not accounted for by alternative diagnoses
- New-onset severe headaches
- Pulmonary congestion or edema
- Renal insufficiency (doubling of baseline creatinine level or increasing to or above 1.1 mg/dL in women without other renal disease)
- Increasing proteinuria

Chronic hypertension with superimposed preeclampsia is also further classified as with and without severe features in the same way as preeclampsia in patients without chronic hypertension (ACOG 2013). Recommendations for delivery timing are also the same as for patients without chronic hypertension.

Eclampsia

Eclampsia is characterized by generalized tonic–clonic seizures or coma not attributable to other medical or neurologic problems that can occur before, during, or after labor (Sibai 2017).

Incidence

Occurs in approximately 1 in 2000 to 1 in 3448 pregnancies in the Western world. In developed countries such as the United States, eclampsia is associated with an increased maternal mortality rate of up to 1.8%. Unfortunately, in developing countries, maternal mortality rates are reported as high as 18%. After a woman has experienced an eclamptic seizure, she is at increased risk with subsequent pregnancies for both preeclampsia (25% risk) and eclampsia (2% recurrence risk). The risk is also higher in patients who experience preterm preeclampsia/eclampsia rather than at term (Sibai 2017).

Clinical Picture

Eclamptic seizures are generally self-limited and rarely last longer than 4 minutes. It is common to have significant FHR decelerations during a seizure, but these almost always resolve soon after the seizure ends.

Risk Factors

Patients with preeclampsia are at risk for developing eclampsia. Some risk factors for eclampsia include preexisting heart disease, systemic lupus erythematosus, anemia, nulliparity, premature separation of the placenta, preexisting or gestational diabetes, and urinary tract infections (Liu *et al.* 2011).

Causes

The exact cause of eclampsia is not known, but some theories implicate cerebral vasospasm and hypertensive encephalopathy.

Treatment

The treatment of eclampsia is to stabilize the patient and begin medication to prevent additional seizures. General principles and actions that should be taken include:

Call for assistance. This should include nursing staff, anesthesia support, and additional providers.

Protect the patient and her airway. Roll patient to left side and put any bedrails up to prevent her from falling. Suction oral secretions as needed.

Initiate magnesium sulfate. Magnesium sulfate should be started as soon as possible. It is important to realize that the magnesium does not stop the current seizure (as the loading dose is administered over 15–20 minutes) but it will help prevent additional seizures. In rare cases of prolonged seizures, a dose of lorazepam (Ativan) is sometimes administered. Dosing for magnesium is explained in Table 14.6.

Treat severe hypertension (i.e., > 160/110). Treatment of hypertension (Figure 14.3) is very important in order to prevent complications such as stroke. This is accomplished with medications including:

Table 14.6 Anti-seizure treatment for preeclampsia and eclampsia

IV infusion of magnesium sulfate
4–6 g loading dose diluted in 100 mL of IV fluid over 15–20 minutes
2 g/h in 100 mL for maintenance infusion
Continue magnesium during labor and until 24 hours after delivery
Magnesium sulfate should be started at the time the decision for delivery is made. It is not stopped during a cesarean section
Intermittent IM injections (sometimes used if there is no IV access)
Give 10 g of a 50% magnesium sulfate solution with 5 g into each buttock
Follow this with 5 g of a 50% solution of magnesium sulfate IM every 4 hours
Continue magnesium during labor and until 24 hours after delivery

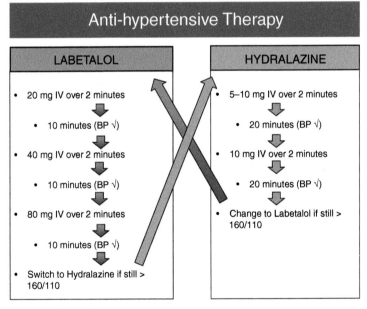

Figure 14.3 Treatment of severe hypertension.

- Hydralazine: 5–10 mg IV every 20 minutes as needed with a total cumulative dose of 20 mg
- Labetalol: 10–20 mg IV then double every 10 minutes as needed up to 80 mg doses with a total cumulative dose of 300 mg
- Nifedipine: 10 mg PO (appropriate agent if no available IV access)

Continue seizure prophylaxis. The recurrence risk of an eclamptic seizure is approximately 10% even in patients receiving magnesium sulfate for seizure prophylaxis. Because of this, after the eclamptic seizure has resolved, all patients should receive magnesium sulfate seizure prophylaxis (at 2 g/h unless there is evidence of renal insufficiency, in which case a lower dose is used and serum magnesium levels are monitored) for at least 24 hours after delivery has been accomplished. Multiple randomized trials have compared magnesium sulfate to phenytoin for prevention of recurrent seizures in eclampsia, and have found that magnesium sulfate is associated with lower rates of recurrent seizures and lower maternal mortality rates (Sibai 2017).

Consider delivery. Delivery is indicated after a patient experiences an eclamptic seizure regardless of gestational age. This does not necessarily mean that a cesarean section must be performed. In general, induction of labor is reasonable, but factors such as an unfavorable cervix, early gestational age, and the fetal status must be taken into consideration. Cesarean section is generally recommended if the patient is < 30 weeks' gestation or has a Bishop score < 5.

Monitor patients for development of complications. Women diagnosed with eclampsia are also at higher risk for other comorbidities including placental abruption, disseminated intravascular coagulopathy, pulmonary edema, acute renal failure, and cardiopulmonary arrest (Liu *et al.* 2011).

Prognosis

Maternal mortality rates of 0% to nearly 14% have been reported, with perinatal mortality ranging from 5.6% to 11.8% (Liu *et al.* 2011).

Preterm Labor

Preterm labor refers to cervical dilation to at least 2 cm with regular uterine contractions prior to 37 weeks' gestation. It is a leading cause of neonatal morbidity and mortality and accounts for up to 70% of deaths among infants without congenital anomalies (ACOG 2016b). Although this is a very common problem, accounting for 50% of all preterm deliveries, the approaches to its management vary widely, though there is some general agreement on the basic treatment approach (ACOG 2016b).

Incidence

The preterm delivery rate in the United States is approximately 12%, and spontaneous preterm labor is responsible for at least half of all preterm births (ACOG 2016b).

Clinical Picture

Patients with preterm labor will often present with abdominal cramping, which they may or may not identify as being a result of uterine contractions. Other possible presenting complaints may include back pain, vaginal spotting or bleeding, pelvic pressure, or increased vaginal discharge.

Risk Factors/Causes

There are multiple risk factors for preterm labor. Some of these are:

- **African-American race.** African-American women on average have a preterm delivery rate of up to 18.4%, versus 11.6% for Caucasian women (Simhan *et al.* 2017).
- **Age.** Low and high extremes of age are risk factors for preterm delivery.
- **Tobacco use.** Women who smoke during pregnancy have a 10% increase in the risk of preterm delivery (McCowan *et al.* 2009).
- **Previous preterm delivery.** This increases the risk of subsequent preterm delivery approximately 1.5–2-fold (ACOG 2012).
- **Multiple gestation.** Women with multifetal gestations are six times more likely to give birth prematurely and 13 times more likely to give birth prior to 32 weeks' gestation (ACOG 2016a).
- **Infection.** Several different infections, such as *Ureaplasma urealyticum, Mycoplasma hominis, Fusobacterium* species, *Bacteroides* species, and *Gardnerella vaginalis*, have been associated with preterm delivery.
- **Uterine malformations.** Anomalies such as a unicornuate or bicornuate uterus increase the risk of preterm delivery 25–50% (Simhan *et al.* 2017).
- **Low socioeconomic status.** This has been associated with preterm delivery, although there are often other associated risk factors.
- **Periodontal disease.** A meta-analysis of 17 studies concluded that periodontal disease was associated with preterm labor with an odds ratio of 2.83 (Vergnes and Sixou 2007).

Workup and Evaluation

Whenever a woman calls with complaints that may be related to preterm labor, she should be told to come to labor and delivery for evaluation. When she arrives she should be placed on the monitor, both to check the FHR tracing and to monitor for contractions. She should then be asked about the following:

- When the symptoms began
- Vaginal bleeding
- Rupture of membranes
- History or presence of any risk factors for preterm labor (as above)

After the history has been taken, an examination and tests should be performed, to include the following:

- Speculum examination with collection of the following:
  - Fetal fibronectin (fFN) swab (prior to any other object placed in the vagina)
  - Vaginal cultures for gonorrhea, chlamydia if patient is symptomatic or has risk factors
  - Wet prep or BD Affirm for bacterial vaginosis if symptomatic
  - Rectovaginal swab for group B streptococcus (GBS) if not performed in the last 5 weeks, with penicillin sensitivities if applicable

- Ultrasound examination of the cervical length if the cervix is not dilated
- Digital examination of the cervix
- Urine specimen for urinalysis and culture
- Send a urine drug screen if patient has risk factors

(Hobel 2016, Simhan *et al.* 2017)

Treatment

The treatment of preterm labor depends on the presence or absence of contractions as well as the condition of the cervix. If any evidence of infection is found during the initial examination, for example, bacterial vaginosis, vaginal candidiasis, or a urinary tract infection, then these should be treated.

The most important interventions for preterm labor that have been shown to decrease perinatal morbidity and mortality are:
1. Transfer of the preterm labor patient to an institution with a neonatal intensive care unit
2. Administration of glucocorticoids to the mother
3. Treatment with antibiotics for group B beta-hemolytic streptococcus
4. Administration of magnesium sulfate for fetal neuroprotection for gestational age < 32 weeks

(Simhan *et al.* 2017)

If the patient is found to be in preterm labor, then tocolysis is undertaken, most often with nifedipine, indomethacin, or magnesium sulfate. In addition, a course of glucocorticoids, either dexamethasone or betamethasone, is started, and antibiotics, usually penicillin G or ampicillin, are started until the results of the GBS culture are available.* A list of common medications as well as dosages and specific indications that may be used for tocolysis can be found in Table 14.7.

The reason for beginning tocolysis is that these medications have been shown to prolong pregnancy for 2–7 days, which allows for a full course of glucocorticoids to be administered and potential maternal transfer if indicated (ACOG 2016b). It is important to remember, however, that there is no consensus on exactly when to begin tocolysis, and that no evidence-based guidelines exist for making this decision.

The most common first-line choices for tocolysis are magnesium sulfate, terbutaline, or nifedipine, with nifedipine becoming the first choice at many institutions. Each of these is given by itself and the contraction pattern is monitored. If there is no significant response, then indomethacin is sometimes added for 48 hours if the patient is at less than 32 weeks' gestation. If the patient progresses and enters active labor, then tocolysis is generally discontinued and preparations are made for delivery. If the patient responds to the medication, then it is usually continued for 24–48 hours as long as the uterine contractions do not persist.

The purpose of the glucocorticoids is that they have been shown to promote fetal lung maturity and decrease the risk of severe respiratory distress after delivery, intraventricular hemorrhage, and necrotizing enterocolitis (Roberts *et al.* 2017).

- If the cervical examination and TV sonogram are equivocal (e.g., cervix is dilated 2 cm and/or cervical length is 2–3 cm) or give conflicting results (e.g., cervix is < 3 cm but has demonstrated change from a previous examination but cervical length is > 3 cm) then the patient should be observed as well and the fetal fibronectin (see Chapter 2) results used to determine treatment. Also, in the presence of more than four contractions per hour, a dose of subcutaneous terbutaline may be given to see if this will stop the contractions.
- If the patient's contractions become stronger or she demonstrates cervical change during observation, she is treated for preterm labor.

---

* Antibiotics should be discontinued if the GBS culture is negative and preterm labor is the only reason for the antibiotics being given.

Table 14.7 Common medications for tocolysis

Medication	Dose	Mechanism of action	Side effects	Contraindications
Calcium-channel blockers (CCBs) (nifedipine)	20–30 mg PO loading dose followed by 10–20 mg q3–8h up to 48 hours (max dose 180 mg/day)	Blocks influx of Ca^+ ions through the cell membrane. Inhibits release of intracellular calcium from sarcoplasmic reticulum, thus increasing calcium efflux from the cell. Decreased intracellular $Ca\pm$ results in myometrial relaxation	Dizziness, flushing, hypotension. Suppression of heart rate, contractility, and systolic pressure when combined with magnesium sulfate. Abnormalities in hepatic enzymes	Hypotension. Aortic insufficiency
NSAIDs (indomethacin)	50–100 mg PO loading dose followed by 25 mg PO q4–6h	Reversibly binds to cyclooxygenase, decreasing production of prostaglandins and reducing uterine contractions	Nausea, reflux, gastritis, emesis. Possible platelet dysfunction in patients with underlying hematologic disorder	Platelet dysfunction. Bleeding disorder. Hepatic dysfunction. Gastric ulcers. Renal dysfunction. Asthma (if hypersensitive to aspirin)
Beta-adrenergic receptor agonists (terbutaline)	0.25 mg SQ q20–30 min up to four doses or until contractions decrease	Stimulates beta receptors on the myometrium, leading to smooth muscle relaxation	Tachycardia, hypotension, tremors, palpitations, dyspnea, chest pain, pulmonary edema, hypokalemia or hyperglycemia	Maternal cardiac disease. Poorly controlled diabetes
Magnesium sulfate	6 g IV loading dose over 20 minutes followed by 2 g/h	Decreases intracellular Ca^+ concentration, thereby inhibiting myometrial contractile response	Flushing, diaphoresis, nausea, loss of deep tendon reflexes, respiratory depression, cardiac arrest	Myasthenia gravis

(ACOG 2016b, Simhan et al. 2017)

228

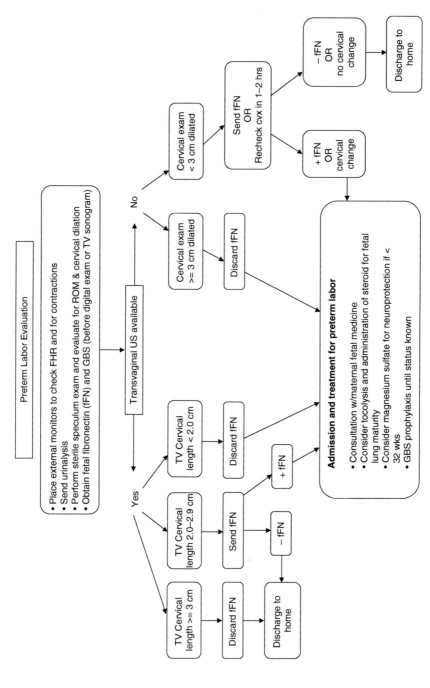

Figure 14.4 Preterm labor evaluation and treatment. FHR, fetal heart rate; GBS, group B streptococcus; ROM, rupture of membranes; TV, transvaginal; US, ultrasound.

See Figure 14.4 for an algorithm for evaluation and treatment of preterm labor.

The important thing to remember about preterm labor is that there is significant variation in how physicians approach and treat these patients. The recommendations in the treatment algorithm are based on the current literature and the fact that preterm delivery before 34–35 weeks is very unlikely (only 1–3%) in women evaluated for preterm labor who have intact membranes, cervical dilation of less than 3 cm, a cervical length of > 3 cm, and within 14 days of a negative fFN (Iams 2003).

Patients who experience a preterm delivery either secondary to spontaneous preterm labor or after PPROM should be counseled about receiving progesterone treatment in future pregnancies in order to decrease the risk of recurrence (ACOG 2012).

Preterm Premature Rupture of Membranes (PPROM)

Preterm premature rupture of membranes (PPROM) is defined as rupture of the amniotic sac prior to 37 weeks' gestation. Appropriate diagnosis is important to allow time for administration of antibiotics and corticosteroids to improve maternal and fetal outcomes.

Incidence

PPROM complicates approximately 1% of all pregnancies and is responsible for 10–20% of all preterm (< 37 weeks) deliveries (Mercer 2017).

Clinical Picture

Patients presenting with PPROM generally present with the same complaints as term patients present with spontaneous rupture of membranes (SROM). They complain of either a large gush of fluid or a continuous leakage of fluid from the vagina (see *Rule Out Ruptured Membranes* in Chapter 4).

Risk Factors

There are many risk factors associated with PPROM. These include the following:

- Smoking during pregnancy
- Previous preterm delivery
- Low body mass index (BMI < 19)
- Multiple gestation
- Polyhydramnios
- Sexually transmitted disease during pregnancy
- Cerclage or previous cervical conization
- Amniocentesis*
- Vaginal bleeding during pregnancy
- Pulmonary disease in pregnancy
- Lower socioeconomic status

(Simhan *et al.* 2014, ACOG 2016c, Mercer 2017)

---

* In most cases where PPROM occurs after amniocentesis, the membranes actually reseal with reaccumulation of the normal amniotic fluid volume. The perinatal survival rate following PPROM after amniocentesis is approximately 91% (ACOG 2016c).

Causes

The exact cause of PPROM is not always evident, although infection or inflammation is often implicated.

Complications

Maternal. With PPROM, there is an increased risk of intra-amniotic infection (15–25%) and placental abruption (2–5%) (ACOG 2016c). Maternal sepsis is, fortunately, a rare event, and occurs in only about 1% of cases.

Fetal. When preterm delivery occurs, the risk of perinatal sepsis is twofold higher if PPROM occurred when compared to preterm labor with intact membranes (Mercer 2014). The fetal survival rate depends greatly on both the gestational age at the time of PPROM and the presence or absence of infection. The rate of pulmonary hypoplasia after rupture of membranes prior to 24 weeks varies between 10% and 20%, and this is associated with high neonatal mortality rates (ACOG 2016c). However, if rupture occurs after 23–24 weeks, alveolar growth has already begun and outcomes are better.

Recurrence

The risk of recurrence for PPROM is three times higher than in women whose neonates are born at term. Patients with a history of preterm delivery should be offered progesterone supplementation in future pregnancies starting at 16–24 weeks to reduce the risk of recurrence (ACOG 2012, 2016c).

Treatment

After the diagnosis has been made (see *Rule Out Ruptured Membranes* in Chapter 4), the treatment depends on the gestational age of the fetus. The patient should be admitted and continuous monitoring started. If there is evidence of fetal distress or intra-amniotic infection, then delivery is indicated regardless of gestational age.

Corticosteroids are administered if the gestation is less than 37 weeks, but plans for delivery are not delayed to complete both doses if it is more than 34 weeks. Magnesium sulfate is administered for fetal neuroprotection in women less than 32 weeks' gestation, as multiple randomized controlled trials have shown a reduced risk of cerebral palsy after receiving magnesium sulfate (ACOG 2016c). Antibiotics are given as well, which have been shown to both increase the latency period from PPROM to delivery and reduce major infant morbidity, to include death, respiratory distress syndrome (RDS), early sepsis, and significant intraventricular hemorrhage (IVH) or necrotizing enterocolitis (NEC) (Mercer 2014).

In addition to corticosteroids and antibiotics, some physicians consider the use of tocolytics in PPROM when it occurs < 34 weeks in order to attempt to gain at least 48 hours to complete a course of corticosteroids. There is currently no convincing evidence that this is either beneficial or harmful to either the mother or fetus, though it may result in a small increase in pregnancy prolongation. Tocolysis has not been proven to prolong pregnancy or improve neonatal outcomes in a patient with ruptured membranes in active labor (ACOG 2016c).

In general, delivery is indicated whenever fetal lung maturity is demonstrated (done by testing amniotic fluid either from an amniocentesis or by sampling pooled fluid from the vagina) or the patient reaches 34 weeks. The reason for this is that after 34 weeks conservative management is associated with an increased risk of intra-amniotic infection and reduced umbilical cord pH, and has not been shown to improve neonatal outcomes (Mercer 2014, ACOG 2016c).

After approximately 24 hours, if the patient is stable and the FHR tracing is reassuring, the fetal status may be followed with a biophysical profile done at least twice weekly and often every other day. If, at any time, there is evidence of intra-amniotic infection, fetal distress, or placental abruption, then delivery is also indicated (ACOG 2016c). See Figure 14.5 for a treatment algorithm for PPROM.

Shoulder Dystocia

This complication occurs when the shoulders fail to deliver either spontaneously or with gentle downward traction after the fetal head has delivered. It is usually caused by the anterior shoulder being wedged behind the pubic symphysis. When this occurs, it is imperative to have a well-rehearsed plan of action so that the fetus can be delivered in the most expedient and safest manner possible. Since some maneuvers to relieve shoulder dystocia require multiple clinical providers, every member of the care team should be familiar with their role.

Although there are well-known risk factors for a shoulder dystocia, most cases are unanticipated. While it is reasonable to offer a prophylactic cesarean delivery if the estimated fetal weight is > 5000 g in a non-diabetic patient or > 4500 g in a diabetic patient, elective induction of a patient with presumed macrosomia in an effort to avoid shoulder dystocia is not currently supported by the literature or ACOG.

Most cases of shoulder dystocia will resolve with only a few maneuvers, but complications, such as a brachial plexus injury, can occur in anywhere from 5.2% to 20% of cases. Fortunately, less than 20% of all brachial plexus injuries result in permanent damage to the child (ACOG 2017b).

Incidence

0.2–2% of vaginal deliveries of vertex fetuses.

Clinical Picture

After delivery of the head, the shoulders fail to deliver spontaneously or with gentle downward traction. Prior to delivery of the head, it may be noted to retract back significantly after each push (Turtle sign).

Risk Factors

- Prior shoulder dystocia (recurrence risk 1–16.7%)
- Diabetes
- Fetal macrosomia (> 4000 g)
- Maternal obesity
- Multiparity
- Post-term gestation

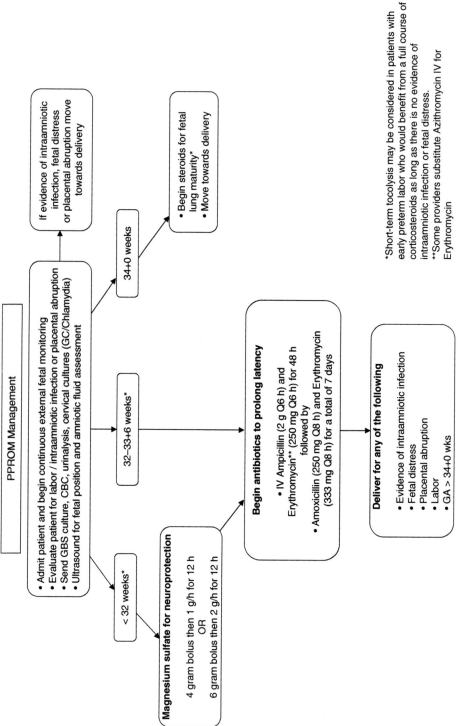

Figure 14.5 Treatment algorithm for PPROM.

PPROM Management

- Admit patient and begin continuous external fetal monitoring
- Evaluate patient for labor / intraamniotic infection or placental abruption
- Send GBS culture, CBC, urinalysis, cervical cultures (GC/Chlamydia)
- Ultrasound for fetal position and amniotic fluid assessment

If evidence of intraamniotic infection, fetal distress or placental abruption move towards delivery

34+0 weeks

- Begin steroids for fetal lung maturity*
- Move towards delivery

32–33+6 weeks*

< 32 weeks*

Magnesium sulfate for neuroprotection

4 gram bolus then 1 g/h for 12 h
OR
6 gram bolus then 2 g/h for 12 h

Begin antibiotics to prolong latency

- IV Ampicillin (2 g Q6 h) and Erythromycin** (250 mg Q6 h) for 48 h followed by
- Amoxicillin (250 mg Q8 h) and Erythromycin (333 mg Q8 h) for a total of 7 days

Deliver for any of the following

- Evidence of intraamniotic infection
- Fetal distress
- Placental abruption
- Labor
- GA > 34+0 wks

*Short-term tocolysis may be considered in patients with early preterm labor who would benefit from a full course of corticosteroids as long as there is no evidence of intraamniotic infection or fetal distress.
**Some providers substitute Azithromycin IV for Erythromycin

- Previous history of a macrosomic fetus
- Prolonged second stage
- Operative vaginal delivery

Treatment

The goal of maneuvers is to relieve the shoulder dystocia and prevent fetal and maternal injury. There are multiple possible maneuvers that can be attempted. They are listed here in the order that they are generally implemented, but there will be some variation between providers.

1. **McRoberts maneuver.** It is generally agreed that this is the initial maneuver of choice. It involves hyperflexion and abduction of the mother's legs back to flatten the lumbar lordosis and potentially free the impacted shoulder. After this maneuver is done, delivery should again be attempted with gentle traction to deliver the anterior shoulder.
2. **Suprapubic pressure.** This is usually performed at the same time as the McRoberts maneuver. An assistant stands up on a stool or high enough to provide downward pressure just above the pubic symphysis in an attempt to dislodge the anterior shoulder laterally toward the fetal sternum. (Note that pressure is not applied directly downward, but at an angle to help rotate and dislodge the anterior shoulder.) It is important to remember **not** to apply fundal pressure, as this has been shown to make the situation worse rather than better.
3. **Delivery of the posterior shoulder.** A hand is placed into the posterior portion of the vagina and the posterior elbow/wrist grasped and swept across the body to deliver the posterior arm. When this occurs, the anterior shoulder will almost always deliver easily. If you are not able to gain access because there is minimal room posteriorly, an episiotomy may be cut to create additional room. Additionally, a 12 or 14 French Foley catheter can be used to create a sling around the posterior shoulder, assisting in delivery of the posterior arm with traction (ACOG 2017b).

The use of the above three maneuvers will resolve approximately 95% of shoulder dystocias within 4 minutes (ACOG 2017b).

If these are not successful, additional maneuvers that can be used include:

4. **Rotational maneuvers: ***
   - Modified Woods screw maneuver. This maneuver is meant to turn the shoulders to an oblique position in order to deliver the child. It is performed by applying pressure behind the posterior shoulder and rotating the child to release the anterior shoulder from behind the symphysis.
   - Rubins maneuvers. This maneuver involves attempting to disimpact the anterior shoulder by transabdominal manipulation and then placing a hand vaginally behind the anterior shoulder to move it to an oblique angle for delivery.
5. **Generous episiotomy.** There is little evidence to support the routine use of episiotomy with a shoulder dystocia. However, if it is difficult to perform the rotational maneuvers or deliver the posterior shoulder, then an episiotomy may be made.

---

* These maneuvers may be described differently in different texts. Just remember that the goal of rotational maneuvers is to move the anterior shoulder out from behind the pubic symphysis.

6. **Gaskin all-fours maneuver.** This maneuver involves having the patient move from her back to a position on her hands and knees and then attempting to deliver the fetus. It may, however, be a very difficult position for the patient to adopt if she has a functioning epidural.

7. **Replacement of the fetal head (Zavanelli maneuver).** This is a last-ditch maneuver if all reasonable efforts have failed to deliver the fetal shoulder. In doing this, the cardinal movements of labor are reversed and the fetal head is rotated back to the midline, flexed, and replaced into the vagina and upward while the mother is quickly moved to have an emergency cesarean section. Terbutaline may be used for uterine tocolysis if needed to make this easier. The risk of significant fetal morbidity and mortality is increased greatly when this has to be performed (Kwek and Yeo 2006).

8. **Abdominal rescue.** This refers to an operative approach where a laparotomy is made and then the provider attempts to manually dislodge the anterior shoulder from above to allow for a vaginal delivery.

9. **Fracture of the clavicle.** The fetal clavicle can be fractured by placing two fingers underneath it and pulling outward. It should not be pushed toward the fetus, as angulation in this manner can result in a fetal pneumothorax. This is actually much more difficult than it sounds, but may allow for compression of the fetal shoulder toward the thorax if successful.

10. **Symphysiotomy.** This is a maneuver used almost exclusively in developing countries when all options have failed and there is no option for operative intervention with abdominal rescue or a Zavanelli maneuver. It involves making an incision in the ligament of the pubic symphysis and is only used in the most extreme circumstances if all other options have failed.

After the delivery of the fetal shoulders, regardless of what maneuvers are required, you should collect a section of the umbilical cord for cord gases.

After everything is over, it is imperative to sit down with the parents to explain exactly what occurred and what maneuvers were done to deliver their child. Additionally, parents should be counseled regarding the risk of recurrence with a future pregnancy. It is also extremely important to debrief with everyone involved in the delivery and review the timing of what occurred so that documentation will be consistent. A detailed note in the chart should include the following elements:

- All providers present at the delivery
- Classify complication as a shoulder dystocia
- Which shoulder was anterior
- How long it took to deliver (head-to-body interval)
- Infant birth weight
- Apgar scores
- Umbilical cord gases
- Mention if the infant is moving extremities after the delivery
- All maneuvers used in the correct order

Umbilical Cord Prolapse

Umbilical cord prolapse occurs when the umbilical cord falls through the cervix into the vagina ahead of the presenting fetal part after the membranes have ruptured. It is an obstetric emergency that requires prompt intervention, as the umbilical vessels contained in the umbilical cord are typically compressed when this happens, which can result in fetal distress and even demise secondary to hypoxemia.

Incidence

This complication occurs in 0.14–0.62% of all deliveries, and the risk of fetal death is less than 10% (Holbrook and Phelan 2013). Fetal lie changes the risk, with cord prolapse occurring in 0.14% of deliveries when the fetus is in the vertex position and 2.5–3.0% when the fetus is breech (Vasquez and Desai 2018).

Clinical Picture

An acute and severe fetal bradycardia or severe repetitive variable decelerations are almost always seen. These are usually in contrast to a normal and reassuring FHR tracing prior to the event. It may also occur immediately after the patient reports rupture of membranes. When a cervical examination is performed in an attempt to determine the etiology of the fetal distress, the umbilical cord is palpable in the vagina.

Risk Factors

- Preterm delivery
- Birth weight < 2500 g
- Fetal malpresentation (breech, transverse)
- Multiple gestation
- Multiparity
- Polyhydramnios
- Rupture of membranes
- Manual rotation of the fetal head
- Amniotomy

Causes

The ultimate cause of umbilical cord prolapse in any situation is something that allows the cord to descend ahead of the presenting part. While there are risk factors, as outlined above, this complication may occur spontaneously or when any of several routine obstetric procedures are performed. Some of these iatrogenic causes include:

- Artificial rupture of membranes*
- Fetal scalp electrode (FSE) placement
- Intrauterine pressure catheter (IUPC) placement
- Amnioinfusion

---

* Because amniotomy may precipitate a cord prolapse, it is imperative that the fetal position be known and the presenting part is well applied to the cervix, in order to decrease the risk.

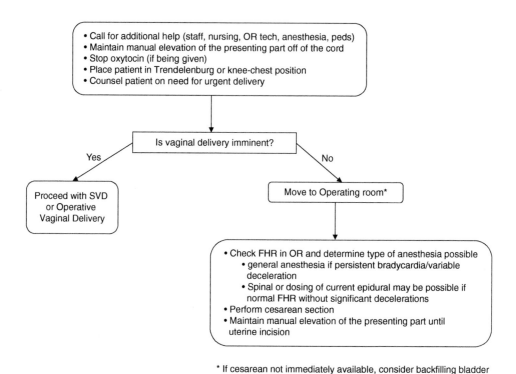

Figure 14.6 Umbilical cord prolapse treatment. FHR, fetal heart rate; OR, operating room; SVD, spontaneous vaginal delivery.

Treatment

Whenever the umbilical cord is palpated in the vagina, the examiner should not remove his or her hand, but rather attempt to elevate the presenting part off of the umbilical cord. You should inform the rest of the care team that you have a cord prolapse, and assemble the team for the operating room. As you do this, also take time to counsel the patient about the complication and explain that it is necessary to deliver the baby urgently by cesarean section. Once in the operating room, recheck the FHR and talk with anesthesia about how quickly you need to proceed with the operation. If the FHR is reassuring, you may be able to use a spinal instead of a general anesthesia. It is important to remember that the initial examiner's hand remains in the vagina until the baby is delivered by cesarean section.

Of note, if cord prolapse is noted but vaginal delivery is imminent, it may be possible to proceed quickly with a vaginal or operative delivery.

If there is any delay in performing the cesarean section you can consider administering terbutaline to decrease uterine contractions or filling the bladder with 500 mL of fluid to elevate the presenting part off the cord (Holbrook and Phelan 2013).

See Figure 14.6 for a treatment algorithm for umbilical cord prolapse.

Uterine Inversion

This is a relatively uncommon occurrence, but when it occurs immediate intervention is necessary to prevent disastrous hemorrhage. It can be a result of overzealous traction on the umbilical cord after delivery, usually in the setting of abnormal placentation. Suprapubic pressure applied during delivery of the placenta is a measure used to try and prevent uterine inversion.

Incidence

1 in 2000 to 1 in 20,000 deliveries (Coad *et al.* 2017).

Clinical Picture

Presence of a beefy red mass of tissue with the delivery of the placenta or inability to palpate the uterine fundus during a postpartum hemorrhage may be an indicator of a uterine inversion.

Risk Factors
- Fundal pressure
- Fundal placentation
- Excessive umbilical cord traction
- Use of oxytocin
- Abnormal placentation (placenta accreta, increta, percreta)

(Coad *et al.* 2017)

Treatment
- Call for help (staff/anesthesia).
- Immediately attempt to manually replace the uterus.*
- Bolus IV fluids/IV access (2 large-bore IVs).
- Crossmatch blood (at least 2 units to start).
- If unable to replace uterus, give agent to relax uterus. Options:
  - Terbutaline 0.25 mg IV
  - Nitroglycerin 50–100 mcg IV (this will result in uterine relaxation within 30 seconds and will last approximately 1 minute)
  - Halogenated anesthetic agent

(Thorp and Laughon 2014, ACOG 2017c)

If these attempts are unsuccessful, then the patient should be moved as an emergency to the operating room, where a laparotomy is performed. The round ligaments are used for traction to restore the uterus to its normal position with what is called the Huntington maneuver. If this maneuver fails because the uterine fundus if trapped within the cervix, the Haultain procedure may be attempted. This entails making a longitudinal incision through the inverted fundus to allow for reinversion. Once successful, this incision is then closed similarly to a hysterotomy made during a cesarean section.

---

* Replacing the uterus involves applying gentle manual pressure to the most distal part of the uterus that is seen and pushing it back into the vagina and through the cervix. Once the uterus is back in position, a fist is kept inside the uterus, and uterotonics are given to make sure the uterus contracts.

Uterine Rupture

Uterine rupture occurs in approximately 1 in 7643 deliveries and is associated with significant morbidity and mortality for both mother and fetus. The amount of fetal and maternal distress and blood loss depends on the time it takes to make the diagnosis, as well as the size and location of the defect. If the uterus ruptures laterally, where the uterine vessels are located, then blood loss may be rapid and severe. If uterine rupture is not diagnosed quickly, then fetal demise is likely.

Incidence

- 1 in 7643 of all deliveries
- 0.5–1.0% of patients with a previous low transverse cesarean section attempting vaginal delivery (see *Vaginal Birth After Cesarean* in Chapter 10)
- In patients with a prior classical incision, a T-shaped uterine incision, or a previous rupture, the risk of subsequent rupture is much higher:
  - Low vertical incision: 0.8–1.1%
  - Classical or T-shaped incision: 4–9%
  - Prior uterine rupture: 6–32%

(Hobel and Lamb 2016, Landon and Grobman 2017)

Clinical Picture

While the clinical presentation of a uterine rupture may occur suddenly or develop over a period of time, some common findings often include the following:

- Fetal distress with either a prolonged bradycardia or variable decelerations that progress to late decelerations and bradycardia
- Loss of uterine contraction strength on IUPC
- Loss of fetal station (fetal vertex not palpable or much higher than previous exam)
- Sudden onset of focal pain (even if the patient has a functioning epidural)
- Vaginal bleeding (common, but not required for diagnosis)
- Maternal hypovolemia, hypotension, shock

(Al-Zirqi *et al.* 2017)

Risk Factors

- Grand multiparity
- Malpresentation
- Abnormal placentation
- Previous classical uterine incision
- Prior myomectomy with entry into uterine cavity
- Use of prostaglandins in a patient with previous cesarean section
- Maternal age > 35 years
- Fetal weight > 4000 g
- Induction of labor
- Fetal or uterine anomalies
- Previous cesarean delivery for dystocia
- Interval of < 16 months between this labor and previous cesarean section

(Dow et al. 2009, Al-Zirqi *et al.* 2017)

Treatment

A uterine rupture is an obstetrical emergency and requires delivery by cesarean section immediately and repair of the rupture. Time is of the essence, as the fetus is usually in significant distress. Steps that should be taken immediately include the following:

- Call for staff backup/OR technician/anesthesiologist/pediatrician.
- Call for blood products (PRBCs/platelets) and antibiotics on the way to the OR.
- Deliver the fetus by emergency cesarean section.*
- Control bleeding; perform hysterectomy if unable to salvage uterus.

Postpartum

Patients with a previous uterine rupture should not be allowed to labor in subsequent pregnancies.

References

ACOG (2006). Mode of term singleton breech delivery. *ACOG Committee Opinion* #340, July 2006, reaffirmed 2016.

ACOG (2012). Prediction and prevention of preterm birth. *ACOG Practice Bulletin* #130, October 2012, reaffirmed 2016.

ACOG (2013). Hypertension in pregnancy: executive summary. American College of Obstetricians and Gynecologists; Task Force on Hypertension in Pregnancy. *Obstet Gynecol* 122: 1122–31.

ACOG (2014). Antepartum fetal surveillance. *ACOG Practice Bulletin* #145, July 2014, reaffirmed 2017.

ACOG (2016a). Multifetal gestations: twin, triplet, and higher-order multifetal pregnancies. *ACOG Practice Bulletin* #169, October 2016.

ACOG (2016b). Management of preterm labor. *ACOG Practice Bulletin* #171, October 2016.

ACOG (2016c). Premature rupture of membranes. *ACOG Practice Bulletin* #172, October 2016.

ACOG (2017a). Intrapartum management of intraamniotic infection. *ACOG Committee Opinion* #340, August 2017.

ACOG (2017b). Shoulder dystocia. *ACOG Practice Bulletin* #178, May 2017.

ACOG (2017c). Postpartum hemorrhage. *ACOG Practice Bulletin* #183, October 2017.

Al-Zirqi I, Daltveit AK, Forsén L, Stray-Pedersen B, Vangen S (2017). Risk factors for complete uterine rupture. *Am J Obstet Gynecol* 216: 165.e1–8.

Ananth CV, Savitz DA, Williams MA (1996). Placental abruption and its association with hypertension and prolonged rupture of membranes: a methodologic review and meta-analysis. *Obstet Gynecol* 88: 309–18.

Atkinson AL, Santolaya-Forgas J, Matta P, Canterino J, Oyelese Y (2015). The sensitivity of the Kleihauer–Betke test for placental abruption. *J Obstet Gynaecol* 35: 139–41.

Belfort MA (2017). Overview of postpartum hemorrhage. *UpToDate*. www.uptodate.com/co ntents/overview-of-postpartum-hemorrhage (accessed May 2018).

Callaghan WM, Kuklina EV, Berg CJ (2010). Trends in post-partum hemorrhage: United States, 1994–2006. *Am J Obstet Gynecol* 202: 353. e1–6.

Chapman E, Reveiz L, Illanes E, Bonfill Cosp X (2014). Antibiotic regimens for management of intra-amniotic infection. *Cochrane Database Syst Rev* (12): CD010076.

Chen KT (2018). Postpartum endometritis. *UpToDate*. www.uptodate.com/contents/post partum-endometritis (accessed May 2018).

Coad SL, Dahlgren LS, Hutcheon JA (2017). Risks and consequences of puerperal uterine inversion in the United States, 2004 through 2013. *Am J Obstet Gynecol* 217: 377.e1–e6

---

* General anesthesia will often be required in this situation.

Creswell JA, Ronsmans C, Calvert C, Filippi V (2013). Prevalence of placenta praevia by world region: a systematic review and meta-analysis. *Trop Med Int Health* **18**: 712–24.

Cunningham FG, Leveno KJ, Bloom SL, *et al.* (2014). Hypertensive disorders. In *Williams Obstetrics*, 24th edn. New York: McGraw-Hill.

Del Priore G, Jackson-Stone M, Shim EK, *et al.* (1996). A comparison of once-daily and 8-hour gentamicin dosing in the treatment of postpartum endometritis. *Obstet Gynecol* **87**: 994–1000.

Dola CP, Garite TJ, Dowling DD, *et al.* (2003). Placenta previa: does its type affect pregnancy outcome? *Am J Perinatol* **20**: 353–60.

Dow M, Wax JR, Pinette MG, Blackstone J, Cartin A (2009). Third-trimester uterine rupture without previous cesarean: a case series and review of the literature. *Am J Perinatol* **26**: 739–44.

Faro S (2005). Postpartum endometritis. *Clin Perinatol* **32**: 803–14.

Gilbert WM (2017). Amniotic fluid disorders. In Gabbe SG, Niebyl JR, Simpson JL, *et al.* (eds.), *Obstetrics: Normal and Problem Pregnancies*, 7th edn. Philadelphia, PA: Elsevier, pp. 786–94.

Hickok DE, Gordon DC, Milberg JA, Williams MA, Daling JR (1992). The frequency of breech presentation by gestational age at birth: a large population-based study. *Am J Obstet Gynecol* **166**: 851–2.

Higgins RD, Saade G, Polin RA, Grobman WA, *et al.* (2016). Evaluation and management of women and newborns with a maternal diagnosis of chorioamnionitis: summary of a workshop. *Obstet Gynecol* **127**: 426–36.

Hobel CJ (2016). Obstetric complications. In Hacker, NF, Gambone JC, Hobel CJ (eds.), *Hacker & Moore's Essentials of Obstetrics and Gynecology*, 6th edn. Philadelphia, PA: Elsevier, pp. 155–69.

Hobel CJ, Lamb AR (2016). Obstetric hemorrhage. In Hacker NF, Gambone JC, Hobel CJ (eds.), *Hacker & Moore's Essentials of Obstetrics and Gynecology*, 6th edn. Philadelphia, PA: Elsevier, pp. 136–46.

Holbrook BD, Phelan ST (2013). Umbilical cord prolapse. *Obstet Gynecol Clin North Am* **40**: 1–14.

Iams JK (2003). Prediction and early detection of preterm labor. *Obstet Gynecol* **101**: 402–12.

Kim CJ, Romero R, Chaemsaithong P, Chaiyasit N, Kim YM (2015). Acute chorioamnionitis and funisitis: definition, pathologic features, and clinical significance. *Am J Obstet Gynecol* **213** (4 Suppl.): S29–52.

Kwek KK, Yeo GS (2006). Shoulder dystocia and injuries: prevention and management. *Curr Opin Obstet Gynecol* **18**: 123–8.

Landon MB, Grobman WA (2017). Vaginal birth after cesarean delivery. In Gabbe SG, Niebyl JR, Simpson JL, *et al.* (eds.), *Obstetrics: Normal and Problem Pregnancies*, 7th edn. Philadelphia, PA: Elsevier, pp. 444–55.

Liu S, Joseph KS, Liston RM, *et al.* (2011). Incidence, risk factors, and associated complications of eclampsia. *Obstet Gynecol* **118**: 987–94.

Lockwood CJ, Russo-Stieglitz K (2017). Placenta previa: epidemiology, clinical features, diagnosis. *UpToDate.* www.uptodate.com/con tents/placenta-previa-epidemiology-clinical-fea tures-diagnosis-morbidity-and-mortality (accessed May 2018).

Mackeen AD, Packard RE, Ota E, Speer L (2015). Antibiotic regimens for postpartum endometritis. *Cochrane Database Syst Rev* (2): CD001067.

Markham KB, Funai EF (2014). Pregnancy-related hypertension. In Creasy RK, Resnik R, Iams JD, *et al.* (eds.), *Creasy and Resnik's Maternal–Fetal Medicine: Principles and Practice*, 7th edn. Philadelphia, PA: Elsevier Saunders, pp. 756–81.

McCowan LME, Dekker GA, Chan E, *et al.* (2009). Spontaneous preterm birth and small for gestational age infants in women who stop smoking early in pregnancy: prospective cohort study. *BMJ* **338**: b1081.

Mercer BM (2014). Premature rupture of the membranes. In Creasy RK, Resnik R, Iams JD, *et al.* (eds.), *Creasy and Resnik's Maternal–Fetal Medicine: Principles and Practice*, 7th edn. Philadelphia, PA: Elsevier Saunders, pp. 663–72.

Mercer BM (2017). Premature rupture of the membranes. In Gabbe SG, Niebyl JR, Simpson JL, *et al.* (eds.), *Obstetrics: Normal and Problem*

Pregnancies, 7th edn. Philadelphia, PA: Elsevier, pp. 647–60.

Mitra AG, Whitten MK, Laurent SL, Anderson WE (1997). A randomized, prospective study comparing once-daily gentamicin versus thrice-daily gentamicin in the treatment of puerperal infection. *Am J Obstet Gynecol* **177**: 786–92.

NHLBI (2012). What are the risks of a blood transfusion? US Dept of Health and Human Services, National Institutes of Health, National Heart, Lung, and Blood Institute. www.nhlbi.ni h.gov/node/3593 (accessed May 2018).

Norwitz ER (2016). Overview of the etiology and evaluation of vaginal bleeding in pregnant women. *UpToDate.* www.uptodate.com/con tents/overview-of-the-etiology-and-evaluation-of-vaginal-bleeding-in-pregnant-women (accessed May 2018).

Oberg SA, Hernandez-Diaz S, Palmsten K, Almqvist C, Bateman BT (2014). Patterns of recurrence of postpartum hemorrhage in a large, population-based cohort. *Am J Obstet Gynecol* **210**: 229.e1–8.

Oyelese Y (2010). Evaluating and management of low-lying placenta or placenta previa on second trimester ultrasound. *Contemporary OB/GYN* **55**: 30–3.

Oyelese Y, Smulian J (2006). Placenta previa, placenta accreta, and vasa previa. *Obstet Gynecol* **107**: 927–41.

Roberts D, Brown J, Medley N, Dalziel SR (2017). Antenatal corticosteroids for accelerating fetal lung maturation for women at risk of preterm birth. *Cochrane Database Syst Rev* (3): CD004454.

Rossen J, Okland I, Nilsen OB, Eggebo TM (2010). Is there any increase of postpartum hemorrhage, and is severe hemorrhage associated with more frequent use of obstetric interventions? *Acta Ostet Gynecol Scand* **89**: 1248–55.

Sibai BM (2017). Preeclampsia and hypertensive disorders. In Gabbe SG, Niebyl JR, Simpson JL, et al. (eds.), *Obstetrics: Normal and Problem Pregnancies*, 7th edn. Philadelphia, PA: Elsevier, pp. 661–705.

Simhan HN, Berghella V, Iams JD (2014). Preterm labor and birth. In Creasy RK, Resnik R, Iams JD, et al. (eds.), *Creasy and Resnik's*

Maternal–Fetal Medicine: Principles and Practice, 7th edn. Philadelphia, PA: Elsevier Saunders, pp. 624–53.

Singla AK, Lapinski RH, Berkowitz RL, Saphier CJ (2001). Are women who are Jehovah's Witnesses at risk of maternal death? *Am J Obstet Gynecol* **185**: 893–5.

Simhan HN, Iams JD, Romero R (2017). Preterm labor and birth. In Gabbe SG, Niebyl JR, Simpson JL, et al. (eds.), *Obstetrics: Normal and Problem Pregnancies*, 7th edn. Philadelphia, PA: Elsevier, pp. 615–46.

Spong CY, Mercer BM, D'alton M, et al. (2011). Timing of indicated late-preterm and early-term birth. *Obstet Gynecol* **118**: 323–33.

Stout MJ, Scifres CM, Stamilio DM (2013). Diagnostic utility of urine protein-to-creatinine ratio for identifying proteinuria in pregnancy. *J Matern Fetal Neonatal Med* **26**: 66–70.

Thorp JM, Laughon SK (2014). Clinical aspects of normal and abnormal labor. In Creasy RK, Resnik R, Iams JD, et al. (eds.), *Creasy and Resnik's Maternal–Fetal Medicine: Principles and Practice*, 7th edn. Philadelphia, PA: Elsevier Saunders, pp. 673–703.

Tikkanen M (2011). Placental abruption: epidemiology, risk factors, and consequences. *Acta Obstet Gynecol Scand* **90**: 140–9.

Tita AT (2017). Intra-amniotic infection (clinical chorioamnionitis or triple I). *UpToDate.* www.uptodate.com/contents/intra-a mniotic-infection-clinical-chorioamnionitis-or-triple-i (accessed May 2018).

Tita AT, Andrews WW (2010). Diagnosis and management of clinical chorioamnionitis. *Clin Perinatol* **37**: 339–54.

Vasquez V, Desai S (2018). Labor and delivery and their complications. In Walls RM, Hockberger RS, Gausche Hill M, et al. (eds.), *Rosen's Emergency Medicine: Concepts and Clinical Practice*, 9th edn. Philadelphia, PA: Elsevier. pp. 2296–312.

Vergnes JN, Sixou, M (2007). Preterm low birth weight and maternal periodontal status: a meta-analysis. *Am J Obstet Gynecol* **196**: 135. e1–7.

Appendix A: Medication Database

Meghan Yamasaki and Shad Deering

Introduction

Every effort has been made to ensure the accuracy of the information and dosing regimens for the medications included in this text. It is, however, still the provider's responsibility to use clinical judgment and consult with the pharmacy or other appropriate sources regarding dosage and contraindications based on the clinical situation, because dosage recommendations may change over time and inadvertent errors in the text can occur and the authors cannot be held responsible for any errors found in this book.

Analgesics

Butorphanol

Other names	Stadol
Indications	Pain relief during latent labor
Contraindications	Known allergy
Dosage	1–2 mg
Dosage interval	q4h
Route of administration	IV or IM
Adverse reactions	Pruritis, respiratory depression, decreased FHR variability, increased BP, nausea, emesis
Breastfeeding	This medication is not usually given in the postpartum period.
Notes	The onset of action of this medication is within minutes when given IV. When administered IM, the onset of analgesia is usually within 30 minutes. It has been reported to increase blood pressure and should not be administered to patients with hypertension or preeclampsia. A 2 mg dose of butorphanol is equivalent to approximately 10 mg of morphine.
Mechanism of action	This medication is a mixed opioid agonist/antagonist.

Fentanyl

Other names	Sublimaze
Indications	Analgesia in labor, pain control postpartum for some procedures (e.g., manual extraction of placenta)
Contraindications	Known allergy, respiratory depression
Dosage	50–100 mcg
Dosage interval	q1–2h
Route of administration	IV/IM
Adverse reactions	Respiratory depression (less likely than with morphine), mild bradycardia
Breastfeeding	This medication is generally not given in the postpartum period.
Notes	This medication is nearly 100 times more potent than morphine, but is less likely to result in respiratory depression, although this complication may still occur. Its onset of action is almost immediate when given IV.
Mechanism of action	This medication is an opioid receptor agonist.

Ketorolac

Other names	Toradol
Indications	Postpartum or postoperative pain control
Contraindications	Known allergy to ketorolac or NSAIDs, actively bleeding ulcer
Dosage	30 mg IV/IM (maximum 120 mg/day), 10–20 mg PO (maximum 40 mg/day)
Dosage interval	q6h (IV/IM), q4–6h (PO)
Route of administration	IV/IM/PO
Adverse reactions	Gastrointestinal distress or bleeding, tinnitus
Breastfeeding	This medication is compatible with breastfeeding.
Notes	This medication is a non-steroidal anti-inflammatory drug (NSAID) that is very helpful with postoperative pain management, as it may be given parenterally and you do not have to wait for the patient's bowel function to return.
Mechanism of action	This medication inhibits cyclooxygenase and therefore prostaglandin synthesis.

Morphine

Other names	N/A
Indications	Pain relief during latent labor
Contraindications	Known allergy, respiratory depression
Dosage	2–5 mg (IV), 10 mg (IM)
Dosage interval	q4h
Route of administration	IV/IM
Adverse reactions	Pruritis, respiratory depression, decreased FHR variability, nausea, emesis

Breastfeeding	Compatible with breastfeeding, but studies indicate that a significant amount of narcotics may be transferred to the infant.
Notes	The onset of analgesia from IV morphine is approximately 5 minutes, and 30–40 minutes from an IM dose. The half-life of the drug in the neonate is approximately 7 hours.
Mechanism of action	This medication is an opioid receptor agonist.

Nalbuphine

Other names	Nubain
Indications	Pain relief during latent labor
Contraindications	Known allergy
Dosage	10 mg
Dosage interval	q3–4h
Route of administration	IV or IM
Adverse reactions	Pruritis, respiratory depression, decreased FHR variability, sedation, nausea, emesis
Breastfeeding	Generally used only in the antepartum period.
Notes	This medication takes effect within minutes when administered IV, and within 15 minutes when given IM. It has a half-life in the neonate of around 4 hours.
Mechanism of action	This medication is a partial opioid agonist.

Percocet

Other names	Endocet, oxycodone+acetaminophen
Indications	Postoperative pain relief
Contraindications	Known allergy, respiratory depression
Dosage	1–2 tablets (2.5 mg oxycodone/325 mg acetaminophen)
Dosage interval	q4–6h
Route of administration	PO
Adverse reactions	Pruritis, nausea, emesis
Breastfeeding	Compatible with breastfeeding, with minimal risk for adverse effects during nursing. Recommended that infants be monitored for sedation or changes in feeding patterns.
Notes	This medication is commonly used for post-cesarean pain control when the patient is tolerating a regular diet.
Mechanism of action	This medication is a mixture of oxycodone and acetaminophen. The oxycodone is an opioid receptor agonist. There are different strengths that may be carried on formulary, with the most common being Percocet 2.5/325 or 5/325, meaning that each tablet contains either 2.5 mg or 5 mg of oxycodone and 325 mg of acetaminophen.

Antibiotics

Ampicillin

Other names	N/A
Indications	Treatment of intra-amniotic infection and endometritis
Contraindications	Known allergy
Dosage	2 g
Dosage interval	q6h
Route of administration	IV
Adverse reactions	Anaphylaxis, urticaria, gastrointestinal upset
Breastfeeding	Compatible with breastfeeding, although potential for modification of infant bowel flora, allergic response, and interference with infant culture results if required.
Notes	This antibiotic is part of the first-line treatment for intra-amniotic infection (see Chapter 14). It is also added to the standard antibiotic regimen for postpartum endometritis after 24 hours if the patient remains febrile, in order to provide coverage for enterococcus.
Mechanism of action	The amino side group allows this drug to penetrate Gram-negative organisms. It then inhibits the crosslinking of bacteria cell wall components.

Azithromycin

Other names	Zithromax, Zmax
Indications	Patients undergoing non-elective cesarean delivery during labor or after rupture of membranes
Contraindications	Allergy to azithromycin
Dosage	500 mg
Dosage interval	Once
Route of administration	IV
Adverse reactions	Nausea, vomiting, diarrhea, abdominal discomfort, rarely QT prolongation
Breastfeeding	Considered safe in breastfeeding.
Notes	This medication is used concurrently with the standard cesarean antibiotic prophylaxis, typically cefazolin. Ideally, both are given within 1 hour of skin incision.
Mechanism of action	This drug inhibits RNA-dependent protein synthesis by penetrating the cell wall and binding to the 50S ribosomal subunit.

Clindamycin

Other names	Cleocin
Indications	Treatment of postpartum endometritis (in addition to gentamycin) Third-line treatment choice for Group B streptococcus Intra-amniotic infection

Contraindications	Allergy to clindamycin
Dosage	900 mg
Dosage interval	q8h
Route of administration	IV
Adverse reactions	Abdominal cramps, diarrhea, elevation of liver function tests, pseudomembranous colitis
Breastfeeding	Considered safe in breastfeeding.
Notes	This medication covers Gram-positive organisms, and most anaerobes. It does not penetrate the CSF, but it is actively transported into abscesses.
Mechanism of action	This drug binds to the 50s ribosomal subunit interface of bacteria and causes abnormal reading of mRNA, and therefore defective bacterial proteins.

Dicloxacillin

Other names	Dynapen
Indications	Treatment of mastitis, superficial nipple infections
Contraindications	Allergy to penicillin
Dosage	500 mg
Dosage interval	q6h
Route of administration	PO
Adverse reactions	Hypersensitivity reactions
Breastfeeding	Considered safe.
Notes	This is the first choice of antibiotics for the treatment of mastitis.
Mechanism of action	The amino side group allows this class of drugs to penetrate Gram-negative organisms, then it inhibits crosslinking of bacteria cell wall components.

Gentamycin

Other names	Garamycin
Indications	Treatment of intra-amniotic infection and postpartum endometritis
Contraindications	Allergy to gentamycin, renal failure (must reduce dosage)
Dosage	5 mg/kg q24h (ONLY FOR POSTPARTUM USE) or 2 mg/kg loading dose followed by 1.5 mg/kg q8h
Dosage interval	Either q8h or q24h, as above
Route of administration	IV
Adverse reactions	Neurotoxicity, ototoxicity, vertigo, nephrotoxicity
Breastfeeding	Considered safe. Small amounts of the medication are excreted into breast milk.
Notes	In the postpartum period, 24-hour dosing regimen may be used. Prior to delivery, the q8h dosing should be used. This medication is an aminoglycoside that covers Gram-negative bacteria.

| Mechanism of action | The antibiotic binds at the 30s/50s interface and causes incorrect reading of mRNA and defective bacterial proteins. |

Penicillin G

Other names	N/A
Indications	Treatment for GBS prophylaxis in labor
Contraindications	Allergy to penicillin
Dosage	5 million units initially, then 2.5 million units with subsequent doses
Dosage interval	q4h
Route of administration	IV
Adverse reactions	Hypersensitivity reactions, rare neurologic toxicity, neutropenia, nephrotoxicity
Breastfeeding	Considered safe. Small amounts are excreted into breast milk. No adverse effects reported.
Notes	This is the first-line therapy for GBS prophylaxis in labor because it is not as broad spectrum as other antibiotics commonly used, such as ampicillin.
Mechanism of action	B-lactam binds penicillin binding proteins and prevents cross-linking of bacterial cell wall components.

Antivirals

Acyclovir

Other names	Zovirax
Indications	Active herpes simplex virus (HSV 1 or 2)
Contraindications	Allergy to acyclovir, renal failure
Dosage	Primary outbreak: 200 mg q4h × 10 days
	Recurrent outbreak: 200 mg q4h × 5 days. Chronic treatment: 400 mg q12h, or 200 mg 3–5 times a day up to 12 months
Dosage interval	See above
Route of administration	IV or PO
Adverse reactions	Skin irritation, crystalline nephropathy possible if given rapidly IV
Breastfeeding	Considered safe.
Notes	This medication is used for the treatment of both primary and secondary HSV outbreaks as well as for prophylaxis against recurrence.
Mechanism of action	This medication is metabolized to a triphosphate analog that inhibits DNA polymerase. It binds to viral thymidine kinase as well.

Valacyclovir

Other names	Valtrex
Indications	Herpes simplex virus (HSV 1 or 2)
Contraindications	Can interact with nephrotoxic medications
Dosage	Primary outbreak: 1 g q12h
	Secondary outbreak: 500 mg q12h
	Suppression therapy: 1 g q24h
Dosage interval	See above
Route of administration	PO
Adverse reactions	Gastrointestinal upset, headaches, hemolytic uremic syndrome, or thrombotic thrombocytopenic purpura are possible at very high doses.
Breastfeeding	Considered safe.
Notes	This medication is used both for the treatment of herpes outbreaks and for prophylaxis during pregnancy to prevent outbreaks near term which would preclude a vaginal delivery.
Mechanism of action	This medication is metabolized to acyclovir.

Zidovudine

Other names	Azidothymidine, Retrovir; formerly known as AZT
Indications	Given during labor in HIV-positive patients
Contraindications	Allergy to zidovudine
Dosage	2 mg/kg IV bolus followed by infusion of 1 mg/kg/h until delivery
Dosage interval	Continuous infusion
Route of administration	IV
Adverse reactions	Headaches, nausea, anemia, neutropenia, myalgias
Breastfeeding	This medication is excreted in high enough concentrations into breast milk to decrease the viral load, but breastfeeding in HIV-positive women is generally not encouraged in the US.
Notes	This medication is used during labor to decrease the risk of HIV transmission from mother to fetus.
Mechanism of action	This is a thymidine analog that is a reverse transcriptase inhibitor.

Seizure Prophylaxis/Treatment

Lorazepam

Other names	Ativan
Indications	Status epilepticus, eclampsia (for the acute seizure)
Contraindications	Acute narrow-angle glaucoma
Dosage	4 mg IV (dilute first) over 2 minutes
Dosage interval	May repeat after 10–15 minutes if needed
Route of administration	IV/IM

Adverse reactions	Ataxia, CNS depression, respiratory depression
Breastfeeding	Effects are unknown. American Academy of Pediatrics states effects may be concerning if prolonged use occurs.
Notes	This is a benzodiazepine. The onset of action is rapid (i.e. < 5 minutes). It is metabolized in the liver. Diazepam (Valium) is similar to lorazepam, but has a longer half-life.
Mechanism of action	This medication enhances GABA-mediated chloride influx, which results in neuronal inhibition. The exact mechanism by which it exerts its anticonvulsant effects is not clear.

Magnesium Sulfate

Other names	N/A
Indications	Seizure prophylaxis with preeclampsia, treatment of eclampsia
Contraindications	Myasthenia gravis
Dosage	Prophylaxis: 4–6 g bolus over 15–20 minutes, then 2 g/h Eclampsia: 6 g over 15–20 minutes followed by 2 g/h
Dosage interval	Prophylaxis: continuous infusion Eclampsia: continuous infusion
Route of administration	IM/IV
Adverse reactions	Respiratory depression, CNS depression, hypotension, muscle weakness (see *Magnesium Sulfate Toxicity* in Chapter 14)
Breastfeeding	Compatible with breastfeeding
Notes	See Chapter 14 for a discussion of preeclampsia/eclampsia. If given IV, the onset of action is within seconds, if IM the onset is approximately 1 hour. Because of this, the medication is rarely given IM. For seizure prophylaxis, in the very rare situation that IV access is not continuously available, the following regimen may be given: 10 g of a 50% magnesium sulfate solution into the buttocks (5 g into each buttock) then 5 g of a 50% magnesium sulfate solution into the buttocks every 4 hours after the initial IM doses
Mechanism of action	Magnesium sulfate decreases neuromuscular conduction as well as the release of acetylcholine, and results in vasodilation as well. It is thought that its anticonvulsant properties are a result of a direct action on the cerebral cortex.

Phenytoin

Other names	Dilantin
Indications	Seizure prophylaxis, eclampsia
Contraindications	Heart block, sinus bradycardia, anticonvulsant hypersensitivity syndrome
Dosage	10–15 mg/kg (slow IV infusion, not more than 50 mg per minute), followed by maintenance doses of 100 mg IV q6–8h

Dosage interval	q6–8h
Route of administration	IV
Adverse reactions	Nystagmus, ataxia, bone marrow suppression, hepatotoxicity, CNS depression, arrhythmias, hypotension
Breastfeeding	There are conflicting reports on the safety of phenytoin with breastfeeding, but at least one source does not recommend breastfeeding, as low concentrations of the drug are secreted into human milk.
Notes	This medication is metabolized in the liver. It has many drug interactions, which should be checked as soon as possible. This medication is not as effective as magnesium sulfate in the prevention of eclamptic seizures and should only be used for this when magnesium is not available or is contraindicated.
Mechanism of action	Phenytoin reduces the flux of sodium, calcium, and potassium across neuronal membranes.

Hemorrhage

Carboprost

Other names	Hemabate, PGF2-alpha
Indications	Postpartum hemorrhage due to uterine atony
Contraindications	Asthma
Dosage	0.25 mg
Dosage interval	0.25 mg q15 minutes up to 8 doses
Route of administration	IM/into myometrium
Adverse reactions	Bronchoconstriction, fevers, chills, nausea, vomiting, diarrhea, pulmonary vasoconstriction
Breastfeeding	This medication is generally used for the acute treatment of postpartum hemorrhage, and is not usually continued after this.
Notes	This medication may be given either after a vaginal delivery or during a cesarean section for uterine atony. It may also be injected directly into the myometrium during a cesarean section. It is important not to administer this drug to patients with asthma, as it may result in significant respiratory distress from bronchoconstriction.
Mechanism of action	This medication is 15-methyl-prostaglandin F2-alpha, which is a synthetic prostaglandin that stimulates the uterus to contract.

Methylergonovine

Other names	Methergine
Indications	Postpartum hemorrhage
Contraindications	Hypertension, preeclampsia/eclampsia
Dosage	0.2 mg
Dosage interval	q2–4h

Route of administration	IM
Adverse reactions	Hypertension, can cause fatal poisoning in patients sensitive to ergot alkaloids, chest pain, dizziness, tinnitus, diarrhea, palpitations, headache
Breastfeeding	May be used during breastfeeding. Small amount of the drug appears in the milk, but no adverse effects have been reported.
Notes	Remember not to give this to preeclamptic/hypertensive patients, as it will increase blood pressure and may precipitate a hypertensive crisis or stroke. It should not be given as an IV bolus.
Mechanism of action	This medication induces uterine smooth muscle contractions, which allows the uterus to clamp down if it is atonic and hemorrhaging.

Misoprostol

Other names	Cytotec
Indications	Postpartum hemorrhage, labor induction (see next section)
Contraindications	Asthma (causes bronchoconstriction), VBAC
Dosage	Postpartum hemorrhage: 400–1000 mcg
Dosage interval	Single dose
Route of administration	Per rectum for postpartum hemorrhage (can be per vagina, but if there is significant bleeding it will come out too quickly)
Adverse reactions	Diarrhea, abdominal pain, nausea, fevers, chills
Breastfeeding	Contraindicated per manufacturer instructions because of the potential for severe diarrhea in the infant.
Notes	This medication is given when uterine atony is the presumed cause of a postpartum hemorrhage.
Mechanism of action	This medication is a prostaglandin E analog that stimulates uterine contractions.

Oxytocin

Other names	Pitocin
Indications	Postpartum hemorrhage due to uterine atony, labor induction/augmentation (see next section)
Contraindications	Contraindications to labor augmentation/induction
Dosage	See Chapter 7 (Table 7.3) for dosing regimens
Dosage interval	Continuous IV drip
Route of administration	IV
Adverse reactions	Uterine hyperstimulation (with fetal distress possible), water intoxication with large doses for a prolonged period of time, postpartum atony
Breastfeeding	Because the half-life is so short, and it is only administered immediately postpartum, usually after delivery of the placenta, oxytocin does not create issues with breastfeeding.

Notes	Pitocin is a synthetic form of oxytocin, a natural hormone in the body. If it seems odd that this medication is given for postpartum atony, when this is a potential complication of the medication, don't worry. A prolonged induction with oxytocin is a risk factor for postpartum atony (remember that the uterus is a muscle that can fatigue like any other muscle). The oxytocin will stimulate the uterus to contract, which will hopefully correct uterine atony and bleeding. If it does not, then other medications/interventions are required (see Chapter 14). When given for atony, no more than 30–40 units are added to 1 liter of crystalloids.
Mechanism of action	Oxytocin receptors are present in the uterus near term, and stimulation of these will cause the uterus to contract.

Tranexamic Acid

Other names	TXA, Cyklokapron, Lysteda
Indications	Postpartum hemorrhage, prophylactically for high-risk patients
Contraindications	Hypersensitivity to tranexamic acid, subarachnoid hemorrhage, active thromboembolic disease, acquired color vision defect
Dosage	1 g
Dosage interval	Initial infusion over 10 min, then additional 1 g if bleeding does not improve after 30 min or stops and restarts within 24 hours
Route of administration	IV
Adverse reactions	Hypotension, dizziness, nausea, diarrhea
Breastfeeding	Tranexamic acid is secreted in breast milk. Breastfeeding is not recommended by the manufacturer.
Notes	Tranexamic acid may be used prophylactically in certain patient populations, including those who refuse blood products, those who are fully anticoagulated at the time of delivery, or those at high risk for postpartum hemorrhage.
Mechanism of action	Antifibrinolytic that inhibits the activation of plasminogen to plasmin, thereby preventing the breakdown of fibrin.

Labor Induction/Augmentation

Dinoprostone

Other names	PGE2, Prostin E2, Cervidil
Indications	Cervical ripening
Contraindications	Previous cesarean section, hypersensitivity to prostaglandins, contraindications to labor induction
Dosage	Dinoprostone gel: 0.5 mg / 2.5 mL syringe Cervidil vaginal insert: 0.3 mg/h released
Dosage interval	Usually single dose (vaginal insert left in place for 12 hours, gel may be repeated q6h for a maximum of 3 doses)
Route of administration	Vaginal

Adverse reactions	Nausea, emesis, fevers
Breastfeeding	This medication is used for labor induction and is not an issue in the postpartum period.
Notes	If the dinoprostone gel is used, then the fetus must be continuously monitored for at least 2 hours. If the vaginal insert is placed, then the fetus must be monitored for as long as it is left in. Oxytocin should not be given until 6–12 hours after the dose of dinoprostone.
Mechanism of action	This drug is a synthetic prostaglandin that stimulates uterine contractions as well as "softens" the cervix to prepare it for labor (see Chapter 7).

Misoprostol

Other names	Cytotec
Indications	Labor induction, postpartum hemorrhage
Contraindications	Asthma (relative contraindication, <2% risk of asthma exacerbation), VBAC
Dosage	Labor induction: 25–50 mcg
Dosage interval	q4–6h
Route of administration	Per vagina (can be rectal for postpartum hemorrhage)
Adverse reactions	Diarrhea, abdominal pain, nausea, uterine hyperstimulation (with fetal distress)
Breastfeeding	Contraindicated per manufacturer instructions because of the potential for severe diarrhea in the infant.
Notes	The most common dosing regimen for labor induction is 25 mcg q4–6h. This lower-dose regimen decreases the incidence of uterine hyperstimulation that can occur. Additional doses should generally not be given if the patient is contracting more than three times in 10 minutes.
Mechanism of action	This medication is a prostaglandin E analog that stimulates uterine contractions.

Oxytocin

Other names	Pitocin
Indications	Labor induction/postpartum hemorrhage
Contraindications	Contraindication to labor induction, fetal distress
Dosage	1–40 mU/min for labor (see Table 7.3 for high- and low-dose options)
Dosage interval	Continuous IV drip
Route of administration	IV
Adverse reactions	Uterine hyperstimulation (with fetal distress possible), water intoxication with large doses for a prolonged period of time, postpartum atony

Breastfeeding	Because the half-life is so short, and it is only administered immediately postpartum, usually after delivery of the placenta, oxytocin does not create issues with breastfeeding.
Notes	Pitocin is a synthetic form of oxytocin, a natural hormone in the body. It takes approximately 40 minutes to reach a steady-state concentration, but the half-life of oxytocin is only 3–5 minutes, which is important to remember if you turn off the infusion as an intervention for fetal distress.
Mechanism of action	Oxytocin receptors are present in the uterus near term, and stimulation of these will cause the uterus to contract.

Tocolytics

Indomethacin

Other names	Indocin
Indications	Preterm labor at < 32 weeks gestation
Contraindications	Aspirin allergy, gestational age > 32 weeks
Dosage	50 mg loading dose, followed by 25 mg doses
Dosage interval	q6h
Route of administration	PO/PR
Adverse reactions	Oligohydramnios, fetal renal failure
Breastfeeding	This medication is used for tocolysis and is not an issue in the postpartum period.
Notes	This medication is given for no more than 48–72 hours because of the potential for oligohydramnios and fetal effects.
Mechanism of action	This medication is a prostaglandin synthesis inhibitor. It is thought to stop uterine contractions by inhibiting the synthesis of prostaglandins, which are implicated in causing contractions.

Magnesium Sulfate

Other names	N/A
Indications	Preterm labor (fetal neuroprotection, second-line tocolytic), seizure prophylaxis with preeclampsia, treatment of eclampsia
Contraindications	Myasthenia gravis
Dosage	4–6 g bolus, followed by 2–4 g/h
Dosage interval	Continuous IV drip
Route of administration	IV for preterm labor
Adverse reactions	Respiratory depression, CNS depression, hypotension, muscle weakness (see *Magnesium Sulfate Toxicity* in Chapter 14)
Breastfeeding	Compatible with breastfeeding

Notes	See Chapter 14 for a discussion of preeclampsia/eclampsia. If given IV, the onset of action is within seconds; if IM, the onset is approximately 1 hour. (Magnesium is almost never given IM for preterm labor.) These patients must be closely monitored to ensure they have adequate urine output (because magnesium sulfate is excreted by the kidneys) and for evidence of pulmonary edema or cardiovascular toxicity. If the patient's serum creatinine is > 1.3 mg/dL, then the continuous infusion dose (usually 2–4 g/h) should be cut in half and serum magnesium levels monitored closely.
Mechanism of action	Magnesium sulfate decreases neuromuscular conduction, decreases the release of acetylcholine, and results in vasodilation as well.

Nifedipine

Other names	Procardia
Indications	Preterm labor/preterm contractions
Contraindications	Hypotension
Dosage	10–20 mg
Dosage interval	q4–6h
Route of administration	PO
Adverse reactions	Hypotension, edema, dizziness, nausea, pulmonary edema, reflex tachycardia
Breastfeeding	This medication is used for tocolysis and should not be an issue in the postpartum period.
Notes	This medication is often used for preterm contractions in the same situation as terbutaline. The side effects of nifedipine are often better tolerated than the tachycardia and palpitations that may occur with terbutaline.
Mechanism of action	This is a calcium-channel blocker. The theory behind this drug as a tocolytic is that by blocking the influx of calcium into the uterine muscle cells, it will decrease contractions, which are dependent on the calcium.

Terbutaline

Other names	Brethine, Bricanyl
Indications	Tocolysis, uterine hyperstimulation
Contraindications	Cardiac arrhythmias, myocardial ischemia or chest pain, pulmonary edema, poorly controlled hyperthyroidism, poorly controlled diabetes
Dosage	0.125–0.25 mg (intermittent IV/SQ dosing)
	5–10 mcg/min (continuous IV)
	2.5–5.0 mg (PO)

Dosage interval	IV drip: continuous SQ or IV intermittent: q3–4h PO: q4–6h
Route of administration	IV/SQ/PO
Adverse reactions	Hypotension, tachycardia, arrhythmias, pulmonary edema, nausea, tremor, headache, myocardial ischemia
Breastfeeding	This medication is used for tocolysis and is not an issue in the postpartum period.
Notes	This medication is most often given SQ or IV for the initial evaluation of preterm labor or while intervening for fetal distress caused by uterine contractions, which can be stopped for a short period of time with this drug. It can also be given PO for maintenance tocolysis. It is not used as a continuous drip in many hospitals at this time. Sometimes a subcutaneous pump is used to deliver a more constant dose to patients requiring long-term tocolysis. The risk of pulmonary edema must always be kept in mind, especially with multiple gestations. The SQ or IV doses of 0.125–0.25 mg are used during labor when uterine hyperstimulation is present and immediate relaxation of the uterus is required because of fetal distress. In these cases, the IV route is preferred as the onset of action is much faster.
Mechanism of action	This is a beta-2 adrenergic agonist that decreases smooth muscle contractions through these actions. Although this medication is selective for the beta-2 receptors, beta-1 receptors in the heart are also stimulated, which causes the tachycardia seen with its administration.

Fetal Indications

Betamethasone

Other names	Celestone
Indications	Risk of premature delivery
Contraindications	Hypersensitivity
Dosage	12 mg
Dosage interval	q24h for a total of 2 doses
Route of administration	IM
Adverse reactions	Hyperglycemia, anaphylaxis, adrenal insufficiency
Breastfeeding	N/A
Notes	Recommend course of steroids for patients between 24^{+0} and 33^{+6} weeks EGA if at risk of preterm delivery. An additional "rescue" course may be considered if at least 14 days since initial course. Additionally, steroids may also be considered for patients between 34^{+0} and 36^{+6} weeks EGA who have never received steroids and are at risk of preterm delivery.

An alternative steroid is dexamethasone. Dexamethasone dosing includes 6 mg IM given q12h for a total of 4 doses.

Mechanism of action   Corticosteroid that increases fetal organ maturation. Regarding lung maturity, betamethasone increases the production of type I and II pneumocytes.

Magnesium Sulfate

Other names   N/A

Indications   Preterm labor (fetal neuroprotection, second-line tocolytic), seizure prophylaxis with preeclampsia, treatment of eclampsia

Contraindications   Myasthenia gravis

Dosage   4–6 g bolus, followed by 2–4 g/h (2 g/h for neuroprotection)

Dosage interval   Continuous IV drip

Route of administration   IV for fetal neuroprotection/preterm labor

Adverse reactions   Respiratory depression, CNS depression, hypotension, muscle weakness (see *Magnesium Sulfate Toxicity* in Chapter 14)

Breastfeeding   N/A

Notes   Use of magnesium sulfate for fetal neuroprotection is recommended between 24^{+0} and 31^{+6} weeks EGA. See Chapter 14 for a discussion of preeclampsia/eclampsia. If given IV, the onset of action is within seconds, if IM the onset is approximately 1 hour. (Magnesium is almost never given IM for preterm labor.) These patients must be closely monitored to ensure they have adequate urine output (because magnesium sulfate is excreted by the kidneys) and for evidence of pulmonary edema or cardiovascular toxicity. If the patient's serum creatinine is > 1.3 mg/dL, then the continuous infusion dose (usually 2–4 g/h) should be cut in half and serum magnesium levels monitored closely.

Mechanism of action   Exact mechanism is unknown. However, it is theorized that the neuroprotective effect is derived from stabilization of neuronal membranes as well as protection against oxidative stress.

Appendix B: Sample Notes and Orders

Allison Eubanks and Shad Deering

Basic Principles

1. Always label your notes with the date and time they are written. If you need to add any information later, always start a new note and notate the date and time. Do not go back in the chart to change information: it gives the appearance of hiding something, even when that is not the intention.
2. If anything is handwritten, make sure to write legibly. Nothing is defensible if it cannot be read.
3. Sign your name at the end of the note.

Notes are generally in the **SOAP** format, which includes the following:

Subjective: this entails how the patient is feeling and what complaints or symptoms they are experiencing. Try and use as much of the patient's wording as possible.

Objective: this is where you record the vital signs, fetal heart rate, and contraction information, as well as laboratory data.

Assessment: make an assessment on the condition of the fetus/maternal condition in a few sentences.

Plan: outline a clear plan for each of the patient's conditions that needs to be addressed.

This format will give you an outline to clearly and consistently relay the maternal and fetal condition and what, if any, additional interventions need to occur.

In the notes contained here, when there are multiple options in parentheses, choose the most appropriate for the situation.

Labor and Delivery Triage

Most hospitals have a standard form on which to triage patients who present to labor and delivery. The format will vary depending on the hospital forms. A triage note is essentially a mini-history and physical, and your main goal is to determine first if the woman and fetus are stable, and, secondly, whether the patient needs to be admitted to the hospital. Always make sure that you have asked the following FOUR QUESTIONS:

- Are you having any vaginal **BLEEDING?**
- Are you feeling any **CONTRACTIONS?** (include time of onset/frequency/intensity)
- Do you feel like you broke your **WATER?** (include time/color of fluid)
- Have you felt your baby **MOVING?** (if not, then how long since the baby moved?)

You will insert the answers to these questions into your note. An example of this is shown in the *Admission H&P* note.

Notes
Admission H&P

Every patient admitted to labor and delivery will need a complete history and physical exam. If you cannot locate the patient's regular chart, which happens all too often, you can get almost everything you need by just talking to her. An exception to this is prenatal laboratory tests, which you will need and can obtain either by locating the chart or from the computer system if your hospital has one.

Basic Outline

S: The patient is a ____ year-old G_P_ _ _ _ at ____ weeks by (sure LMP/unsure LMP/ 1st-trimester US/2nd-trimester US). She presents with a chief complaint of ____ (contractions /ROM/bleeding/etc.). She reports ____ (put answers to the FOUR QUESTIONS here).

Her prenatal course has been complicated by:

PMH: (chronic hypertension, diabetes, autoimmune disorders, previous VTE, etc.)

PSH: (abdominal surgeries, any uterine surgeries)

OB: G_ P_ _ _ _ (include the year, birth weight, mode of delivery, complications)

GYN: (regular menses, history of PID/STDs, fibroids, polyps, endometriosis, abnormal Pap smears, cervical dysplasia, procedures or surgeries on uterus)

ALL: (list with reactions)

SOC: (tobacco use ±, include packs per day [ppd], alcohol use, drug use)

FAM: (congenital diseases or defects, bleeding disorders)

MED: (include doses)

O: Pulse, blood pressure (BP), temperature (temp), respiratory rate (RR)

FHR: Baseline = (130s, 150s, etc.)

Variability = (marked/moderate/minimal/absent)

Accelerations = (present/absent: 15 × 15 or 10 × 10 depending on gestational age)

Decelerations = (present/absent, late/prolonged/variable/early/recurrent/periodic)

FHR category = (I / II / III)

TOCO: contractions are every ___ minutes and occurring (regularly/irregularly)

HEENT:

LUNGS:

HEART:

ABD:

EXT:

GU: V/V (vulva/vagina)

Cervix: dilation/effacement/station

EFW: _____ g by (Leopold's maneuvers/ultrasound)

PRESENTATION: (vertex/breech/transverse) by ultrasound

Pelvis is (adequate/inadequate) by clinical pelvimetry

PRENATAL LABS:

Hct	Hgb	Platelets
Sickdex	Urinalysis	GC/Chlamydia
HIV	Hepatitis B	Blood type
Rubella	GBS	Antibody screen
Amnio	Pap	

   Rhogam given (include if applicable): (gestational age)

US exams:

   Date:

   GA (by LMP/US):

   EFW:

   Placenta location: (anterior/posterior/marginal/low lying/previa)

   Abnormalities:

A: Patient is a _____ year-old G_P_ _ _ _ at _____+_____ weeks with a prenatal course complicated by (gestational diabetes, chronic hypertension, fetal renal pelviectasis, etc.) who presents to labor and delivery for:

1. (List diagnoses, such as latent labor, active labor, signs and symptoms of preeclampsia, premature rupture of membranes, preterm labor)
2. (Support above diagnosis with findings from history and physical: labs show _____, exam significant for – cervical dilation/pooled amniotic fluid/severe lower extremity swelling, etc.)

P: 1. (Admit to labor and delivery)
2. (Continuous fetal monitoring)
3. (Counseled and consented for delivery)
4. (Anesthesia and pediatrics as needed)
5. (Penicillin prophylaxis started for GBS+ status)
6. (Address each diagnosis above here. See example note)

Admission H&P Example

S: The patient is a 25 y/o G4P2012 at 38^{+2} weeks by sure LMP and 1st-trimester US. She presents with a chief complaint of regular uterine contractions since 0600 this morning

She reports regular uterine contractions every 5 minutes

She denies any vaginal bleeding

She denies any ROM

She reports good FM

Her prenatal course has been complicated by her Rh-negative status and mild asthma for which she was treated with salbutamol inhalers PRN this pregnancy without problems

PMH: Asthma since age 14, no history of intubations/hospitalizations

PSH: Appendectomy at age 12, D&C at age 21

OB: G4P2012

      G1: 2006 – SVD at term, 3400 g male, uncomplicated

      G2: 2008 – first-trimester spontaneous abortion with a D&C

      G3: 2010 – SVD at term, 3600 g female, uncomplicated

      G4: current pregnancy

GYN: regular menses since age 13, no history of STD/PID, no abnormal Paps

ALL: Percocet (nausea/vomiting/hives)

SOC: denies tobacco/alcohol/illicit drug use

FAM: no family history of DM/HTN/cancer, no history of congenital defects, no history of bleeding disorders

MED: PNV daily, salbutamol MDI q4h PRN for asthma exacerbation (has only required this approximately 1 ×/month, last use 5 weeks ago)

O: Pulse 77, BP 125/87, temp 37.0 °C, RR 12

FHR: baseline = 140s with moderate variability and + accelerations 15 × 15, no decelerations, reassuring non-stress test

TOCO: contractions are every 3–4 minutes and regular

HEENT: WNL

LUNGS: CTA bilaterally with no expiratory wheezes noted.

HEART: RRR with normal S1/S2

ABD: gravid, uterus is NTTP

EXT: NTTP, 1+ bilateral pedal edema with no cords palpable

GU: V/V: normal vaginal discharge, no lesions noted

Cervix: 4/75/–1

EFW: 3800 g by Leopold's maneuvers

PRESENTATION: vertex by ultrasound

PRENATAL LABS:

Hct – 33.5%	Hgb – 11.0	Platelets – 256
Sickdex – n/a	Urinalysis – neg	GC/Chlamydia – neg
HIV – neg	Hepatitis B – neg	Blood type – A neg
Rubella – immune	GBS – neg	Antibody screen – neg
Amnio – n/a	Pap	

Rhogam given: 28^{+2} weeks

US EXAMS:

Date: 1/16/18

GA by 1st-trimester US = 11^{+3} weeks

EFW = n/a

Placenta = anterior

Abnormalities = none

Date: 4/9/18

GA = 23^{+3} weeks

EFW = 330 g

Placenta = anterior

Abnormalities = none

A: The patient is a 25 y/o G4P2012 at 38^{+2} weeks with prenatal course complicated by Rh-negative status and mild asthma without regular medications or exacerbations who presents in active labor with SVE 4/75/–1 at 12:30pm. NST reactive and reassuring. She denies ROM, vaginal bleeding, and reports active fetal movement.

P: 1. Labor

   - Admit to labor and delivery
   - Manage labor, no augmentation required at this time
   - Consented for delivery
   - Anesthesia and pediatrics PRN
   - GBS-negative, no antibiotic prophylaxis

   2. Continuous fetal monitoring
   3. Asthma

   - Check pulse oximeter now
   - Use salbutamol MDI as needed – keep at bedside
   - Will ensure no Hemabate given for uterine atony

Cesarean Counseling Note
Basic Outline

The patient was counseled regarding our recommendation to proceed with a cesarean section for the following indication: _____

Risks and benefits of the procedure were discussed. These included, but were not limited to:

- Hemorrhage with the need for transfusion of blood products
- Risk of adverse reaction or infection from blood products, should they be required, including adverse reaction to the transfusion or infection with HIV/hepatitis/other infections
- Infection after the procedure requiring intravenous antibiotics and longer stay in the hospital
- Damage to bowel, bladder, or other abdominal organs with need for further surgery to repair/remove damaged organs
- Need to remove the uterus if severe bleeding encountered, which would preclude any future childbearing*
- Risk of maternal or fetal death

The patient and her partner verbally acknowledged that they understood the indication for the procedure, as well as the risks and benefits.

The consent form was signed, witnessed, and placed on the chart.

Vaginal Delivery Note

If you think of a delivery note as a narrative of how the delivery occurred, it will be easier to remember all the essential elements. This note should be written after every vaginal delivery (both spontaneous and operative).

Basic Outline

The patient progressed to ____/____/____ (dilation/effacement/station: +1/+2/+3 or at whatever station she began to push) (with/without) oxytocin and (with/without) epidural anesthesia and with good maternal effort delivered a viable (male/female) infant over an (intact perineum/midline episiotomy/mediolateral episiotomy) with Apgars of ____/____.

The infant presented in (OA/OP/LOA/LOP/ROA/ROP) position and restituted (LOA/LOP/ROA/ROP).

(No nuchal cord was present/A loose nuchal cord was manually reduced/delivered through/A tight nuchal cord was manually/surgically reduced/delivered through.)

The anterior then posterior shoulders delivered without difficulty. (If there is a shoulder dystocia, see the addendum below for how to document this.) The rest of the body delivered easily. After (30 seconds/1 minute) the cord was clamped × 2 and cut by provider/father and the infant (placed on the maternal abdomen/handed to the nurses/pediatricians for baby care). Oxytocin infusion was started with delivery of the posterior shoulder.

The placenta delivered (spontaneously/by manual extraction) and inspection of the placenta demonstrated that it was (intact/fragmented). The cord insertion appeared (normal/velamentous/circumvallate/etc.) with 3 vessels.

Fundus noted to be firm with bimanual massage and oxytocin. The cervix was inspected and (lacerations/no lacerations) were noted. The sidewalls were inspected and (lacerations/no lacerations) were noted. The perineum was inspected with findings of (describe any lacerations or extension of the episiotomy here).

---

* This sounds extreme, and the last part probably even obvious, but it needs to be spelled out clearly in case there are complications.

Describe how each laceration, if any, was repaired, including the type of suture used. (For example: Repair performed using 3–0 Vicryl in running, locked fashion/figure-of-eight suture/simple interrupted suture. Skin reapproximated in running, subcuticular fashion.)

At the end of the repair, all tissues noted to be hemostatic. All lap and needle counts correct × 2.

EBL for the delivery was _____ mL.

Delivering physicians: (staff), (resident).

Delivery Note Example

The patient progressed to C/C/+2 with oxytocin augmentation and epidural anesthesia and with good maternal effort delivered a viable female infant over an intact perineum with Apgars of 9/9.

The infant presented in OA position and restituted ROA. A loose nuchal cord was delivered through.

The anterior then posterior shoulders delivered without difficulty. The rest of the body delivered easily. After 1 minute, the cord was clamped × 2 and cut by father and the infant was placed on the maternal abdomen. Oxytocin infusion was started with delivery of the posterior shoulder.

The placenta delivered spontaneously and inspection of the placenta demonstrated that it was intact. The cord insertion was normal with 3 vessels.

Fundus noted to be firm with bimanual massage and oxytocin. The cervix was inspected and no lacerations were noted. The sidewalls were inspected and no lacerations were noted. The perineum was inspected with findings of a second-degree laceration. Repair performed using 3–0 Vicryl in running, locked fashion. Skin reapproximated in running, subcuticular fashion. At the end of the repair, all tissues noted to be hemostatic. All lap and needle counts correct × 2.

EBL for the delivery was 200 mL.

Delivering physicians: Joe Smith (Staff), Jean Smith (Resident)

Shoulder Dystocia Delivery Addendum*

After delivery of the fetal head, which presented in the (OA/OP/LOA/LOP/ROA/ROP) position, with appropriate downward traction in the standard fashion, the anterior shoulder (left shoulder/right shoulder) did not deliver spontaneously. At this time, additional staff, including pediatrics, was requested, and McRoberts position employed, along with suprapubic pressure. With these maneuvers, the anterior shoulder delivered, followed by the posterior shoulder and the rest of the infant. The normal 3-vessel cord was clamped × 2 and cut and the infant handed to pediatrics. The infant was noted to be moving both arms and had no bruising noted. The time from delivery of the fetal head to delivery of the shoulders was 30 seconds.

---

* Insert this after the part of the note describing the delivery of the fetal head. Insert a description of additional maneuvers as needed. Make sure you indicate which shoulder was anterior and how long it took to deliver the shoulder.

Labor Progress Note
This is a note that you will write whenever you check on a patient during labor to determine how she is progressing.

Basic Outline
S: Patient reports feeling ____ with (adequate/marginal/inadequate) pain control

O: Pulse, BP, temp, RR

FHR: baseline (130s, 150s, etc.) with (increased/average/minimal/absent) variability and (accelerations/decelerations)

FHR is category I/II/III

TOCO: contractions are every ____ minutes and occurring (regularly/irregularly)

Cervical exam: ____/____/____ (dilation/effacement/station)

Fetal head position is: (OA/OP/LOA/LOP/ROA/ROP)

Medications: Oxytocin is at mU/min (if patient is on oxytocin)

Antibiotics (ampicillin 2 g IV q6h)

Other medications

A: ____ y/o G_P_ _ _ _ at ____ + ____ weeks in labor.

Labor is (progressing appropriately/protracted)

FHR is category I/II/III

P: Depends on FHR category

If Category I
Category I tracing with no evidence of interruption in fetal oxygenation pathway due to absence of decelerations and can rule out fetal acidemia due to moderate variability and spontaneous accelerations.
- FHR strip review q2h
- SVE as indicated
- Continue to titrate oxytocin per protocol

If Category II
Category II: minimal variability. Category II tracing with no evidence of interruption in fetal oxygenation pathway due to absence of decelerations. Although periods of minimal variability, can rule out fetal acidemia due to periods of moderate variability and spontaneous accelerations.
- Strip review q2h
- SVE as indicated
- Continue to titrate oxytocin per protocol (if patient on oxytocin)

Category II: decelerations. Category II tracing with evidence of interruption in fetal oxygenation pathway due to presence of non-recurrent decelerations; however, can rule out fetal acidemia due to moderate variability and spontaneous accelerations.
- Strip review q2h
- SVE as indicated
- Continue to titrate oxytocin per protocol

Category II: decelerations with minimal variability. Category II tracing with evidence of interruption in fetal oxygenation pathway due to presence of non-recurrent decelerations. Although periods of minimal variability, can rule out fetal acidemia due to periods of moderate variability and spontaneous accelerations.

- Strip review q2h
- SVE as indicated
- Continue to titrate oxytocin per protocol

Labor Progress Example

S: Patient reports feeling well with adequate pain control.

O: Pulse 95, BP 130/75, temp 37.1 °C, RR 10

FHR: baseline = 140s with average variability and intermittent mild variable decelerations with spontaneous recovery

FHR is overall reassuring. Category II with decelerations

TOCO: contractions are every 5 minutes and occurring regularly

Cervix: 5/90/–1

Fetal head position = LOA

Medications: oxytocin is at 6 mU/min, PCN G 2.5 million units IV q4h

A: 27 y/o G3P1011 at 38^{+2} weeks in active labor

Labor is progressing appropriately

The FHR is overall reassuring with mild variable decelerations, category II

P: Category II tracing with evidence of interruption in fetal oxygenation pathway due to presence of non-recurrent decelerations. Can rule out fetal acidemia because of moderate variability and spontaneous accelerations.

- Strip review q2h
- SVE as indicated
- Continue to titrate oxytocin per protocol
- Will place IUPC and start amnioinfusion for variable decelerations

Labor/Fetal Intervention Note
Basic Outline

S: Went to see patient secondary to (FHR decelerations, bradycardia, complaint of SROM, complaint of increasing pain)

O: Pulse, BP, temp, RR

FHR: baseline = (130s, 150s, etc.) with (marked/moderate/minimal/absent) variability and (accelerations/decelerations)

FHR is overall (reassuring/non-reassuring/ominous) and category I/II/III

TOCO: contractions are every ____ minutes and occurring (regularly/irregularly)

Cervical exam: ____/____/____ (dilation/effacement/station)

Fetal head position is: (OA/OP/LOA/LOP/ROA/ROP)

Interventions:

AROM performed with (clear fluid/thin meconium/moderate meconium/thick meconium)

Internal monitors placed (IUPC/FSE)

(e.g., Terbutaline 0.25 mg IV given × 1)

(e.g., O_2 by facemask administered to mother)

Maternal position changed to (side, knee–chest, etc.)

FHR recovered after _____ minutes

A: _____ y/o G_P_ _ _ _ at _____ + _____ weeks in labor with the following issues:

Labor is (progressing appropriately/protracted)

FHR is overall (reassuring/non-reassuring/ominous) and category (I/II) with (variable decelerations/late decelerations/accelerations) and (increased/average/decreased/absent) variability

P: Continue to monitor labor progress and intervene as needed

Continue to monitor FHR (if overall reassuring)

Labor/Fetal Intervention for Distress: Example

S: Went to see patient secondary to late FHR deceleration with nadir to the 80s last 3 minutes.

O: Pulse 100, BP 110/78, temp 37.2 °C, RR 12

FHR: baseline = 130s with moderate variability prior to deceleration

TOCO: contractions are every 2 minutes and occurring regularly

Cervical exam: 6/100/0

Fetal head position is: ROA

Interventions:

Oxytocin (previously at 10 mU/min) stopped

AROM performed with clear fluid noted

Internal monitors placed (IUPC and FSE)

Terbutaline 0.25 mg IV given × 1

O_2 by face mask administered to mother

Maternal position changed to knee–chest

With the above interventions, the FHR recovered back to a baseline of 120s–130s and moderate variability

A: 22 y/o G1P0 at 37^{+0} weeks in labor with the following issues:

Labor is progressing appropriately

S/P late deceleration which responded to conservative measures. FHR tracing is currently reassuring

P: Continue to monitor labor progress and intervene as needed. Will continue to hold oxytocin at this time and monitor. Consider restarting in approximately 30 minutes if FHR tracing continues to be reassuring.

Continue to closely monitor FHR tracing.

Labor/Fetal Intervention for Pain Control: Example

S: Went to see patient secondary to complaint of feeling increased pain with contractions. Patient requesting additional pain relief.

O: Pulse 105, BP 114/88, temp 37.2 °C, RR 14

    FHR: baseline = 120s with moderate variability and no decelerations

    FHR tracing is overall reassuring and category I

    TOCO: contractions are every 4–5 minutes and occurring regularly

    Cervical exam: 5/C/0

    Fetal head position is: LOA

A: 32 y/o G3P2002 at 40^{+2} weeks in labor with the following issues:

    Labor is progressing appropriately

    FHR tracing is overall reassuring and category I

    Increased pain with contractions

P: After discussing options for pain control with patient, she desires an epidural. Will contact anesthesia to see patient. Category I tracing with no evidence of interruption in fetal oxygenation pathway due to absence of decelerations and can rule out fetal acidemia due to moderate variability and spontaneous accelerations.

    Continue to monitor labor progress and intervene as needed.

    Continue to monitor FHR tracing.

Magnesium Sulfate Note

In general, when patients are on magnesium sulfate, it will be either for neuroprophylaxis or for seizure prophylaxis for preeclampsia. It is important to check on these patients approximately every 4 hours to ensure that they do not have signs or symptoms of magnesium toxicity and good urine output (since it is excreted by the kidneys).

Basic Outline

S: The patient reports feeling ____. She denies any (bleeding/ROM). She also denies any (shortness of breath/chest pain/nausea/vomiting/visual changes/blurry vision/right upper quadrant pain/lower extremity pain). Patient does currently complain of (shortness of breath/chest pain/nausea/vomiting/blurry vision)*

O: Pulse, BP, temp, RR

    Urine output = ____ mL/hour over the past 4 hours

    FHR: baseline = (130s, 150s, etc.) with (marked/moderate/minimal/absent) variability and (accelerations/decelerations).

    FHR tracing is overall (reassuring/non-reassuring/ominous)

    TOCO: contractions are every ____ minutes and occurring (regularly/irregularly)

    LUNGS: (check for evidence of pulmonary edema, crackles)

---

* It is important to know what the normal side effects of magnesium sulfate are, as well as those that are potential signs of toxicity (see Chapter 14). Also, for patients who are being treated for preeclampsia, it is important to ask the following questions. These symptoms can be signs of worsening preeclampsia, which may change management:

- Do you have a headache?
- Do you have any right upper quadrant pain?
- Are you seeing any flashing lights?

HEART: (ensure regular rate, rhythm)

EXT: (check DTRs in upper/lower extremities)

Cervix: (only perform if there is suspicion that the patient is changing her cervix)

Current magnesium dose: _____ grams/hour

Magnesium level: _____ at _____ (time, if drawn)

A: _____ y/o G _ P _ _ _ _ at _____ + _____ weeks receiving magnesium sulfate at _____ g/h for (seizure prophylaxis/neuroprophylaxis) currently (with/without) evidence of magnesium toxicity.

P: (if stable without signs of toxicity) Continue magnesium sulfate at current dose and continue to monitor.

(if unstable or with signs of toxicity) Take appropriate measures such as decreasing or stopping the infusion and/or administering calcium gluconate. See Chapter 14.

Magnesium Sulfate Note: Example

S: The patient reports feeling relatively well. She denies any bleeding/ROM. She also denies any shortness of breath/chest pain/nausea/vomiting/RUQ pain/LE pain. Patient does currently complain of some blurry vision and hot flushes.

O: Pulse 80, BP 120/68, temp 36.9 °C, RR 14

Urine output = 60 mL/h over the past 2 hours

FHR: baseline = 140s with minimal variability, no decelerations, and accelerations

FHR tracing is overall reassuring and category I

TOCO: contractions are every 10 minutes and occurring irregularly. They have decreased in frequency over the past 2 hours.

LUNGS: CTA bilaterally

HEART: RRR with normal S1/S2

EXT: DTRs 2+ upper and lower extremities

Current magnesium dose: 2 g/h

A: 38 y/o G2P0010 at 32^{+2} weeks receiving magnesium sulfate at 2 g/h for preterm labor and neuroprophylaxis currently without evidence of magnesium toxicity.

P: Will continue magnesium sulfate at current dose and continue to monitor closely for signs/symptoms of toxicity. If contractions continue to decrease, will consider decreasing dose of magnesium sulfate.

Operative Note for Cesarean Delivery

An operative note is done after a cesarean delivery. Make sure that, under "procedure," you specify the type of uterine incision – i.e., low transverse cesarean section, low vertical cesarean section, classical cesarean section – as these all have implications for future deliveries (see Chapter 10).

Basic Outline

Memory aid: $P^3SSAAFFEUDC^3$

- Preoperative diagnosis
- Postoperative diagnosis
- Procedure
- Surgeons: (staff), (resident), (medical student)

- Specimens
- Anesthesia
- Antibiotics
- Findings
- Fluids
- EBL
- UO
- Drains
- Complications
- Condition
- Count

Cesarean Delivery: Example

Preop diagnosis: term IUP at 37^{+5} weeks, arrest of dilation

Postop diagnosis: SAA

Procedure: PLTCS

Surgeons: (staff), (resident), (medical student)

Specimens: placenta to pathology, cord gases

Anesthesia: epidural

Antibiotics: cefazolin 2 g IV

Findings: viable male infant with Apgars 8/9, weight = 3560 g, normal appearing uterus, bilateral fallopian tubes and ovaries

Fluids: 1200 mL LR

EBL: 850 mL

UO: 400 mL clear, yellow urine

Drains: Foley to gravity

Complications: none

Condition: stable to recovery room

Count: sponge, needle, instrument count correct × 2

Postpartum Notes

These notes will be written daily on all patients who deliver. While they have similar components, there are some important differences depending on the type of delivery and any complications that may have occurred.

Basic Outline

S: The patient reports feeling _____ this morning. She has had (minimal/average/heavy) lochia overnight using approximately _____ pad(s) every _____ hours. She describes her pain as (well controlled, marginally controlled, poorly controlled.) She denies any (nausea/vomiting/fevers/chills) overnight and tolerated a (regular/clear liquid) diet. She (is/is not) able to urinate with minimal discomfort and (has/has not) ambulated overnight.

The patient is (breastfeeding/bottle-feeding) and the infant is feeding (well/poorly) and otherwise (doing well/having issues being addressed by the pediatricians*).

---

* If the baby is having problems, note exactly what these issues are in the chart.

O: Pulse, BP, Tcurr, Tmax, RR

    HEART:

    LUNGS:

    BREASTS: (lactating/engorged/note any erythema or infection)

    ABD: uterus is (firm/soft) at U ($\pm$ 1, 2, 3, . . .: see Chapter 2)

    GU: (this is generally only if there is a specific complaint or the patient had a significant laceration and repair)

    EXT:

    Labs: (note if any labs drawn)

    Meds: (note medication/dosage/route/schedule)

    Rubella: (immune/non-immune)

    Rh: (positive/negative)

A: ____ y/o G _ P _ _ _ _ postpartum day # ____ with the following issues:

    Lochia is currently (appropriate/heavy)

    Pain control is currently (adequate/inadequate)

    (Note other issues such as fevers, nausea, etc.)

P: Continue to monitor lochia (or order a CBC if it is extremely heavy)

    Continue current medications for pain (or additional meds as needed)

    Continue routine postpartum care

    (Address other issues here)

Consults

Spontaneous Vaginal Delivery: Example

S: The patient reports feeling well this morning. She has had average lochia overnight using approximately one pad every 4–5 hours. She describes her pain as well controlled on ibuprofen. She denies any nausea/vomiting/fevers/chills overnight and tolerated a regular diet without difficulty. She is able to urinate with minimal discomfort and has ambulated overnight.

    The patient is breastfeeding and the infant is feeding well and being seen by the pediatricians for some mild jaundice.

O: Pulse 90, BP 127/87, Tcurr 37.0 °C, Tmax 37.2 °C, RR 12

    HEART: RRR

    LUNGS: CTA bilaterally

    BREASTS: lactating with no evidence of infection

    ABD: uterus is firm at U − 1

    GU: episiotomy repair intact without erythema or evidence of infection

    EXT: NTTP, trace bilateral LE edema

    Labs: none pending

    Meds: ibuprofen 800 mg PO q8h

    Rubella: non-immune

    Rh: positive

A: 21 y/o G1P1001 postpartum day #2 with the following issues:

    Lochia is currently appropriate

    Pain control is currently adequate

    Patient is rubella non-immune

    Patient is currently doing well

P: Continue to monitor lochia

    Continue current medications for pain

    Continue routine postpartum care

    Ensure patient receives rubella vaccine prior to discharge

    Anticipate discharge tomorrow

Cesarean Delivery: Example

S: The patient reports feeling well this morning. She has had minimal lochia overnight using approximately one pad every 6 hours. She describes her pain as marginally controlled at this time. She has taken one Percocet overnight for pain. She denies any nausea, vomiting, fevers, or chills and tolerated ice chips overnight. She currently has a Foley catheter in place. She also denies any lightheadedness/dizziness. She has not been up to ambulate yet.

    The patient is bottle-feeding and the infant is doing well.

O: Pulse 88, BP 124/76, Tcurr 37.2 °C, Tmax 37.3 °C, RR 12

    Urine output = 800 mL overnight (66 mL/h)

    HEART: RRR

    LUNGS: CTA bilaterally

    BREASTS: lactating without any erythema or evidence of infection

    ABD: uterus is firm at U, incision is C/D/I without erythema or drainage

    Abdomen is non-distended and appropriately tender to palpation with no rebound/ guarding, normoactive bowel sounds

    GU: deferred

    EXT: NTTP

    Labs: preop Hct = 34.6, postop Hct = 27.8

    Meds: Percocet 2.5/325 1–2 tab PO q4–6h PRN, ibuprofen 800 mg PO q8h

    Rubella: immune

    Rh: positive

A: 36 y/o G3P2012 postop day #1 with the following issues:

    Lochia is currently appropriate

    Patient is hemodynamically stable (adequate UO, stable VS, appropriate Hct)

    Pain control is currently poor, but patient has not taken full doses of her current meds

    No evidence of infection at this time

P: Continue to monitor for bleeding/infection

    Discontinue Foley catheter, will check due to void in 4–6 hours

Continue current medications for pain, giving two additional Percocet now, and then ensure patient takes ibuprofen on schedule and does not get behind on her pain control

Continue routine postoperative care

Patient to ambulate today with assistance

Advance diet to regular as tolerated

Vaginal Birth After Cesarean (VBAC) Counseling Note
Basic Outline

The patient is a ____ y/o G _ P _ _ _ _ at ____ weeks by (LMP/US). She had a previous cesarean section for ____ (list indication) and this was documented as a (low transverse cesarean section/low vertical cesarean section). She currently desires to attempt a vaginal delivery with this pregnancy.

Patient was counseled regarding the potential risks and complications of a VBAC, to include but not limited to uterine rupture (risk of less than 1%) with fetal distress and the need for an emergency cesarean section. Risks of this complication include bleeding, transfusion, hysterectomy, and poor fetal outcome. She also understands that there is a chance she will require a cesarean section during labor for normal obstetric indications. The patient verbalized understanding that she has the option to have a repeat cesarean section at this time and that she understands the potential risks and desires to proceed with VBAC attempt.

VBAC Counseling Note: Example

The patient is a 34 y/o G2P1 at 38^{+0} weeks by LMP and 8-week sonogram who presents with SROM that occurred at approximately 0530 today. She had a previous cesarean section for a breech presentation and this was documented as a low transverse cesarean section. She currently desires to attempt a vaginal delivery with this pregnancy.

Patient was counseled regarding the potential risks and complications of a VBAC to include but not limited to less than 1% risk of uterine rupture with fetal distress and the need for an emergency cesarean section. Risks of this complication include bleeding, transfusion, hysterectomy, and poor fetal outcome. She also understands that there is a chance she will require a cesarean section during labor for normal obstetric indications. The patient verbalized understanding that she has the option to have a repeat cesarean section at this time and that she understands the potential risks and desires to proceed with VBAC attempt.

Orders
Admission Orders

Any time a patient is admitted to labor and delivery, orders will be required so that the nursing team knows what the plan will be. At your institution, you will likely have a standard set of admission orders. Become familiar with these and make sure they address all of the items included in these examples.

Basic Outline
Memory aid: **ADC VANDIMFL**
- Admit: admit to labor and delivery. Attending is ____
- Diagnosis: (term IUP in labor/PTL/PROM/SROM/etc.)
- Condition: (stable/unstable/critical)

- Vital signs: as per protocol, likely q4h in latent labor
- Allergies: specify allergies (NKDA if none)
- Nursing: notify physician for:

  - temperature > 38.0 °C
  - SBP > 140 < 90
  - DBP > 90 < 50
  - pulse > 105

- Diet: (NPO/clear liquids/regular diet/etc.)
- IV fluids LR or NS at 125 mL/h (if the patient is NPO)
- I/O: (this is not usually required for most patients unless they are on magnesium sulfate or postop)
- Medications: (antibiotics if GBS-positive, evidence of intra-amniotic infection, or other indications)
- Fetal monitoring: (continuous FHR monitoring/continuous TOCO)
- Labs: type and screen, CBC

Sample Admission Orders
- Admit: admit to labor and delivery. Attending is Dr. Smith
- Diagnosis: term IUP in labor
- Condition: stable
- Vital signs: as per protocol
- Allergies: clindamycin – hives
- Nursing: notify physician for:

  - temp > 38.0 °C
  - SBP > 140 < 90
  - DBP > 90 < 50
  - pulse > 105

- Diet: clear liquids
- IV fluids: heplock
- I/O: N/A
- Medications: penicillin G 5 million units IV now, then 2.5 million units IV q4h during labor for GBS prophylaxis
- Fetal monitoring: continuous FHR monitoring/continuous TOCO
- Labs: type and screen, CBC × 1 on admission

Magnesium Sulfate Orders
For Preeclampsia
- Start magnesium sulfate infusion now with 6 g IV over 20 minutes followed by continuous infusion of 2 g/h
- Please place Foley catheter
- Strict I/O
- Notify physician for urine output < 30 mL/h
- VS as per protocol
- Continuous fetal monitoring

For Neuroprotection/Tocolysis

- Start magnesium sulfate infusion now with (4 or 6) g IV over 20 minutes followed by continuous infusion of (2–4) g/h
- Please place Foley catheter
- Strict I/O
- Notify physician for urine output < 30 mL/h
- VS as per protocol
- Continuous fetal monitoring

Oxytocin Orders

Low-dose Protocol

- Please start oxytocin at 1 mU/min, may increase dose by 2 mU/min every 30 minutes to a maximum of 20 mU/min
- If uterine hyperstimulation or fetal distress present, notify physician and stop oxytocin infusion
- Continuous FHR monitoring
- Continuous TOCO monitoring

High-dose Protocol

- Please start oxytocin at 6 mU/min, may increase dose by 6 mU/min every 20 minutes to a maximum of 20 mU/min
- If uterine tachysystole or fetal distress present, notify physician and stop oxytocin infusion
- Continuous FHR monitoring
- Continuous TOCO monitoring

Resuming High-dose Oxytocin after Uterine Tachysystole

- May restart oxytocin at half of dose it was being given when stopped
- May increase oxytocin dose by 2 mU/min every 20–40 minutes to a maximum of 20 mU/min
- If uterine hyperstimulation or fetal distress present, notify physician and stop oxytocin infusion

Postoperative Orders

- Admit: transfer to recovery when stable
- Diagnosis: S/P PLTCS/RLTCS
- Vital signs: as per protocol
- Allergies: specify allergies (NKDA if none)
- Nursing: Foley catheter to gravity
- Strict I/O
- Diet: regular
- IV fluids: lactated Ringer's at _____ mL/h (normal rate is approx. 125 mL/h)
- Meds: (antibiotics, pain medications*)
- Labs: CBC in a.m.

---

* Pain medication immediately postoperatively will usually be covered either by the anesthesiologist with a longer-acting medication in an epidural, or with a PCA device. Check with your institution for whose responsibility it is to order PCAs.

- Notify physician for:
  - temp > 38.0 °C
  - SBP >140 < 90
  - DBP > 90 < 50
  - pulse > 105
  - urine output < 30 mL/h

Postpartum Orders
- Admit: transfer to postpartum when stable
- Diagnosis: S/P SVD
- Vital signs: as per protocol
- Allergies: specify allergies (NKDA if none)
- Nursing: Foley catheter to gravity (if in place)
- Strict I/O
- Diet: regular
- IV fluids: lactated Ringer's at _____ mL/h (normal rate is approx. 125 mL/h)
- Meds: usually acetaminophen/ibuprofen/ bowel regimen/witch-hazel/protofoam
- Labs: CBC in AM if concerned for heavy blood loss
- Notify physician for:
  - temp > 38.0 °C
  - SBP >140 < 90
  - DBP > 90 < 50
  - pulse > 105
  - urine output < 30 mL/h

Additional Orders for Patients with Third/Fourth-Degree Lacerations
- Ice pack to perineum × 24–48 hours
- Stool softeners (see what your hospital carries, commonly Colace and MiraLAX)
- Sitz baths bid

Dictation
Cesarean Delivery Dictation
It is important to dictate the operative note on a cesarean delivery as soon after the procedure as possible so that you remember exactly what you did, especially if anything was out of the ordinary routine.

Basic Outline
- Date of operation
- Preoperative diagnosis
- Postoperative diagnosis
- Procedure performed
- Surgeons
- Staff
- Anesthesia
- Estimated blood loss
- Intravenous fluids

- Urine output
- Fetal sex/weight
- Apgars
- Antibiotics given
- Indications for procedure
- Procedure. This is where you will describe the procedure in detail. In the narrative below, where there are options the choices are shown in (parentheses).
- After informed consent was obtained from the patient, she was taken to the operating room where an (epidural/spinal/general) anesthetic was administered. The FHR in the operating room was _____ bpm prior to the procedure. A Foley catheter was then placed and the patient prepped and draped in the normal, sterile fashion. After anesthesia was determined to be adequate, a Pfannenstiel skin incision was made using a scalpel and the incision carried down to the underlying fascia, which was scored on the right and left of the midline. The fascia was then incised in a curvilinear fashion on either side using Mayo scissors. Two Kocher clamps were then used to grasp the anterior edge of the fascia and the rectus muscles were separated both sharply and bluntly from the fascia. The Kocher clamps were then placed on the inferior edges of the fascia and the muscles again dissected away from the fascia. The rectus muscles were then split bluntly in the midline. The peritoneum was identified and (entered bluntly/tented up and entered sharply with Metzenbaum scissors). The peritoneal incision was (sharply/bluntly) extended and the bladder blade placed to provide exposure of the lower uterine segment. The vesicouterine fold was (identified as clear of the lower uterine segment / over the lower uterine segment requiring a bladder flap). (*bladder flap* – The vesicouterine fold was elevated using pickups and incised using Metzenbaum scissors. This incision was extended in a curvilinear manner in each direction. The bladder flap was then created bluntly without difficulty.) A (low transverse/low vertical/classical uterine incision) was then made with a scalpel and carried down in layers until the uterine cavity was entered. The incision was then extended (bluntly/sharply) with bandage scissors. The fetus presented in the (vertex/breech/transverse) position. The fetal (vertex/buttocks) was brought through the incision with appropriate fundal pressure, the rest of the infant delivered and then the umbilical cord was doubly clamped and cut and the infant handed off to pediatrics after delayed cord clamping. Apgars were _____ / _____.
The placenta was then (manually removed/spontaneously expressed) and the uterus cleared of all clots and debris. Good uterine tone was noted with oxytocin titrated by anesthesia. The uterus was exteriorized and the incision was repaired in (one/two) layer(s) with 0-Vicryl suture without difficulty and good hemostasis was noted.
The uterus, fallopian tubes, and ovaries were visualized and were normal in appearance. The uterus was then replaced into the abdomen and the gutters cleared of all clots and debris. (If the bladder flap or peritoneum is closed, then note this here.) The uterine incision was again visualized and noted to be hemostatic. The fascia was then closed with two running sutures of 0-Vicryl/PDS without difficulty. The subcutaneous tissue was then irrigated and good hemostasis obtained. The subcutaneous layer was closed with (simple interrupted/a running) suture(s) of 3-0 Vicryl. The skin was then closed with (staples/subcutaneous sutures using 4-0 Vicryl/Monocryl/etc.). The incision was covered with a sterile pressure dressing and all clots were expressed from the uterus. The patient was taken to the recovery room in stable condition. Sponge, needle, and instrument counts were correct × 2.

Cesarean Delivery Dictation: Example

This is Dr. Jon Smith dictating operative report on patient Jane Doe, medical record 123-45-6789.

Date of operation: 12/12/17

Preoperative diagnosis: intrauterine pregnancy at 39^{+5} weeks. Arrest of dilation

Postoperative diagnosis: same as above

Procedure performed: primary low transverse cesarean section

Surgeons: Jon Smith, Bill Smith (resident), Will Smith (medical student)

Staff: Jon Smith

Anesthesia: epidural

Estimated blood loss: 1000 mL

Intravenous fluids: 1500 mL LR

Urine output: 400 mL

Fetal sex/weight: male/3500 g

Apgars: 9/9

Antibiotics given: cefazolin 2 g

Indications for procedure: Patient is a 25 y/o G1P0 at 39^{+5} weeks' gestation who presented to labor and delivery in active labor. She progressed to 7/C/0 and despite more than 2 hours of adequate contractions as documented by an intrauterine pressure catheter, failed to make any further cervical change. The patient was counseled regarding conservative management versus a cesarean delivery, including the risks of bleeding, transfusion, infection, damage to the bowel/bladder, hysterectomy, and death, and she and her partner verbalized understanding.

Procedure: After informed consent was obtained from the patient, she was taken to the operating room where an epidural anesthesia was found to be adequate. The FHR in the operating room was 150 bpm without evidence of decelerations prior to procedure. A Foley catheter was then placed and the patient prepped and draped in the normal, sterile fashion. After anesthesia was determined to be adequate, a Pfannenstiel skin incision was made using a scalpel and the incision carried down to the underlying fascia, which was scored right and left of the midline. The fascia was then incised in a curvilinear fashion on either side using Mayo scissors. Two Kocher clamps were then used to grasp the anterior edge of the fascia and the rectus muscles were separated both sharply and bluntly from the fascia. The Kocher clamps were then placed on the inferior edges of the fascia and the muscles again dissected away from the fascia. The rectus muscles were then split bluntly in the midline and the peritoneum was entered bluntly. The peritoneal incision was bluntly extended and the bladder blade placed to provide exposure of the lower uterine segment. The vesicouterine fold was elevated using pickups and incised using Metzenbaum scissors. This incision was extended in a curvilinear manner in each direction. The bladder flap was then created bluntly without difficulty. A low transverse uterine incision was then made with a new scalpel and carried down in layers until the uterine cavity was entered. The incision was then extended bluntly. The fetus presented in the vertex position. The fetal vertex was brought through the incision with appropriate fundal pressure and the infant was bulb-suctioned and then the umbilical cord doubly clamped and cut and the infant handed off to pediatrics. Apgars were 8/9. The placenta was then spontaneously expressed and the uterus cleared of all clots and debris. Good uterine tone was noted with oxytocin titrated by anesthesia. The uterus was exteriorized and the incision was repaired in two layers with 0-Vicryl suture without difficulty and good hemostasis was noted. The uterus, fallopian tubes, and ovaries were visualized and were normal in appearance. The uterus was then replaced into the abdomen and the gutters cleared of all clots and debris. The uterine incision was again visualized and noted to be hemostatic. The fascia was then closed with a running-locked suture of 0-Vicryl without difficulty. The subcutaneous tissue was then irrigated and good hemostasis obtained. The subcutaneous layer was closed with three interrupted sutures of 3-0 Vicryl. The skin was then closed with staples. The incision was covered with a sterile pressure dressing and all clots were expressed from the uterus. The patient was taken to the recovery room in stable condition. Sponge, needle, and instrument counts were correct × 2.

Appendix C: Cesarean Talk-through

Allison Eubanks and Shad Deering

Introduction

While you will probably assist on many cesarean sections before performing one, it is imperative that you know, without hesitation, the steps involved and how to perform each of them, so that you are prepared when you do get the chance. This includes everyone on the operative team, so that every member of the team can anticipate what the next step is. When starting to learn about the procedure, it is helpful to "talk through" the operation in sequence, asking for instruments and verbalizing what steps you are taking. This will help ingrain the procedure in your mind, make your staff more comfortable in the OR when they hear you say what you are going to do, and make the operative dictation much easier.

If you pay attention to your attending in the OR before you do the procedure, you will find there are always some small variations, such as different sutures, or different ways to close certain layers. Make mental notes of these for when you operate with them. Do what your attending is comfortable with, and, as you become more senior, decide what you think works best and incorporate it into your practice.

Here, we present a practice talk-through in which you call for instruments and say what steps you are taking. Please refer to the section at the end of this appendix for illustrations of the common instruments used during a cesarean section.

Note: By convention, the primary surgeon stands on the patient's right side.

Preoperative Preparation

The patient is lying on the OR table with a left hip roll, the abdomen is prepped, and the patient is draped. Before starting, check the following:

1. Bovie (electrocautery) is functioning and the patient has a grounding pad on the thigh.
2. Suction is on the field and functioning.
3. Foley catheter is in place.
4. Antibiotic prophylaxis has been ordered (usually 2 g cefazolin).
5. Compression stockings or pneumatic compression devices are on and functioning.
6. Lights are focused on the area where the incision will be made.
7. All necessary personnel (nurse, pediatrics, anesthesia provider, patient's partner) are present or standing by.

Time Out

If you have not already done this, conduct a surgical pause, also known as a time out, before you start the procedure. At a minimum, this generally consists of identifying the patient and confirming the procedure to be performed with agreement between the patient and the OR team. Check and see if your institution has a formal time out procedure/checklist.

Procedure

In the following talk-through, the **bold text** indicates where you call for instruments. The *italics* indicate what you are saying and what you are doing.

"Allis clamp"

"Testing anesthesia level" — Clamp the skin at the planned incision line and by the umbilicus. If the patient's anesthesia is adequate, this will not hurt. If it is not adequate, she will let the anesthesia provider know and you wait for the problem to be corrected.

"Marking pen" — Using the marking pen, you will draw your planned incision. Start at the midline and make a vertical line to mark the center – this will aid in your repair, as well. Then, 2 finger breadths above the pubic symphysis, you will make lateral marks about 6–8 cm away from the midline with a slight turn towards the patient's shoulders, following Langer's lines.

"Two dry laps" — Place one laparotomy sponge above the planned incision site and one below to provide traction and countertraction as you make the incision.

"Scalpel" — This will usually be a #10 blade.

"Start time" — Say this as you make your incision, so the circulating nurse can note it.

"Making incision to fascia" — After getting through the skin, concentrate on the middle 6–8 cm of the incision and go down to the fascia.

"Scoring fascia" — Score the fascia on either side of the midline so you can see the rectus muscles.

"Pickups with teeth and Mayo scissors"

"Extending fascial incision" — Do this by lifting up with your pickups, sliding the scissors under the fascia to separate the fascia from the muscle, then incising with your Mayo scissors (tips curved towards patient's head).

"Two Kocher clamps"

"Placing clamps on anterior fascia" — Place one clamp on the superior edge of the fascia on either side of the midline and lift up for exposure.

"Mayo scissors"

"Dissecting fascia from rectus"

This can be done both bluntly with a dry lap and with the Mayo scissors, or with a scalpel, incising the rectus muscle where it is attached in the midline to the fascia.

"Placing clamps on inferior fascia"

Place clamps on inferior edge of fascia, one on each side of the midline.

"Dissecting fascia from rectus"

Again, do this bluntly and sharply down to the pubic symphysis. Ask for Mayo scissors or scalpel if needed.

"Removing clamps"

Remove Kocher clamps and give them back to the OR technician.

"Two hemostats and Metzenbaum scissors"

"Identifying peritoneum"

Identify the peritoneum in the midline, as high as possible to avoid the bladder. Place the hemostats approximately 1 cm apart and elevate them to ensure there is no bowel, bladder, or anything else below the area you are going to incise.

"Incising peritoneum"

Make small incision in peritoneum with Metzenbaum scissors.

"Extending peritoneal incision"

This can be done bluntly by stretching, or with Metzenbaum scissors.

"Bladder blade and large Rich retractor"

A Rich may also be called a Richardson retractor.

"Placing bladder blade and Rich"

Place the bladder blade so you can see the lower uterine segment, and the large Rich superiorly so you have adequate visualization.

"Smooth pickups and Metzenbaum scissors"

You should be more specific on the pickups, depending on what your institution carries. Either Russian or De Bakey pickups are appropriate.

"Identifying bladder flap"

Identify the vesicouterine fold where the bladder reflection is and elevate the serosa just above this in the midline. If making a bladder flap, make a curvilinear incision in both directions with scissors, with the curved end of the scissors pointed towards the patient's head. (If not making a bladder flap, then proceed to the step of replacing the bladder blade.)

"Kelly clamp"

"Making bladder flap"

Clamp the Kelly onto the inferior edge of the incision and, with your fingers always on the uterus, push gently down to push the bladder away from the uterus.

"Removing clamp"

Remove the Kelly clamp and hand it back to the OR technician.

"Replacing bladder blade"

Place the bladder blade in between the bladder and the uterus, using the Kelly clamp for exposure.

"Palpating uterus"	Palpate the uterus to determine if it is rotated significantly and find the midline where you will make your incision. Ensure your skin and fascial incisions are appropriately sized for the anticipated size of the baby. Also, palpate the lower uterine segment to feel for how thick the segment is in anticipation of your incision. Remember, a laboring patient will have very little tissue between your scalpel and the baby.

"Scalpel"

"Uterine incision"	Make a small U-shaped incision in the lower uterine segment above your bladder flap. After the first pass, palpate the incision and use suction to visualize the area. Make successive passes, with care to NOT CUT THE BABY! If you are going layer by layer, often the membranes will push out at some point.
"Scalpel back"	Once you are through the initial lower uterine segment, hand the scalpel back to the OR technician safely.
"Extending uterine incision"	Extend the uterine incision superior-laterally in a curvi-linear fashion by one of two methods: 1. Insert the index fingers at each corner and pull upwards in the same direction as you would cut with bandage scissors. 2. If unable to extend bluntly, then call for "**bandage scissors**" and place your left hand inside the uterus between the scissors and the baby and extend the incision superiorly and laterally. You may then need to repeat this on the other side.
"Allis clamp"	If the membranes are bulging at this point, ask for an Allis clamp to rupture the membranes. Call out the color of the fluid for pediatrics. Ensure your assistant has the suction ready.
"Placing hand in uterus"	Place your right hand into the uterus and grasp the infant's head, and bring it to the level of the hysterotomy while maintaining proper head flexion.
"Remove bladder blade"	Your assistant will remove the bladder blade to allow you more room for the fetal head to deliver.
"Fundal pressure"	With this, your assistant will provide fundal pressure, which will allow you to deliver the baby. You may also apply the fundal pressure with your left hand, rather than have your assistant do it. At the same time as fundal pressure is applied, elevate the fetal head through the incision with the right hand. Make sure not to flex your wrist significantly during delivery as this can cause an unwanted extension of the uterine incision.

"Bulb suction"

"Suctioning baby"   Suction out the infant's mouth and nares.

"Waiting to clamp cord" Delay cord clamping for 30–60 seconds if fetal status allows, as you would during a vaginal delivery, if this is your hospital's policy.

"Kelly clamps × 2"

"Clamping and cutting umbilical cord." Doubly clamp and ligate the umbilical cord as you would during a vaginal delivery.

NOTE: This is the time to obtain an additional portion of the umbilical cord for gases if the situation warrants – e.g., if the cesarean was done for fetal distress or the fetus is very premature.

"Baby to peds"   Hand the infant to the waiting pediatrician.

"Delivering placenta"   Provide moderate traction on the umbilical cord with the remaining Kelly clamp to deliver the placenta.
If this does not work, then the placenta can be manually removed by inserting one hand into the uterus and finding the plane between the membranes and the uterus.

"Ring forceps"

"Removing membranes"   As the placenta comes out of the uterus, the membranes will trail and you will use the ring forceps to grasp them and help remove them.

"1 wet and 2 dry laps"

"Exteriorizing uterus"   Palpate around the uterus to ensure there are no extensive adhesions that would prevent exteriorization. If not, grasp the fundus with the thumb and fingers of one hand and exteriorize the uterus. Wrap the fundus with the wet lap and use your left hand to provide traction.

"Removing clots from uterus" Use the dry laps to clean out the interior of the uterus to make sure there are no membranes or clots left in the cavity.

"Checking uterine tone" As you clean out the uterus, ensure it clamps down appropriately so that hemorrhage from uterine atony does not occur. If the uterus will not firm up, you must take action to prevent hemorrhage.

"Please give oxytocin"   This lets the anesthesia provider know you would like oxytocin, usually titrated by anesthesia protocol. This is run into the patient's IV fluids to help with uterine tone.

"Bladder blade"   Replace the bladder blade to keep the bladder away from your sutures as you repair the uterine incision.

"Ring forceps" or **"Pennington clamp"**	Use these to grasp each lateral angle of the incision as needed. You may also use them to clamp off bleeding areas of the incision until you can incorporate them with your suture. You can also use an Allis clamp for the angles.
"Inspecting incision"	Look at the incision to make sure you do not have an extension laterally into the uterine vessels or inferiorly into the cervix.
"Suture, 0-Vicryl on a CTX, and Russian forceps"	This is a common suture used for uterine closure. You may prefer chromic, Monocryl, or another suture.
"Repairing uterine incision"	Begin at the opposite side and close the incision, sewing towards yourself. With the first bite, make sure you have palpated with your fingers laterally to where you are placing the suture to ensure you do not accidentally incorporate the uterine artery or ureter. This is a running, locked suture.
"Suture, 0-Vicryl on CTX"	Again, you may prefer chromic or another suture, and some providers do not place a second layer, although there is now data that suggest this is helpful in that it increases the thickness of the lower uterine segment in subsequent pregnancies.
"Placing imbrication layer"	This is a method by which the initial uterine incision is oversewn. It can be done in either a horizontal or a vertical fashion depending on provider preference and room from bladder.
"Inspecting incision"	After the uterine incision is closed, observe it to check for obvious bleeding. If there is significant bleeding from an area, call for a suture and repair it. If not, then proceed to the next step.
"Inspecting cul-de-sac and anatomy"	Push the uterus forwards and look into the cul-de-sac, checking for clots and debris. If there is a significant amount of either, use a lap to remove it. Look at the exterior of the uterus, ovaries, and fallopian tubes for any abnormalities that will need to be dictated in the operative report. Some providers choose to irrigate the posterior cul-de-sac with the Poole suction tube.
"Inspecting incision"	Look again at the uterine incision to ensure there is no active bleeding. If there is, then call for a suture and repair it; otherwise, proceed to the next step.
"Replacing uterus"	Remove the bladder blade, then turn the uterus at a slight angle and place it back into the abdominal cavity.
"Bladder blade"	Replace the bladder blade and look at the incision again.

"Medium Rich retractor, clean wrung-out lap sponge, and irrigation"

Place the retractor at one corner of the incision under the peritoneum and retract upwards. The other person will then use either a clean lap or irrigation, or both, and clean out the lateral gutter on that side of the uterus. This is then repeated on the opposite side.

"Inspecting incision and fascia"

Look one last time at your incision, especially the lateral angles, to ensure there is no significant bleeding. Also be sure to inspect the upper abdominal fascia to ensure there are no holes larger than 1 cm that need to be closed.

"Medium Rich retractor, pickups with teeth, and 0-Vicryl suture"

Insert the retractor at one corner of the incision above the fascia and visualize the corner of the fascial incision. Use the pickups to grasp the angle and place your suture there. This is generally a simple running suture. You can continue until you are approximately halfway, then stop and tie or run the suture for the entire incision. It may be helpful to place a Kocher on the corners to better identify the apex.

NOTE: Many providers prefer a PDS suture for repeat cesarean sections.

"Irrigation and clean lap"

Irrigate the subcutaneous tissue, then place the lap sponge in the incision. As you remove the lap, look for bleeding in the subcutaneous tissue. If there is any, cauterize the area using electrocautery.

"Is the count correct?"

Ask this question now, as your circulating nurse should have either completed or at least started to recount all instruments, lap sponges, and needles that were placed on the field during the operation. If the count is incorrect, you must locate any missing items before closing.

"Plain gut/3–0 Vicryl and Adson pickups"

If the patient has subcutaneous tissue that is over 2 cm thick, it has been shown that closing this layer with either a simple running suture or interrupted sutures decreases incidences of hematomas and seromas. It can also help release tension on the skin closure and enhance the healing process.

"Staples and two Adson pickups" or **"4–0 Vicryl suture and Adson pickups"**

You will ask for either of these depending on your preference for closing the skin. Staples are generally used in obese patients or in patients with concern for infection or poor healing.

Also, other sutures than Vicryl may be used. If you do use suture, you will usually place steri-strips afterwards. It is important to line up the center of the incision, using either the mark you made at the initial incision or the patient's own linea nigra, on both the superior and inferior edges.

"Sterile towel"	Place the sterile towel over the closed incision.
"Taking down drapes"	Hold the towel on the incision as the anesthesia providers take down the drapes.
"Wet and dry laps"	Clean off any remaining prep from the abdomen, taking care not to rub so hard as to open the incision.
"Sterile bandage and tape"	Place the bandage on the incision and then cover with tape, placing pressure on the incision.
"Evacuating clots"	Place one hand on the abdomen and palpate the fundus and the other into the vagina after moving the patient's legs. Check uterine tone and evacuate clots from the vagina.
"Wet and dry towel"	Use these to clean the perineum and remove the clots you expressed.

When you have completed the operation, remove your gown, put on non-sterile gloves, and assist the nurses in taking the patient to the recovery room. After doing this, talk with the anesthesia provider and ask about the following information for your operative report:

- Estimated blood loss
- Urine output
- Fluids given during the procedure

Next, talk to your nurse and ask for these items:

- Apgar scores
- Birth weight
- Infant gender (if you do not remember)

For an example of how to dictate an operative note, please refer to Appendix B, *Sample Notes and Orders*.

Instruments for Cesarean Section

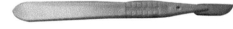

Figure C.1 Scalpel, usually #10 blade.

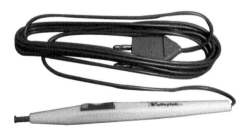

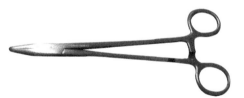

Figure C.3 Needle driver.

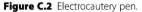
Figure C.2 Electrocautery pen.

Clamps

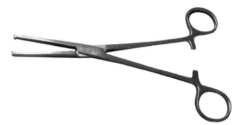

Figure C.4 Kocher – used on fascia for dissection or location of apexes before closing.

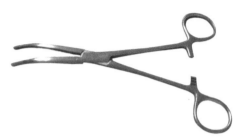

Figure C.5 Kelly – used on bladder flap or to identify peritoneum, also used to clamp fetal umbilical cord.

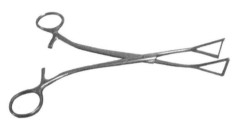

Figure C.6 Pennington – used on uterus to identify edges and control bleeding while closing the hysterotomy.

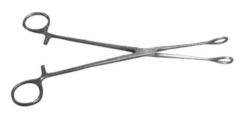

Figure C.7 Ring forceps – used to help remove all trailing membranes from the placenta in the uterus. Can also be used in place of the Pennington to identify edges of the hysterotomy and control bleeding while closing.

Pickups

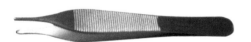

Figure C.8 Adson – used mostly for skin closure.

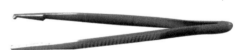

Figure C.9 Bonney – used for fascial closure.

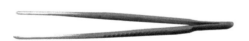

Figure C.10 De Bakey – can be used on uterus, good for grabbing vessels that require cauterization.

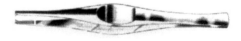

Figure C.11 Ferris Smith – used for fascial closure.

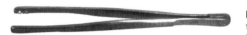

Figure C.12 Russian – smooth pickups that work well on the uterus for closing the hysterotomy and making the bladder flap without causing much damage.

Retractors

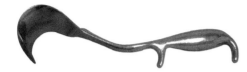

Figure C.13 Bladder blade.

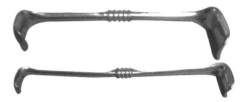

Figure C.14 Richardson–Eastman.

Scissors

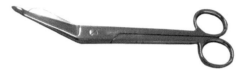

Figure C.15 Bandage – can be used to extend hysterotomy or to complete a Maylard incision if the baby cannot be delivered through tight rectus muscles; also used to cut the umbilical cord.

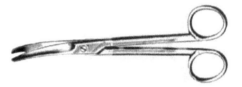

Figure C.16 Mayo – used on thicker tissue such as fascia.

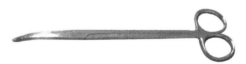

Figure C.17 Metzenbaum – used on thinner tissue such as peritoneum.

Suction Devices

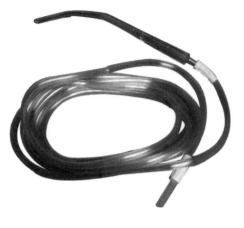

Figure C.18 Yankauer.

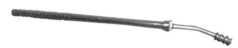

Figure C.19 Poole.

Index